DERMATOLOGY - LABORATORY AND CLINICAL RESEARCH

SCARS AND SCARRING

CAUSES, TYPES AND TREATMENT OPTIONS

DERMATOLOGY - LABORATORY AND CLINICAL RESEARCH

Additional books in this series can be found on Nova's website under the Series tab.

Additional e-books in this series can be found on Nova's website under the e-book tab.

DERMATOLOGY - LABORATORY AND CLINICAL RESEARCH

SCARS AND SCARRING

CAUSES, TYPES AND TREATMENT OPTIONS

YONGSOO LEE
EDITOR

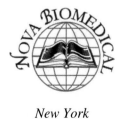

New York

Copyright © 2013 by Nova Science Publishers, Inc.

All rights reserved. No part of this book may be reproduced, stored in a retrieval system or transmitted in any form or by any means: electronic, electrostatic, magnetic, tape, mechanical photocopying, recording or otherwise without the written permission of the Publisher.

For permission to use material from this book please contact us:
Telephone 631-231-7269; Fax 631-231-8175
Web Site: http://www.novapublishers.com

NOTICE TO THE READER

The Publisher has taken reasonable care in the preparation of this book, but makes no expressed or implied warranty of any kind and assumes no responsibility for any errors or omissions. No liability is assumed for incidental or consequential damages in connection with or arising out of information contained in this book. The Publisher shall not be liable for any special, consequential, or exemplary damages resulting, in whole or in part, from the readers' use of, or reliance upon, this material. Any parts of this book based on government reports are so indicated and copyright is claimed for those parts to the extent applicable to compilations of such works.

Independent verification should be sought for any data, advice or recommendations contained in this book. In addition, no responsibility is assumed by the publisher for any injury and/or damage to persons or property arising from any methods, products, instructions, ideas or otherwise contained in this publication.

This publication is designed to provide accurate and authoritative information with regard to the subject matter covered herein. It is sold with the clear understanding that the Publisher is not engaged in rendering legal or any other professional services. If legal or any other expert assistance is required, the services of a competent person should be sought. FROM A DECLARATION OF PARTICIPANTS JOINTLY ADOPTED BY A COMMITTEE OF THE AMERICAN BAR ASSOCIATION AND A COMMITTEE OF PUBLISHERS.

Additional color graphics may be available in the e-book version of this book.

Library of Congress Cataloging-in-Publication Data

Library of Congress Control Number: 2013939636

ISBN: 978-1-62808-005-6

Published by Nova Science Publishers, Inc. † New York

Solely to the One who originally designed existence and non-existence
as well as everything else.

Contents

Preface		ix
Notice		xi
Introduction		1
Chapter 1	Scars and Scarring: Causes, Types, and Treatment Options *Anna Chacon, Katlein França, Jennifer Ledon and Keyvan Nouri*	3
Chapter 2	Psychological Impact of Scars *Katlein França, Anna Chacon, Jennifer Ledon, Jessica Savas and Keyvan Nouri*	25
Pathogenesis of Scarring		39
Chapter 3	Pathogenesis of Scars: An Overview *Chao-Kai Hsu, Julia Yu-Yun Lee and Ming-Jer Tang*	41
Chapter 4	Redox-Signaling during Wound Healing: A Role for Cytoprotective Enzymes in Scar Prevention? *Ditte M. S. Lundvig and Frank A. D. T. G. Wagener*	57
Chapter 5	Moving Beyond Inflammation in Cutaneous Scar Formation *Victor W. Wong and Geoffrey C. Gurtner*	99
Prevention		107
Chapter 6	Prevention of Scars *Rei Ogawa*	109
Treatment Options		121
Chapter 7	Radiation Therapy for Scars *Rei Ogawa*	123
Chapter 8	Surgical Therapy for Scars *Rei Ogawa*	131

| **Chapter 9** | Non/minimally Invasive Treatment Options
Jennifer Ledon, Jessica Savas, Katlein Franca,
Anna Chacon, Yongsoo Lee and Keyvan Nouri | **139** |

New Treatment Options and New Classification of Scars   **169**

Chapter 10	Lasers: Physics and Principles *Yongsoo Lee and Inja Bogdan Allemann*	**171**
Chapter 11	Classification of Scars: Conventional and New *Yongsoo Lee*	**179**
Chapter 12	Treatment Options - Combination Treatments: Combination of Lasers / Combination of Lasers and Surgical Scar Revision *Yongsoo Lee*	**187**
Chapter 13	Recommended Treatment Protocols *Yongsoo Lee*	**203**
Chapter 14	Striae Distensae *J. A. Savas, J. Ledon, K. Franca,* *A. Chacon and K. Nouri*	**211**
Chapter 15	Research on Scar Treatments *Yongsoo Lee*	**223**

Index   **235**

Preface

'Normal' is a statistical term that might have been used since long before the concept of statistics took place in human minds. We humans call something normal when a feature happens in majority of friends or relatives. Later, statisticians defined 'normal' by employing the concept of standard deviations. Anyway, when you say something is normal, most people have the same kind of feature or characteristic. For example, if we observed that all humans only had one eye, it would have been considered normal to have one eye. However, we humans have taken a one-eyed mythical creature a monster because the majority of us have two eyes. The current definition of normal is the definition of last resort, which humans devised in their desperate situation of having nothing with which to compare themselves.

Wrinkles happen to 100% of humans when they age. This is, of course, normal by definition. However, ironically, it is normal for a human being to desire to remove those wrinkles from their skin. Scars also happen in 100% of cases that suffer injuries of more than a certain depth to trigger the emergency repair system of the skin. Even though scars happen normally from a statistical point of view, normal people want them removed from their skin.

What are we pursuing? Are we trying to be normal? Are hypertensive patients taking anti-hypertensive medications every day to be normal? It seems so. However, they are taking the medication wishing to live out a normal life span. Simply, it is disguised to look like they are trying to be normal but they are wishing to live abnormally long by normalizing their blood pressures. Something that is embedded deep in human hearts and minds drive them to pursue something that is not normal. Even though it is perfectly normal to die, humans desire not to die. Likewise, researchers and medical practitioners of aesthetic medicine have been trying to make normal subjects abnormal by making normal (statistical majority) people with wrinkles or scars abnormal (statistical minority) individuals without wrinkles or scars, despite of their aging or injuries.

Our human minds race against the keen reality of the violent stream that conveys the physical body back to a state of organic molecules of post-mortem decomposition. Our minds seem to be programmed to long for beautiful moments of the past as we, from time to time, remember the "good old days". Maybe, our minds have been dreaming of the good old days of perfection with no sorrows, no regrets, no disease, no aging, no injuries, no scarring, no death and no post mortem decomposition, before something seriously had gone wrong.

The editor believes in the concept of a normal need to be refreshed before we contemplate scars and scarring, causes, types and treatment options. Normal probably means the original state that human skin was supposed to be or designed to be.

Despite of the desperate and helpless standing of statistics, as just mentioned, there is no way to demonstrate the relationship between treatments and the outcomes apart from statistics. On top of this, there are unique difficulties encountered in scar treatment research. Without identifying these difficulties and solutions to them, we are just like a blind man who is guided by the blind, in the labyrinth of scar treatments.

Since the beginning of the era that human beings began seeking aesthesis beyond the quest of life prolongation, there have been numerous options invented for scar treatments. Not all but almost all of the useful treatment options up to this point in time are described in this work, along with the latest discoveries of scar pathogenesis. Even combinations of these treatment options and the latest laser treatment options are described with the help of a new scar classification system that is based not only on the morphology and the natural behavior of the scars, but also on the responses of the scars to laser treatments.

It is the editor's hope that this book, *Scars and Scarring: Causes, Types and Treatment Options,* would illuminate the direction of future scar treatment research. He has high hopes that it would provide a greater understanding of scar pathogenesis as well as practical guidance to more successful scar treatments in order that more fellow human beings could be brought back to the original design.

Notice

Medicine is an ever-changing science. As new research and clinical experience broaden our knowledge, changes in treatments and drug therapy are required. The editor and publisher of this work has checked with sources believed to be reliable in their efforts to provide information that is complete and generally in accord with the standards accepted at the time of publication. However, in view of the possibility of human error or changes in medical sciences, neither the editors nor the publisher nor any other party who has been involved in the preparation or publication of this work warrants that the information contained herein is in every respect accurate or complete, and they disclaim all responsibility for any errors or omissions or for the results obtained from use of the information contained in this work. Readers are encouraged to confirm the information contained herein with other sources. For example and in particular, readers are advised to check the product information sheet included in the package of each device and drug they plan to administer to be certain with the information contained in this work is accurate and that changes have not been made in the recommended dose, parameter settings of devices or in the contraindications for administration. This recommendation is of particular importance in connection with new or infrequently used drugs or devices. As the laser or other types of device settings of parameters are highly in need of adjustment depending on the state of the scars or skin at the time of treatment, the practitioner needs to check the state of the patient and the operation manual accompanying the devices. It is solely the practitioner's responsibility to set the parameters of lasers or other types of devices and neither the editors nor the publisher nor any other party involved in the preparation or publication of this work claim any responsibility for the results obtained from use of the information contained in this book.

Introduction

In: Scars and Scarring
Editor: Yongsoo Lee

ISBN: 978-1-62808-005-6
© 2013 Nova Science Publishers, Inc.

Chapter 1

Scars and Scarring: Causes, Types, and Treatment Options

*Anna Chacon[1], Katlein França[1], Jennifer Ledon[1]
and Keyvan Nouri*[*2]

[1]Clinical Research Fellow, Mohs and Laser Unit
University of Miami Miller School of Medicine,
Department of Dermatology and Cutaneous Surgery
Miami, Florida, US
[2]Dermatology, Ophthalmology & Otolaryngology
Louis C. Skinner, Jr., M.D. Endowed Chair in Dermatology
Richard Helfman Professor of Dermatologic Surgery
University of Miami Medical Group
Sylvester Comprehensive Cancer Center/University of Miami Hospital and Clinics
Mohs, Dermatologic & Laser Surgery
Surgical Training
Department of Dermatology & Cutaneous Surgery
University of Miami Leonard M. Miller School of Medicine
Sylvester Comprehensive Cancer Center, Mohs/Laser Unit
Miami, FL, USA

Abstract

In developed nations, about 100 million people will acquire scars after a surgical procedure each year. Although scars rarely pose a significant health risk, patients often

---

[*] Corresponding author: 4Professor of Dermatology, Ophthalmology, and Otolaryngology, Louis C. Skinner, Jr., MD Endowed Chair of Dermatology, Richard Helfman Professor of Dermatologic Surgery, Vice Chairman of the University of Miami Medical Group, Chief of Dermatology Services at Sylvester Comprehensive Cancer Center/University of Miami Hospitals and Clinics, Director of Mohs, Dermatologic & Laser Surgery, Director of Surgical Training, University of Miami Miller School of Medicine, Department of Dermatology and Cutaneous Surgery, 1475 NW 12th Avenue, #2175, Miami, Florida 33136, knouri@med.miami.edu.

experience significant physical, aesthetic, psychological and social distress. The appearance, duration, and improvement of a scar are among the most common concerns that many patients with scars ask their physicians. Scars are the result of injury to the skin from trauma or disease. When wound healing is interrupted from its normal, systematic pattern, abnormal scarring occurs. Scars can be classified as hypertrophic, normotrophic, and atrophic. Raised (or hypertrophic) scars include: keloids and hypertrophic scars. Atrophic scar subtypes include: striae distensae, epidermal and dermal atrophy, and panatrophy.

Other scars may occur as a result of acne, burns, or contractures. There are various treatment options available including ablative and non-ablative lasers and other possibilities, such as dermabrasion, chemical peels, microneedling, intra-lesional therapy, surgery and cryotherapy. This chapter presents causes, types and treatment options for scars.

I. Introduction

What will my scar look like? When will it go away? What can I do to make it look better? These are all common questions that many patients who have suffered a skin injury ask themselves or their physicians.

In developed nations, about 100 million people will acquire scars after a surgical procedure each year; it is estimated that around 11 million people have keloids. [1] Scars are the result of skin injury from trauma or disease. [2] Although scars rarely pose a significant health risk, patients often experience significant physical, aesthetic, psychological and social distress.

These consequences may be associated with substantial financial and emotional costs. Fortunately, there are many treatment options to improve cosmetic and physical appearance, as well as quality of life. Furthermore, these treatment modalities may deter future harmful consequences since scars often act as sites for development of other diseases. [3]

Physicians should consider a patient's history, body site, and tendencies toward scarring; for example, certain locations with greater tension result in a higher risk of scarring. [4] The physician should aim to lessen scar formation and contemplate its severity. This chapter discusses the causes, types, and treatment of scars.

II. Causes

Scars are the result of the skin's response to injury. Wound healing is a series of events that take place after injury to the skin. This process attempts to repair the function of skin as a barrier as well as its tensile strength. Abnormal scarring may occur if wound healing is disrupted from its normal, pre-planned pattern.

Although changes in color and vascularity are often transient in nature, the resulting changes in texture through disruption of collagen may be permanent, especially concerning keloids. [5, 6] The three consecutive, yet overlapping stages that comprise wound healing include: inflammation, granulation, and remodeling. [7] The first stage consists of a response to skin injury containing inflammatory cells. [8]

The first cells present in an injury are neutrophils, which debride bacteria and necrotic tissue and recruit other key inflammatory mediators. [8] Macrophages arrive and promote an environment for granulation tissue formation by elaborating a variety of cytokines such as Vascular Endothelial Growth Factor (VEGF). [7] Fibroblasts arrive, multiply, and deposit collagen – initially type III and afterwards, mostly type I – during the proliferative phase of the wound healing process. Simultaneously, the formation of new capillaries in the wound bed is driven by angiogenic factors. Re-epithelialization also occurs due to migration of keratinocytes across the wound [9]

During the remodeling phase, there is concurrent collagen formation and destruction.[6] Meanwhile, myofibroblasts help to increase the tensile strength. [6] Granulation tissue deposition is reduced as the cells accountable for this process undergo apoptosis. [10]

Hypertrophic scars may result from disruption of this systematic process [10] This disturbance causes an overzealous healing response in which small vessels, collagen fibers, and fibroblasts are arranged in a nodular fashion. [6] The ensuing inadequate replacement of collagen fibers resembles a pitted, dimpled surface.

The purpose of this chapter is to review the causes and types of scars, as well as the strengths and limitations of lasers and other therapies. We will also discuss the different management options used to improve the appearance and symptoms of hypertrophic, keloid, atrophic, striae, and acne scars.

III. Types of Scars

Scars can be classified as hypertrophic, normotrophic, and atrophic. Raised (or hypertrophic) scars include: keloids and hypertrophic scars. Atrophic scar subtypes include: striae distensae, epidermal and dermal atrophy, and panatrophy. Other scars may occur as a result of acne, burns, or contractures.

Hypertrophic Scars

Hypertrophic scars are elevated scars that stay within the borders of the original lesion. Clinically, hypertrophic scars and keloids are very similar but keloids exceed the surrounding boundaries of the original injury. [11] They are usually pink-red, raised, firm, itchy, and tender. Hypertrophic scars and keloids can lead to symptoms such as pain, pruritus, dysesthesias, and the formation of strictures. [12] Common locations include areas of increased pressure or movement, and/or in the site of a burn injury [11, 13].

The pathogenesis may be attributed to excess collagen synthesis along with limited collagen destruction during the remodeling stage of wound healing. [11] Type III collagen is made in greater amounts in hypertrophic scars than in normal, healthy skin. As a result, thick collagen bundles form with fibroblasts arranged in a nodular fashion instead of smoothly [13]

This period of collagen synthesis generally peaks at six months and then starts to decline. Decreased flexibility and extensibility due to altered enzymatic matrix properties contribute to the firm feel of both hypertrophic and keloid scars. These enzymatic alterations include: greater concentrations of glycosaminoglycan, greater percentages of hyaluronic acid and chondroitin sulfate, resembling the characteristics of a tendon. Furthermore, hypertrophic scars have nearly four times as much collagenase activity and less elastic fiber component (0.1%) than normal skin (1-2%). [14]

The typical locations for hypertrophic scars include: the trunk and the extremities. Hypertrophic scars usually take approximately four weeks to appear after trauma or a surgical insult. [13] In most cases, spontaneous regression with maturation, softening, and flattening after the associated insult occurs.

Keloids

Keloids are raised, reddish-purple, nodular scars that invade the surrounding skin in a manner that depends on each particular site. It is difficult to classify a scar as a keloid unless it has been present for more than one year, but there is no specific time interval. The time to appearance after insult may be weeks to months, however, they may also arise spontaneously without a clear inciting event. [13] Clinically, keloids cause much more symptoms than hypertrophic scars including: pain, pruritus, physical discomfort, burning sensations, and dysesthesias. [13]. Keloids are more common among individuals with darker skin types, but can occur in anyone. [13] Other relevant factors include: wound tension, particular locations such as the parasternal area, shoulder, back and earlobe; young age; pregnancy; family history; deep lacerations; severe acne scarring; blood type A; ear piercing; and healing by secondary intention [2]. While clinically similar to hypertrophic scars, keloids are very different microscopically. Collagen synthesis, primarily type I, in keloids may persist for several years, while in most scars the duration is only six months. [2] Collagen fibers are arranged in swirling, nodular whorls with increased hyaluronidase. [13] The exophytic nature of keloids risks greater exposure to minor trauma, abrasions, irritation and interference with surrounding objects and structures. Despite their appearance and pathophysiology, keloids are relatively resistant to malignant degeneration. Possible reasons include increased activity of ALT (alanine transaminase) liver enzyme, which is high in keloids, normal in hypertrophic and regular scars, and low in malignant tumors.

An extended proliferative phase of wound healing leads to the proliferation and growth over time unique to keloids [13]. Keloids usually persist indefinitely unless there is treatment or intervention. They tend to grow over time and in most cases, will recur if excised.

Striae Distensae

Striae distensae, also known as "stretch marks," are linear streaks of wrinkled skin. [13] They are the most common example of atrophic scarring, affecting approximately half of the population. [15] Characteristic settings that play a contributory role include: pregnancy, rapid weight change, puberty and developmental growth, and excessive use of corticosteroids (both oral and topical). [13] The incidence of striae is much greater in women than men, with a 70% incidence in the former vs. 40% for the latter. Pregnancy is a typical precursor; striae distensae affect approximately 90% of pregnant women, particularly during their third trimester [2] Initially, striae distensae appear as reddish-purple, violaceous, urticarial and pruritic streaks (striae rubra). The pathophysiology behind this initial presentation is driven by dermal inflammation combined with mast cell degranulation, elastic tissue destruction, and capillary dilatation. [16] Within a few months, the inflammation subsides, leaving behind hypopigmented, fibrotic, almost parallel lines (striae alba). [16] The appearance of striae alba is due to epidermal atrophy and the linear accumulation of dermal bundles [16]. Although the entire pathophysiology remains undefined, estrogen and mast cell degranulation may play contributory roles. [16]

Atrophic Scars

Atrophic scars are flat, dermal depressions that tend to arise after acute inflammation, trauma, or disease, which causes collagen destruction and dermal atrophy. [13] Their appearance is generally small with an indented center. Contributory factors include: nodulocystic acne, vesicular viral diseases such as childhood varicella, surgery, medications, and trauma [13] On the skin surface, these indented scars bear a resemblance to the depressions of a golf ball. As a result, the irregular tomography of the skin represents a challenge for treatment. [17] Thus, the goals of therapy are aimed at restoration of a smooth, skin surface.

Acne Scars

Scarring may occur as a result of acne lesions retreating from their active phase. The two main types of acne scars are: atrophic and hypertrophic. [17, 18] With respect to the latter subtype, patients may be left with a hypertrophic scar or a keloid.

The atrophic subtype is about three times as common, and is present in approximately 80-90% of individuals who scar after an acne outbreak. [18] Further classifications of atrophic subtype include: ice pick, boxcar, and rolling, in descending order of frequency. [17, 18]

Ice-pick scars are the most common subtype and are usually small (around 2 mm in diameter), sharply demarcated, deep scars. They are wider at the epithelial surface and extend vertically into the dermis or even the subcutaneous tissue, giving a characteristic "V" shape. [18] Rolling scars: tend to be wider, greater than 4-5 mm, and shallower than other acne scars. Their rolling or undulated pattern is characterized by tethering of the dermis to the subcutaneous tissue in otherwise normal skin. The shape that represents this lesion is that of the alphabet letter, "M." [18] Boxcar scars: Boxcar scars are typically oval, round depressions with sharply defined vertical margins. Their depth may vary from superficial (0.1-0.5 mm) or deep (> 0.5 mm), and sometimes resemble residual scarring after a chickenpox infection. Their shape resembles a "U" rather than a "V" since they are typically wider than icepick scars and do not taper [19].

IV. Assessment

Important Scar Variables to Consider

The classification of scars is becoming more important in daily, dermatologic clinical evaluations. Although there is no ideal universal standard, scars need to be approached in a systematic manner. This approach may be guided by specific criteria, such as: color, blood supply, texture, surface area, thickness or height, and pliability.

While there is a wide variety of treatment options such as: cryotherapy, radiation, surgery, pressure therapy, and different types of lasers; a proper assessment may be able to guide treatment modalities.

A. Color

Color may be measured by assessing the mismatch in pigmentation compared to normal skin. Different scales range from subjective measurements stating the degree of mismatch as: none, slight, obvious, or gross; to objective methods using instruments that measure the erythema and melanin indices, to flow Dopplers that measure the amount of blood flow that contributes to a scar's pigmentation. The eye is also a powerful visual tool that can detect the imperfections in scar coloration [20]

B. Vascularity

Vascularity may be evaluated as normal, pink, red, or purple according to the Vancouver Burn Scar Scale among other instruments [21].

C. Scar Thickness and Height

Ultrasound is both reliable and accurate for calculating scar thickness and remains as an effective resource. [22]

D. Pliability

Pliability refers to features of mobility, laxity, stiffness, elasticity, and contraction. Pliability may be measured by attempting to fold the scar and may be graded as: normal, supple, yielding, firm, banding, or a contracture. Scars that overlay joints are more likely to contribute to contractures. Functionality is also an important variable that is reflected by the value of pliability [20]

E. Texture

The surface texture is a difficult parameter to estimate. With age, changes in a scar's surfaces occur, becoming more irregular and raised. Examples of measurement devices that are used for cosmetic purposes include: optical and mechanical profilometers [20].

F. Surface Area

The planimetry, or surface area, is important to assess because scars may contract with time or become hypertrophic in nature. Tracing scars may help estimate the contraction margins, but only short-term during the wound healing process.

Photography is the most common, reliable, and accurate measurement, especially on planar surfaces. [22] Digital photography is the recommendation of choice and the gold standard. [20]

Nevertheless, many of these scales lack correlation with symptoms, such as: pruritus, pain, psychosocial status, aesthetic impact, functionality and/or disability, and future expectations, all of which should be done as part of a comprehensive patient assessment before discussing treatment options.

Important Patient Variables to Consider

When deciding upon treatment modalities, physicians should also consider certain patient variables that may influence treatment outcome.

A. Skin Types

Ethnic makeup is an important consideration since certain phototypes are prone to the development of particular types of scars. [23]. For example, dark-skinned individuals are more predisposed to keloid development. The incidence of keloids in blacks and individuals of Hispanic heritage is approximately 4.5-16%. [24]

Increased levels of hemoglobin in darker-skinned individuals compete with the pigment in the energy absorption from vascular-specific lasers. [25] Consequently, the amount of energy delivered to the scar results in lower yields [25].

Furthermore, laser destruction of melanin in the epidermis may result in accidental hypopigmentation.[25] On the other hand, when using specific laser resurfacing techniques such as, Er:YAG (Erbium: Yttrium-Aluminum-Garnet) or carbon dioxide (CO_2) lasers, the patient should be warned about possible, temporary hyperpigmentation after treatment [26]

B. Coexisting Infectious or Inflammatory Condition

Patients should not undergo laser therapy in the setting of a concurrent infection or inflammatory process. Infections due to bacterial or viral etiologies may spread after laser surgery. [26, 27] Inflammation of the dermis may hinder the healing process and treatment efficacy. Certain skin conditions such as psoriasis, severe acne, and dermatitis may actually worsen after laser therapy. [27]

C. Medications

Many patients who seek laser treatment for atrophic acne scarring usually have a history of severe acne and were (previously or currently) on treatment with isotretinoin. Isotretinoin alters the wound healing environment and impairs collagenase production; thus, concurrent treatment with lasers may in fact lead to unsightly hypertrophic scarring.[27, 28] Current recommendations suggest stopping isotretinoin at least six months before laser therapy. [27]

D. Goals and Expectations

It is important for patients to understand that no treatment is 100% perfect, and there is nothing that can make scars magically disappear. Hence, multiple treatments may be required to improve the outcome and some residual scar tissue may remain [28]

As a result, patients should be advised to maintain compliance regarding appointments and to avoid possible complications that may arise. [28]

V. Non-Laser Therapy

There are various options for the treatment of scars. Several techniques will now be discussed.

Dermabrasion

Dermabrasion is a facial resurfacing technique that promotes re-epithelialization after mechanical ablation of damaged skin. [30] The re-epithelialization process usually takes 5 to 7 days for completion and allows the epidermis to regenerate after the defective dermis and epidermis have been removed. [31] Several methods and instruments are used to perform dermabrasion. [32]

The devices used are usually small, portable and hand-held. End pieces, including wire brushes, diamond fraises and serrated wheels, are attached to the end of the dermabrader to allow precise resurfacing. This technique can be combined with other dermatologic procedures, including chemical exfoliation, soft tissue augmentation and laser procedures and should be performed by a trained and skilled surgeon. [31] It is a less costly procedure when compared to lasers and some chemical peels. It has been used for the treatment of several dermatological conditions like Mohs defects, rhinophyma, actinic keratoses, seborrheic keratoses, angiofibromas, syringomas, solar elastosis, epidermal nevi, and tattoo removal. Dermabrasion is a cost-effective option to treat acne and atrophic scars. [31, 33]

The procedure is contraindicated in patients with recent facial surgery, isotretinoin use within the last 6 to 12 months and active skin infection. Depending on patient expectations and the extent of the procedure, local anesthesia, sedation, or general anesthesia may be considered. [34]

Chemical Peels

Chemical peels are a widely used technique in dermatological practice in which a chemical solution is applied to the skin to promote accelerated exfoliation. The result is thickening of the epidermis, deposition of collagen, reorganization of structural epidermis, and increased dermal volume. [35] The type of peel should be determined according to the skin condition and desired results. Peels are an alternative for patients who cannot afford expensive alternatives.

Repeated sessions are usually necessary to reduce the visibility of deep scars. More superficial scars respond better to this procedure. The most common types of peels used to treat scars are glycolic acid, lactic acid, salicylic acid, and trichloroacetic acid. [36, 37].

Glycolic acid: This type of peel can be used in different concentrations, usually between 20 and 80%. It can be used for the treatment of acne scarring and also for active acne vulgaris [38, 39]

Lactic acid: This peel is less irritating than glycolic acid and its percentages ranges from 10% to 70%. It has larger molecule that allows it to penetrate slowly, reducing treatment-induced inflammation. [40]

Salicylic acid: It is a keratolytic and lipophilic substance typically applied in 20% to 30% formulations and shows good results in the treatment of superficial scars. [38, 41]

Tricholoroacetic acid: It is a synthetically derived peeling agent made of acetic acid and chlorine. The mechanism of action for TCA is the coagulation of proteins and cell necrosis. It is available in different percentages (5-100%) and show good results in the treatment of different types of scars. [42, 43]

Phenol (carbolic acid): It is the deepest type of chemical peel and only a single treatment is required. Recovery time is usually the longest of any peel, sometimes a week or longer. There is a risk of hypopigmentation. [44]

Microneedling

Also known as Collagen Induction Therapy, medical microneedling is a procedure that uses microneedles, arranged on a drum shape instrument to produce channels in dermis to stimulate collagen and proteins. [45] These microneedles are available in a variety of shapes and sizes. The indications of this procedure include treatment of acne, burns, and surgical scars and also has been used widely for facial rejuvenation [46].

The use of topical anesthesia is recommended as some patients may find the procedure to be painful. Rolling should be done 15-20 times in horizontal, vertical, and oblique directions for better results [47]

Microneedling is a simple and inexpensive office procedure and is safe for all skin types. This procedure can be associated to other treatments like subcision, chemical peels, and microdermabrasion [45]

Topical Treatments

Several products are available over-the-counter and by prescription. Scar hydration is an important factor in wound healing and can be achieved with the use of topical creams, gels, and lotions. [48] Antihistamine creams can be effective in the treatment of pruritus. [49] Pressure dressings are commonly used and semi-occlusive silicone-based ointments are used to speed the healing process and to reduce the appearance of scars. [50, 51] Several studies show that onion extract may be an option to improve the global appearance of a scar as well its softness, redness, and texture [52-54].

Injections

Corticoid injections (triamcinolone acetonide 10 mg / 40 mg) are widely used to treat scars. A long-term course under medical supervision can help to flatten and soften the appearance of hypertrophic scars. [55, 56] Steroids inhibit collagen synthesis and also has anti-inflammatory properties. Multiple injections may be required to achieve a desirable effect. [55, 56]

The use of 5-fluorouracil (5-FU) injections has also been reported as an effective treatment for keloids and hypertrophic scars. This drug inhibits fibroblast proliferation in tissue culture and reduces post-operative scarring. This treatment is considered painful so administration of triamcinolone acetonide or a field block of anesthesia can be useful to reduce pain [57].

Studies have also reported the use of bleomycin, a chemotherapy agent, to treat keloids. Due to its side effects and costs, the use of bleomycin is restricted. Interferon has also been reported as an alternative option to treat keloids. Studies suggest that it could be more effective to prevent a scar's recurrence than intra-lesional steroids [58].

Surgical Removal

Scalpels, electrosurgery, and laser surgery can be used to excise scars. These procedures should be associated with other methods, such as pressotherapy, silicone gel sheeting, or intra-lesional corticosteroids to prevent recurrence. [59, 60]

Cryotherapy

Cryotherapy is used to soften and flatten the lesions, but also makes the intra-lesional therapies easier. It is a safe, economic, and easy-to-perform monotherapy to treat keloid lesions and hypertrophic scars. Local anesthesia can be used to minimize pain during the procedure. [61]

VI. Peri-Operative Management with Laser Therapy

Pre-Operative

A good history including onset, location, associated symptoms, changes, and previous attempted therapies is always important irrespective of the treatment choice. Hypertrophic scars should be treated early, preferably within a few months of appearance because there are many blood vessels during this time. Adjustment of laser parameters may be needed for previous attempted therapies such as cryosurgery, which causes fibrosis. Although some experts have found no association regarding scar location, Nouri et al. (2003) found that facial, arm, and shoulder scars have a better response to treatment than those on the anterior chest wall. [29]

Pulsed-dye laser (PDL) for keloids and hypertrophic scars is usually performed in an outpatient setting and does not require anesthesia under normal circumstances. A topical anesthesia, such as lidocaine may be applied within an hour before treatment if requested by the patient. The lesion should be clean, and free of makeup and creams. A photograph may be taken for comparison and to monitor improvement during each treatment session. Each individual present during the procedure should wear eyewear safety at all times to protect the eye from retinal and ocular damage.

Post-Operative

Physicians should educate patients to avoid sun exposure to minimize pigmentary alterations. The site of treatment should be cleansed appropriately and trauma to this area should be avoided. Follow-up treatments with further laser applications may be done in 4-6 weeks.

Potential Complications and Adverse Effects

Purpura is the most commonly reported side effect from laser treatment, appearing immediately and lasting approximately one week. Patients that undergo laser therapy often describe is a common, yet uncomfortable sensation similar to having a rubber band snap on one's skin. Burning or pruritus are also a common symptoms that typically subside within days. If pigmentary alterations occur, patients may be given a bleaching cream.

Prevention

To avoid complications, postponing of further treatment sessions should be done until the affected area has completely healed. Keep the affected area moist with an ointment, such as petroleum jelly, and covered with a non-occlusive bandage to avoid contact and minimize trauma. One may also consider adjusting the laser settings. Subsequent treatment may need deferral to ensure effective targeting of the scar.

VII. Scar-Specific Lasers

Lasers for Hypertrophic Scars and Keloids

The first-line therapy for hypertrophic scars and keloids is PDL, which is usually done in an outpatient setting. [11] If anesthesia is used, a topical lidocaine cream is usually applied approximately 30 minutes before the procedure; for instance, 30% lidocaine powder in a water-cream mixture. Other topical anesthetic options include: lidocaine 2.5% and prilocaine 2.5% cream mixture, or liposomal lidocaine 4% cream. An intra-lesional injection or nerve block may benefit patients with scars in sensitive locations such as the lips, breasts, perineum, and digits [27].

This technique consists of serial, non-overlapping laser pulses that cover the entire area of the scar. [27] Physicians should aim to treat the entire scar during each session. Scar variables that are determining factors for choosing the laser's energy density include: color, location, height, size, and skin type. The level of energy densities and fluences has a positive correlation to the amount of fibrosis in a scar. For instance, scars that are thicker and darker often use higher fluences while less fibrotic scars in sensitive areas, such as the parasternal area and breasts, require lower fluences.

Generally, sessions should commence at low fluences, permitting modification of energy to higher fluences depending on the lesion's response to previous therapy. [27] On that note, if the initial response to treatment is favorable, the energy density should remain constant at the same level for subsequent therapy sessions. If there is minimal response to treatment, consider increasing energy fluences by 10% during the next session. If the patient develops adverse effects such as crusting and vesiculations, consider lowering fluences while paying careful attention to pulse technique to avoid overlap.

Post-operative bruising after PDL treatment generally disappears within 7-10 days. [62] The patient should avoid unnecessary manipulation of the affected area during the healing period. Post-operatively, the patient is allowed to shower and afterwards, to gently "pat dry" the lasered areas. Use of a non-stick bandage to conceal the affected area is appropriate. A follow-up laser therapy session is recommended in 6-8 weeks for evaluation of response to treatment and subsequent laser application if deemed necessary.

The most commonly encountered complication is focal hyperpigmentation of the treated skin. This usually fades by avoiding the sun and using solar protection. If this side effect is present, postpone the next laser session to avoid interfering with a competing laser target, i.e. melanin. To hasten the healing process, consider prescribing a daily or twice daily topical application of hydroquinone.

On occasion, patients may develop an allergic contact dermatitis due to topical antibiotics or irritation from bandages. When a post-treatment rash is present, it is important to determine whether it is normal vs. abnormal, purpuric vs. non-purpuric, and if it is related or unrelated to laser irradiation. For example, if pruritus is involved, the rash may be attributed to contact dermatitis. In this case, topical steroid creams are recommended until symptoms subside and the rash clears. Remember to discontinue use of the offending agent immediately. [27]

Regarding reported results, hypertrophic scars demonstrate a 50-80% improvement rate after two laser sessions. Meanwhile, keloids and severe hypertrophic scars typically require more treatment sessions to achieve optimal outcomes.

Lasers for Striae Distensae

Striae distensae respond better to low-energy densities (3 J/cm2) and 585- or 595-nm pulsed dye lasers [11]. Adjacent targeting may be needed to cover the entire surface area involved, and usually only 1-2 sessions are needed for satisfactory results. [27] After laser irradiation, striae distensae usually do not exhibit bruising comparable to hypertrophic scars or keloids but may appear slightly pink due to tissue vascularity and edema. Superficial crusts and vesicles should not appear when appropriate techniques and fluences are used.

Other lasers such as ablative and non-ablative CO_2 have been applied to scars for treatment. In a study comparing different laser treatments to patients with striae alba, investigators found that both fractional Er:glass laser and ablative fractional CO_2 laser resurfacing significantly improved scars. The abdominal striae in this study demonstrated dramatic improvement both clinically and histologically while undergoing three treatment sessions at 4-week intervals. [63]

Lasers for Atrophic Scars

Carbon dioxide and Er:YAG laser vaporization of facial atrophic scars for recontouring is a very popular procedure among patients. [26, 64-67] Both laser modalities attain foreseeable and reproducible tissue vaporization by way of selective ablation of water-containing tissue, achieving more precision than dermabrasion. [68-74]

During laser resurfacing, destruction of the epidermis and varying portions of the dermis takes place. [75, 76] A study done by Fitzpatrick et al. showed that the depth of vaporization and residual necrosis secondary to CO_2 laser resurfacing was directly proportional to the pulse energy and the number of laser pulses [77].

The Er:YAG pulsed lasers have 10 times more selectivity for water in tissue than CO_2 lasers, resulting in greater tissue vaporization and less residual thermal damage of the dermal layer. [74] There is less overall risk of erythema after Er:YAG treatment; yet, the overall decrease in clinical improvement presents a challenge to the limited photothermal effect on tissue, unique to Er:YAG. [74] In conclusion, the CO_2 laser results in more shrinkage of collagen relative to its counterpart.[26] Still, Er:YAG lasers may be preferable for mild atrophic scars considering the shorter post-operative recovery.

Regardless of which treatment modality is chosen, management goals remain the same: A) to soften the transition between the atrophic scar and normal, surrounding skin; B) to stimulate production of collagen within the area of atrophy [27]. Treat the entire cosmetic subunit to minimize risk of uneven texture or color. For treatment of a single scar, spot resurfacing is strongly suggested. The use of a handheld scanning device is beneficial for decreasing treatment times when lasering large areas. De-epithelialization usually requires 2-3 passes with Er:YAG laser at 5 J/cm2 and one pass with CO_2 laser at 300 mJ. Once this process of de-epithelialization is accomplished, the scar edges can be further recontoured with further vaporizing laser passes. Partially desiccated tissue may be removed with wet gauze (soaked with either saline or water) to prevent charring after each laser pass. [77]

In general, varying patterns of sizes and shapes are used with the computer pattern generator (CPG) scanning device (a.k.a. Coherent UltraPulse) in the context of 300 mJ of energy and 60 watts of power. [27] Dependent on scarring severity and the system being used, scanning devices attached to other CO_2 laser systems, such as Sharplan FeatherTouch or Luxar NovaPulse, may be used at 5-20 watts per scan. [27] The scanning sizes delivered to the affected area range from 4-10 mm in diameter. Each session usually needs 2-3 passes, thus the physician should carefully remove all partially desiccated tissue between passes. After treating the entire cosmetic subunit, the respective scar edges may be recontoured further using spots or scans with a smaller diameter.

Another option for de-epithelialization and contouring of scars is the Er:YAG laser with a 5-mm spot size at 1-3 J (5-15 J/cm2). The Er:YAG laser uses a technique similar to CO_2. Furthermore, wiping between laser passes as a precaution for desiccated tissue is unnecessary because Er:YAG vaporization does not usually produce significant desiccated tissue. Yet, hair-bearing areas will need wiping in order to decrease thermal conduction to skin through seared surface hairs. Bleeding usually occurs with the third laser pass secondary to dermal penetration and the inability of the Er:YAG laser to photocoagulate vessels [26].

The treated skin commonly appears reddened and swollen immediately after treatment when using either CO_2 or Er:YAG laser; these symptoms may worsen during the next 48 hours due to sloughing of coagulated tissue. [77] Several steps that may lessen associated symptoms while appeasing the patient include: semi-occlusive dressings, nightly head elevation, topical emollients, and cooling the affected area with wet compresses. [78] The first post-operative week is essential for monitoring wound healing, response to treatment, and complications, such as rashes and infection.

Re-epithelialization takes 4-7 and 7-10 days for Er:YAG and CO_2 laser resurfacing, respectively [26].

As mentioned previously, transient post-operative hyperpigmentation is a common side effect that may occur with either CO_2 or Er:YAG therapy. This particular complication is more common in patients with darker phototypes and typically occurs around 1-2 months post-laser. [79, 80] Although the hyperpigmentation is generally self-limited, bleaching creams and acid preparations may hasten the resolution. [26] Recommended bleaching creams are those with hydroquinone or arbutin components; suggested acid preparation ingredients are: glycolic, retinoic, azelaic, kojic, or ascorbic. [26] Contrastingly, hypopigmentation is generally a late complication usually observed more than six months after laser and is presumed to be permanent. [26]

Post-operative re-epithelialization of the skin predisposes to infections of bacterial (i.e. staphylococcus, pseudomonas), viral (i.e. HSV), or fungal (i.e. Candida) etiology. [26] However, appropriate antibiotic prophylaxis and suitable wound care significantly reduce the incidence of infection. If a post-operative infection is suspected, it must be diagnosed and treated promptly. [79, 80]

Ectropion and hypertrophic scar formation are the most severe complications of laser treatment, likely due to exceedingly aggressive technique. [79] While ectropion may be corrected surgically, hypertrophic scars resulting from burning may be managed with a 585-nm PDL laser.

Since collagen remodeling usually lasts 12-18 months, consider postponing revisions of the remaining scars until approximately one year later for optimal clinical results. Although the Er:YAG system is efficacious in the treatment of atrophic scars, the CO_2 laser system offers more collagen remodeling. For mild acne scarring and contouring of scars edges, the Er:YAG laser is the recommended option. [74]

Lasers for Acne Scars

With respect to skin remodeling, laser treatment is both safe and efficacious for improving appearance. Apart from lasers, other methods, such as excision, subcision, cryotherapy, punch grafts, fillers, peels, and silicone sheeting compression, may be used to improve acne scars. [81] Punch excisions may be more effective for removal of icepick scars since they usually extend deep into the dermis. [27, 81, 82] In contrast, the treatment goal for rolling scars should target the irregular anchoring of the dermis to the subcutis. [27, 82] Thus, revision with lasers are mostly recommended for superficial acne scars and shallow boxcar lesions. [27, 81, 82]

A beneficial alternative may include ablative laser resurfacing with CO_2 or Er:YAG lasers. After the initial therapy session, the skin should be given a period of 6-8 weeks of healing. Post-operative redness may last up to 12 weeks. For optimal appearance and skin remodeling, the lesion may be treated with additional laser therapy sessions.

As mentioned previously, treatment with CO_2 lasers carry potential side effects such as delayed hypopigmentation, scarring, and increased healing time. [79] Although ablative lasers may be used as a sole treatment for acne scars, potential risks must be considered and discussed with patients before undergoing treatment. CO_2 and ER:YAG lasers may be combined to enhance selectivity of the CO_2 laser since the Er:YAG laser demonstrates preferential uptake. The Erbium laser is more selective, localized, and less destructive to the skin than CO_2 resurfacing because the energy is consumed quickly within the targeted tissue.

To hasten the wound healing process and reduce post-operative CO_2 laser complications, the CO_2 laser may be used to initially treat the scar followed by Er:YAG irradiation for further remodeling. [79] As opposed to ablative laser resurfacing, non-ablative lasers deliver thermal energy and damage the dermis but do not significantly disrupt the epidermis. [66] The respective lasers promote remodeling and generation of collagen, mostly type III. As the wound healing process unfolds, type I collagen becomes more prominent. [66] Clinical improvement usually requires more than one treatment session, yet, the lesion may improve in appearance months later, even after the laser treatments have been fulfilled.

According to Alster and McMeekin, the 585-nm PDL may improve erythematous and hypertrophic acne scars. [83] In this study conducted in 1996, 22 patients demonstrated dramatic improvements in erythema and skin texture after only 1-2 treatments (6-7 J/cm2; 7-mm spot size). The average rate of improvement is approximately 67.5% after 6 weeks of treatment with one PDL session. There was a mean improvement rate of 72.5% 6 weeks later for 8 patients that received an additional PDL session.

The 1064-nm Q-switched neodymium: yttrium-aluminum-garnet (Nd:YAG) laser has also been used to treat atrophic acne scars. [84] During this study, the respective laser was used to treat mild-moderate atrophic scars for five sessions at 3-week intervals at an average fluence of 3.4 J/cm2, 4- to 6- nanosecond pulse duration, and a 6-mm spot size. Approximately four weeks after the fifth laser session, skin roughness improved in texture by 23.3%. The scars improved further with time. Patients showed a 39.2% statistically significant improvement from initial measurements at their 6-month follow-up. As stated earlier, a significant portion of this improvement may be attributed to the ongoing effect of collagen remodeling after the laser treatment sessions have been completed. The 1064-nm Q-switched Nd:YAG laser is both a safe and effective option for mild-moderate atrophic acne scars given its tolerable side effects, such as mild-moderate erythema, petechiae, and discomfort.

Another treatment option for acne scars is the 1320-nm Nd:YAG laser along with its incorporated cryogen cooling spray. In a 2004 study by Sadick and Schecter, 8 patients showed moderate improvement with six monthly sessions of three passes each.[85] A more favorable response was noted in icepick scars without fibrosis compared to those with more fibrous tissue. Seven out of 8 patients demonstrated statistically significant positive results approximately five months and one year after completing laser treatments. Further investigation established that atrophic scars improved the most after only three laser sessions. Meanwhile, there was only a mild response for Asian patients who enrolled in the study. No improvement was seen in 8 patients and only a mild response to treatment was observed in 9 patients out of a total of 27 that underwent treatment. More improvement may be observed if this treatment is combined with another type of therapy, such as surgery or intense-pulsed-light (IPL) source.

A comparable study by Tanzi and Alster (2004) investigated the effectiveness of the 1320-nm Nd:YAG laser compared to 1450-nm diode laser for treatment of atrophic facial scars. [86] A total of 20 patients received three monthly treatments for mild-moderate acne scars. One of the two lasers was randomized for half of each patient's face. The greatest clinical improvement was seen at six months after completion of laser sessions, as expected within the associated period of heightened collagen production during wound healing. Regarding improvement of the appearance of mild-moderate facial atrophic scars, both lasers proved to be safe and non-invasive alternatives. Though the 1450-nm diode laser demonstrated significantly better results, only modest improvements in appearance were seen with both lasers.

Recently developed, fractional lasers deliver high-intensity light fractionated through focused lenses. [87] This technology generates arrays of microscopic columns of thermal injury surrounded by uninjured tissue. These minute columns are called "microscopic thermal treatment zones." The operator may adjust the laser's energy and density of these zones. Other approved uses for fractional laser devices include: skin resurfacing, soft-tissue coagulation, melasma, peri-orbital rhytides, and acne scars. [87]

The reserve of adjacent viable tissue that remains undamaged allows for rapid repair of the epidermis and decreases patient downtime. [87] Thus, for scar treatment, both ablative and non-ablative fractional lasers may be used effectively.

The safety and effectiveness of the non-ablative 1540-nm Er:glass fractional laser for surgical and post-traumatic scars was analyzed in a study by Vasily et al. [88] To assess the impact of fractional treatment and to assess healing post-treatment of scars, a histologic study was conducted to compare the lesions with baseline histologic findings of the scar. These findings showed quick epidermal re-epithelialization approximately 72 hours after treatment. Roughly two weeks after treatment, rearrangement of dermal collagen fibers and scar tissue remodeling was evident. Compared to baseline, 43% of the scars demonstrated 75% or more improvement, while 73% showed 50% or more, respectively. [88]

A combination of dot peeling (focal application of higher trichloroacetic acid concentrations), subcision (subcutaneous incisionless surgery), and fractional laser irradiation may be incorporated as an alternative treatment option. A pilot study investigated the safety and efficacy of this alternative for the treatment of acne scars. In this study, there was a mean decrease of 55.3% in acne scar severity scores. Approximately 80% of patients reported noticeable improvement [82].

A study conducted by Cho et al. (2010) evaluated the safety and efficacy of single-sessions of 1550-nm Er-doped fractional photothermolysis and 10,600-nm CO_2 fractional laser systems for acne scars.[89] This study was randomized, split-face, investigator-blinded with a total of 8 patients who had acne scars. One of the two lasers of the fractional photothermolysis and CO_2 fractional laser systems were randomized for half of each patient's face. Based on clinical evaluation, the fractional photothermolysis system demonstrated 2 ± 0.5 improvement while the CO_2 laser system showed 2.5 ± 0.8 improvement at three months post-treatment [89].

A study in 2008 concluded that lasers may be used to improve the appearance of scars immediately after surgery. [90] As Capon et al. (2010) demonstrated, the 810-nm diode laser improves the appearance of surgical scars immediately in the post-operative period. An important variable in scar improvement is the dose of the laser, which must be well-controlled and adjusted appropriately. The Laser-Assisted Skin Healing (LASH) technique, which modifies wound healing, causes an elevation in skin temperature. An additional suggestion from the authors stated that LASH could also be used for revision of hypertrophic scars. [90] An open study on 24 Japanese patients (ages 15-44) with facial acne scars managed with five sessions of low-energy, double-pass, 1450-nm diode lasers at 4-week intervals, was conducted by Wada and colleagues. [91] Before treatment, the average duration of the acne scars was approximately 4.8 years with a range varying from 1-9 years. Patients were evaluated clinically by physicians and with imaging at baseline, one month after the final laser session, and at a 3-month follow-up. During follow-up, topical agents for acne were allowed. All patients finished the five treatment sessions and 75% demonstrated at least 30% improvement in appearance of acne scars. Intriguingly, approximately 92.9% of the patients in the study that had improved by more than 30% actually maintained effectiveness after three months of follow-up [91].

Conclusion

Understanding the mechanism of formation of scars is important to identify and suggest optimal treatments to patients. Several techniques and lasers devices are available. Laser technology is an efficacious therapy and has been shown successful results in the management of different type of scars.

The appropriate classification of the type is mandatory to determine which laser will be effective. Pulsed dye lasers are the best option for hypertrophic scars, keloids and striae. The use of 585-nm PDL has demonstrated improvements in scar erythema, quality and appearance, starting on the suture removal day. Several laser categories have been used to treat atrophic scars, ablative resurfacing is an effective therapy but the adverse post operatively events and side effects limit its use. Non-ablative resurfacing is safer but may not be as effective as ablative resurfacing. Future perspectives include the use of multiple lasers to optimize results. Other options for treatment that may be less expensive, such as dermabrasion, chemical peels, microneedling, injections, surgery and cryotherapy, were also discussed in this chapter.

References

[1] Sund, B., New developments in wound care. *PJB Publications*, 2000.
[2] Sahl, W.J., Jr. and H. Clever, *Cutaneous scars: Part I. Int. J. Dermatol*, 1994. 33(10): p. 681-91.
[3] Sahl, W.J., Jr. and H. Clever, *Cutaneous scars: Part II. Int. J. Dermatol*, 1994. 33(11): p. 763-9.
[4] Bayat, A. and D.A. McGrouther, *Clinical management of skin scarring. Skinmed,* 2005. 4(3): p. 165-73.

[5] Akaishi, S., R. Ogawa, and H. Hyakusoku, Keloid and hypertrophic scar: neurogenic inflammation hypotheses. *Med. Hypotheses*, 2008. 71(1): p. 32-8.
[6] English, R.S. and P.D. Shenefelt, Keloids and hypertrophic scars. *Dermatol Surg*, 1999. 25(8): p. 631-8.
[7] Habif, T.P., *Surgical Procedures, in Clinical Dermatology*, 4 ed.2009, Elsevier.
[8] Falanga, V. and S. Iwamoto, Wound repair: mechanisms and practical considerations., in *Fitzpatrick's Dermatology in General Medicine*, 7 ed.2008, McGraw-Hill. p. 91-2.
[9] Fonder, M.A., et al., Treating the chronic wound: A practical approach to the care of nonhealing wounds and wound care dressings. *J. Am. Acad. Dermatol*, 2008. 58(2): p. 185-206.
[10] Profyris, C., C. Tziotzios, and I. Do Vale, Cutaneous scarring: Pathophysiology, molecular mechanisms, and scar reduction therapeutics Part I. The molecular basis of scar formation. *J. Am. Acad. Dermatol*, 2012. 66(1): p. 1-10; quiz 11-2.
[11] Alster, T.S. and C. Handrick, Laser treatment of hypertrophic scars, keloids, and striae. *Semin Cutan Med Surg*, 2000. 19(4): p. 287-92.
[12] Phillip CM, S.D., Berlien HP., Laser treatment of scars and keloids - how we do it. *Medical Laser Application*, 2008. 23(2): p. 79-86.
[13] Lupton, J.R. and T.S. Alster, Laser scar revision. *Dermatol Clin*, 2002. 20(1): p. 55-65.
[14] Abergel, R.P., et al., Biochemical composition of the connective tissue in keloids and analysis of collagen metabolism in keloid fibroblast cultures. *J. Invest Dermatol*, 1985. 84(5): p. 384-90.
[15] Klehr, N., Striae cutis atrophicae. Morphokinetic examinations in vitro. *Acta Derm. Venereol* Suppl (Stockh), 1979. 59(85): p. 105-8.
[16] Bak, H., et al., Treatment of striae distensae with fractional photothermolysis. *Dermatol Surg*, 2009. 35(8): p. 1215-20.
[17] Omi, T., et al., Fractional CO2 laser for the treatment of acne scars. *J. Cosmet Dermatol*, 2011. 10(4): p. 294-300.
[18] Fabbrocini, G., et al., Acne scars: pathogenesis, classification and treatment. *Dermatol Res Pract*, 2010. 2010: p. 893080.
[19] Rivera, A.E., Acne scarring: a review and current treatment modalities. *J. Am. Acad. Dermatol*, 2008. 59(4): p. 659-76.
[20] Idriss, N. and H.I. Maibach, Scar assessment scales: a dermatologic overview. *Skin Res Technol*, 2009. 15(1): p. 1-5.
[21] Baryza, M.J. and G.A. Baryza, The Vancouver Scar Scale: an administration tool and its interrater reliability. *J. Burn Care Rehabil*, 1995. 16(5): p. 535-8.
[22] Beausang, E., et al., A new quantitative scale for clinical scar assessment. *Plast Reconstr Surg*, 1998. 102(6): p. 1954-61.
[23] Shah, S. and T.S. Alster, Laser treatment of dark skin: an updated review. *Am. J. Clin. Dermatol*, 2010. 11(6): p. 389-97.
[24] Alster, T.S. and E.L. Tanzi, Hypertrophic scars and keloids: etiology and management. *Am. J. Clin. Dermatol*, 2003. 4(4): p. 235-43.
[25] Alster, T. and L. Zaulyanov, Laser scar revision: a review. *Dermatol Surg*, 2007. 33(2): p. 131-40.
[26] Alster, T.S., Cutaneous resurfacing with CO2 and erbium: YAG lasers: preoperative, intraoperative, and postoperative considerations. *Plast Reconstr Surg*, 1999. 103(2): p. 619-32; discussion 633-4.

[27] Groover I.J., and T. Alster, Laser revision of scars and striae. *Dermatol Ther*, 2000. 13(1): p. 50-9.
[28] Zachariae, H., Delayed wound healing and keloid formation following argon laser treatment or dermabrasion during isotretinoin treatment. *Br. J. Dermatol*, 1988. 118(5): p. 703-6.
[29] Nouri, K., et al., 585-nm pulsed dye laser in the treatment of surgical scars starting on the suture removal day. *Dermatol Surg*, 2003. 29(1): p. 65-73; discussion 73.
[30] Alkhawam, L. and M. Alam, Dermabrasion and microdermabrasion. *Facial Plast Surg*, 2009. 25(5): p. 301-10.
[31] Gold, M.H., Dermabrasion in dermatology. *Am. J. Clin. Dermatol*, 2003. 4(7): p. 467-71.
[32] Emsen, I.M., An Update on Sandpaper in Dermabrasion with a Different and Extended Patient Series. *Aesthetic Plast Surg*, 2008.
[33] Coleman, W.P., 3rd, J.M. Yarborough, and S.H. Mandy, Dermabrasion for prophylaxis and treatment of actinic keratoses. *Dermatol Surg*, 1996. 22(1): p. 17-21.
[34] Harmon, C., and C. Prather., *Dermabrasion Procedures*. Medscape., 2011 Jun 30. Available from www.emedicine.medscape.com
[35] Fabbrocini, G., *Chemical peels*. Medscape., 2012 Jan 26. Available from www.emedicine.medscape.com
[36] Camacho, F.M., Medium-depth and deep chemical peels. *J. Cosmet Dermatol*, 2005. 4(2): p. 117-28.
[37] Rendon, M.I., et al., Evidence and considerations in the application of chemical peels in skin disorders and aesthetic resurfacing. *J. Clin. Aesthet Dermatol*, 2010. 3(7): p. 32-43.
[38] Garg, V.K., S. Sinha, and R. Sarkar, Glycolic acid peels versus salicylic-mandelic acid peels in active acne vulgaris and post-acne scarring and hyperpigmentation: a comparative study. *Dermatol Surg*, 2009. 35(1): p. 59-65.
[39] Fartasch, M., J. Teal, and G.K. Menon, Mode of action of glycolic acid on human stratum corneum: ultrastructural and functional evaluation of the epidermal barrier. *Arch Dermatol Res*, 1997. 289(7): p. 404-9.
[40] Sachdeva, S., Lactic acid peeling in superficial acne scarring in Indian skin. *J. Cosmet Dermatol*, 2010. 9(3): p. 246-8.
[41] Fung, W., et al., Relative bioavailability of salicylic acid following dermal application of a 30% salicylic acid skin peel preparation. *J. Pharm. Sci*, 2008. 97(3): p. 1325-8.
[42] Fabbrocini, G., et al., CROSS technique: chemical reconstruction of skin scars method. *Dermatol Ther*, 2008. 21 Suppl 3: p. S29-32.
[43] Bhardwaj, D. and N. Khunger, An Assessment of the Efficacy and Safety of CROSS Technique with 100% TCA in the Management of Ice Pick Acne Scars. *J.Cutan Aesthet Surg*, 2010. 3(2): p. 93-6.
[44] Kaminaka, C., et al., Phenol peels as a novel therapeutic approach for actinic keratosis and Bowen disease: prospective pilot trial with assessment of clinical, histologic, and immunohistochemical correlations. *J. Am. Acad. Dermatol*, 2009. 60(4): p. 615-25.
[45] Sharad, J., Combination of microneedling and glycolic acid peels for the treatment of acne scars in dark skin. *J. Cosmet Dermatol*, 2011. 10(4): p. 317-23.
[46] Majid, I., Microneedling therapy in atrophic facial scars: an objective assessment. *J. Cutan Aesthet Surg*, 2009. 2(1): p. 26-30.

[47] Badran, M.M., J. Kuntsche, and A. Fahr, Skin penetration enhancement by a microneedle device (Dermaroller) in vitro: dependency on needle size and applied formulation. *Eur. J. Pharm Sci*, 2009. 36(4-5): p. 511-23.

[48] Jackson, B.A. and A.J. Shelton, Pilot study evaluating topical onion extract as treatment for postsurgical scars. *Dermatol Surg*, 1999. 25(4): p. 267-9.

[49] Cheng, B., H.W. Liu, and X.B. Fu, Update on pruritic mechanisms of hypertrophic scars in postburn patients: the potential role of opioids and their receptors. *J. Burn Care Res*, 2011. 32(4): p. e118-25.

[50] Stavrou, D., et al., Silicone-based scar therapy: a review of the literature. *Aesthetic Plast Surg*, 2010. 34(5): p. 646-51.

[51] Shih, R., J. Waltzman, and G.R. Evans, Review of over-the-counter topical scar treatment products. *Plast Reconstr Surg*, 2007. 119(3): p. 1091-5.

[52] Draelos, Z.D., The ability of onion extract gel to improve the cosmetic appearance of postsurgical scars. *J. Cosmet Dermatol*, 2008. 7(2): p. 101-4.

[53] Hosnuter, M., et al., The effects of onion extract on hypertrophic and keloid scars. *J. Wound Care*, 2007. 16(6): p. 251-4.

[54] Perez, O.A., et al., A comparative study evaluating the tolerability and efficacy of two topical therapies for the treatment of keloids and hypertrophic scars. *J. Drugs Dermatol*, 2010. 9(5): p. 514-8.

[55] Roques, C. and L. Teot, The use of corticosteroids to treat keloids: a review. *Int. J. Low Extrem Wounds*, 2008. 7(3): p. 137-45.

[56] Anthony, E.T., et al., The cost effectiveness of intralesional steroid therapy for keloids. *Dermatol Surg*, 2010. 36(10): p. 1624-6.

[57] Fitzpatrick, R.E., Treatment of inflamed hypertrophic scars using intralesional 5-FU. *Dermatol Surg*, 1999. 25(3): p. 224-32.

[58] Berman, B. and M.R. Duncan, Short-term keloid treatment in vivo with human interferon alfa-2b results in a selective and persistent normalization of keloidal fibroblast collagen, glycosaminoglycan, and collagenase production in vitro. *J. Am. Acad. Dermatol*, 1989. 21(4 Pt 1): p. 694-702.

[59] Furtado, F., B. Hochman, and L.M. Ferreira, Evaluating keloid recurrence after surgical excision with prospective longitudinal scar assessment scales. *J. Plast Reconstr Aesthet Surg*, 2012. 65(7): p. e175-81.

[60] Bran, G.M., et al., Auricular keloids: combined therapy with a new pressure device. *Arch Facial Plast Surg*, 2012. 14(1): p. 20-6.

[61] Rusciani, L., et al., Cryotherapy in the treatment of keloids. *J. Drugs Dermatol*, 2006. 5(7): p. 591-5.

[62] Alster, T.S., Improvement of erythematous and hypertrophic scars by the 585-nm flashlamp-pumped pulsed dye laser. *Ann. Plast Surg*, 1994. 32(2): p. 186-90.

[63] Yang, Y.J. and G.Y. Lee, Treatment of Striae Distensae with Nonablative Fractional Laser versus Ablative CO(2) Fractional Laser: A Randomized Controlled Trial. *Ann. Dermatol*, 2011. 23(4): p. 481-9.

[64] Alster, T.S., A.B. Lewis, and A. Rosenbach, Laser scar revision: comparison of CO2 laser vaporization with and without simultaneous pulsed dye laser treatment. *Dermatol Surg*, 1998. 24(12): p. 1299-302.

[65] McDaniel, D.H., K. Ash, and M. Zukowski, Treatment of stretch marks with the 585-nm flashlamp-pumped pulsed dye laser. *Dermatol Surg*, 1996. 22(4): p. 332-7.

[66] Alster, T.S. and T.B. West, Resurfacing of atrophic facial acne scars with a high-energy, pulsed carbon dioxide laser. *Dermatol Surg*, 1996. 22(2): p. 151-4; discussion 154-5.

[67] Walia, S. and T.S. Alster, Prolonged clinical and histologic effects from CO2 laser resurfacing of atrophic acne scars. *Dermatol Surg,* 1999. 25(12): p. 926-30.

[68] Waldorf, H.A., A.N. Kauvar, and R.G. Geronemus, Skin resurfacing of fine to deep rhytides using a char-free carbon dioxide laser in 47 patients. *Dermatol Surg*, 1995. 21(11): p. 940-6.

[69] Alster, T.S., C.A. Nanni, and C.M. Williams, Comparison of four carbon dioxide resurfacing lasers. A clinical and histopathologic evaluation. *Dermatol Surg*, 1999. 25(3): p. 153-8; discussion 159.

[70] Alster, T.S., A.N. Kauvar, and R.G. Geronemus, Histology of high-energy pulsed CO2 laser resurfacing. *Semin. Cutan Med. Surg*, 1996. 15(3): p. 189-93.

[71] Smith, K.J., et al., Depth of morphologic skin damage and viability after one, two, and three passes of a high-energy, short-pulse CO2 laser (Tru-Pulse) in pig skin. *J. Am. Acad. Dermatol*, 1997. 37(2 Pt 1): p. 204-10.

[72] Stuzin, J.M., et al., Histologic effects of the high-energy pulsed CO2 laser on photoaged facial skin. *Plast Reconstr Surg*, 1997. 99(7): p. 2036-50; discussion 2051-5.

[73] Ross, E.V., et al., Long-term results after CO2 laser skin resurfacing: a comparison of scanned and pulsed systems. *J. Am. Acad. Dermatol*, 1997. 37(5 Pt 1): p. 709-18.

[74] Alster, T.S., Clinical and histologic evaluation of six erbium:YAG lasers for cutaneous resurfacing. *Lasers Surg Med,* 1999. 24(2): p. 87-92.

[75] Alster, T.S., On: increased smooth muscle actin, factor XIIIa, and vimentin-positive cells in the papillary dermis of carbon dioxide laser-debrided porcine skin. *Dermatol Surg*, 1998. 24(1): p. 155.

[76] West, T.B., Laser resurfacing of atrophic scars. *Dermatol Clin*, 1997. 15(3): p. 449-57.

[77] Fitzpatrick, R.E., et al., Pulsed carbon dioxide laser, trichloroacetic acid, Baker-Gordon phenol, and dermabrasion: a comparative clinical and histologic study of cutaneous resurfacing in a porcine model. *Arch Dermatol*, 1996. 132(4): p. 469-71.

[78] Alexiades-Armenakas, M.R., J.S. Dover, and K.A. Arndt, The spectrum of laser skin resurfacing: nonablative, fractional, and ablative laser resurfacing. *J. Am. Acad. Dermatol*, 2008. 58(5): p. 719-37; quiz 738-40.

[79] Nanni, C.A. and T.S. Alster, Complications of carbon dioxide laser resurfacing. An evaluation of 500 patients. *Dermatol Surg*, 1998. 24(3): p. 315-20.

[80] Bernstein, L.J., et al., The short- and long-term side effects of carbon dioxide laser resurfacing. *Dermatol Surg,* 1997. 23(7): p. 519-25.

[81] Lim, T.C. and W.T. Tan, Carbon dioxide laser for keloids. *Plast Reconstr Surg*, 1991. 88(6): p. 1111.

[82] Kang, W.H., et al., Atrophic acne scar treatment using triple combination therapy: dot peeling, subcision and fractional laser. *J. Cosmet Laser Ther*, 2009. 11(4): p. 212-5.

[83] Alster, T.S. and T.O. McMeekin, Improvement of facial acne scars by the 585 nm flashlamp-pumped pulsed dye laser. *J. Am. Acad Dermatol,* 1996. 35(1): p. 79-81.

[84] Friedman, P.M., et al., Treatment of atrophic facial acne scars with the 1064-nm Q-switched Nd:YAG laser: six-month follow-up study. *Arch Dermatol*, 2004. 140(11): p. 1337-41.

[85] Sadick, N.S., Update on non-ablative light therapy for rejuvenation: a review. *Lasers Surg Med*, 2003. 32(2): p. 120-8.

[86] Tanzi, E.L. and T.S. Alster, Comparison of a 1450-nm diode laser and a 1320-nm Nd:YAG laser in the treatment of atrophic facial scars: a prospective clinical and histologic study. *Dermatol Surg*, 2004. 30(2 Pt 1): p. 152-7.

[87] Alster, T.S., E.L. Tanzi, and M. Lazarus, The use of fractional laser photothermolysis for the treatment of atrophic scars. *Dermatol Surg,* 2007. 33(3): p. 295-9.

[88] Vasily, D.B., et al., Non-ablative fractional resurfacing of surgical and post-traumatic scars. *J. Drugs Dermatol*, 2009. 8(11): p. 998-1005.

[89] Cho, S.B., et al., Non-ablative 1550-nm erbium-glass and ablative 10 600-nm carbon dioxide fractional lasers for acne scars: a randomized split-face study with blinded response evaluation. *J. Eur. Acad. Dermatol Venereol*, 2010. 24(8): p. 921-5.

[90] Capon, A., et al., Scar prevention using Laser-Assisted Skin Healing (LASH) in plastic surgery. *Aesthetic Plast Surg*, 2010. 34(4): p. 438-46.

[91] Wada, T., et al., Efficacy and safety of a low-energy double-pass 1450-nm diode laser for the treatment of acne scars. *Photomed Laser Surg*, 2012. 30(2): p. 107-11.

In: Scars and Scarring
Editor: Yongsoo Lee

ISBN: 978-1-62808-005-6
© 2013 Nova Science Publishers, Inc.

Chapter 2

Psychological Impact of Scars

Katlein França,[1,] Anna Chacon,[1] Jennifer Ledon,[1] Jessica Savas[1] and Keyvan Nouri[2]*

[1]University of Miami Miller School of Medicine
Department of Dermatology and Cutaneous Surgery, Miami, Florida, US
[2]Dermatology, Ophthalmology & Otolaryngology
Louis C. Skinner, Jr., M.D. Endowed Chair in Dermatology
Richard Helfman Professor of Dermatologic Surgery
University of Miami Medical Group
Sylvester Comprehensive Cancer Center/University of Miami Hospital and Clinics
Mohs, Dermatologic & Laser Surgery
Surgical Training
Department of Dermatology & Cutaneous Surgery
University of Miami Leonard M. Miller School of Medicine
Sylvester Comprehensive Cancer Center, Mohs/Laser Unit
Miami, FL, USA

Abstract

The management of scars is a challenge for professionals since these lesions can greatly impact quality of life. Although scars rarely pose a health risk, patients constantly present not only with physical discomfort, but also aesthetic, social and psychological distress. The psychological management of patients with burn scars is extremely important and has been well described in the literature. Patients may experience post-traumatic stress disorder due the traumatic nature of the burn accident. These lesions are cosmetically disfiguring and may even lead to depression, anxiety and problems with social interaction. Scars can have long-lasting physical and psychosocial effects, even if remedial and cosmetic treatment is sought. Several authors have identified acne scars as an important contributor to low self-esteem, especially within the adolescent age group. Fearing a negative response from other persons may cause timidity, reclusion, and in

---

[*] E-mail: knouri@med.miami.edu

extreme cases, social phobia. Psychological support and the establishment of a good doctor-patient relationship are essential for better comprehensive care of these patients.

Introduction

Scars are areas of fibrosis that occur in normal skin after injuries. Although they are a natural part of the healing process, the scarring process can result in functional, cosmetic and psychological consequences. [1] The management of scars is a challenge for professionals since these lesions can greatly impact quality of life. [2, 3] Different types of skin injuries can lead to scar formation. Burns, surgeries and trauma are the most common causes and are usually associated with a traumatic and psychologically disturbing event. [4,5,6] Cosmetically disfiguring lesions may lead to depression, anxiety and problems with social interaction. [7] These scars can have long-lasting physical and psychosocial effects, sometimes even if remedial and cosmetic treatment is sought. [6] This chapter will discuss the psychological aspects related to disfigurement caused by the different types of scars and will address the psychological and psychopharmacological treatment for these conditions.

Psychosocial Aspects of Disfigurement

Disfigurement is the state of having one's appearance deeply harmed by physical disorders, injuries or birth defects. When visible areas such as the face, hands and arms are affected, it is more difficult for sufferers to cope. [7,8,9,10] The face is considered a psychologically important area of the body and disfigurement of this area can cause severe social consequences for patients. [9,11] Apart from major injuries, minor lesions have been found to cause significant anxiety, depression and low self-esteem. [11,12] A study that evaluated the psychological impact of minor facial injuries and the influence of patient and scar characteristics in relation to self-consciousness and anxiety levels found that larger scar size, living alone and the etiology of injury were significantly related to self-consciousness and anxiety levels. However, gender, age, socioeconomic group, scar location, satisfaction with appearance and number of scars were not. [11] Facial trauma patients also report problems in social, marital and occupational functions. [11] Patients reported high rates of substance abuse, post-traumatic stress disorder symptoms, stigmatization and lower quality of life. [13,14,15] Studies have shown that the general population often tries to avoid making eye contact or having to look at the disfigurement and respond to people with a disfigurement with less trust and respect. [16]

The improvement of quality of life and high standards of care for these patients should be the ultimate goal. [17] Psychosocial rehabilitation should be offered and will be discussed in more details in this chapter. (see section titled "Psychological Treatment")

Burn Scars

Burns can be defined as injuries to tissues caused by contact with heat, flame, chemicals, electricity, or radiation. [18] An extensive burn is one of the most traumatic and devastating injuries that can occur to an individual. [19] All deep burns will heal by scarring. Primarily, scars can only be minimized by various cosmetic procedures and physical therapy, but not completely eliminated. [19] Psychopathological responses may be induced by the traumatic nature of the burn accident and the subsequent painful treatment. [6,20,21] Several authors have studied the occurrence of depression and post-traumatic stress disorder (PTSD) in these patients. Data shows a prevalence of 13-23% and 13-45% of depression and post-traumatic disorder cases, respectively. [20] Other studies have shown different rates of depression affecting burn patients. Rates of moderate to severe depression have been determined by self-reported measures in hospitalized burn patients and the measures range from 10 to 54%. [21,22,23,24]

Post-traumatic stress disorder is a type of anxiety disorder where individuals re-experience the traumatic event in some way. They become sensitive to normal life experiences and tend to avoid people or places that may remind them of the traumatic event. [25] The risk factors related to PTSD are the severity and type of initial symptoms, occurrence of depression, visibility of the burn injury and anxiety. [20]

Diagnostic criteria for PTSD include a history of exposure to a traumatic event meeting two criteria and symptoms from each of three symptom clusters: intrusive recollections, avoidant/numbing symptoms, and hyper-arousal symptoms. A fifth criterion concerns the duration of symptoms and a sixth assesses functioning. [26] (see table 2)

A study involving 52 hospitalized burn patients found that 18 (35.3%) met PTSD criteria at 2 months. High rates of PTSD were also found at 6 months (N = 16, 40.0% of the 40 available patients) and 12 months (N = 14, 45.2% of the 31 available patients). The same study observed that patients with more severe burns were not more likely to develop PTSD. [27]

Corri and colleagues studied the association of PTSD and pain with functioning and disability. The sample was composed of 171 consecutive patients admitted to a regional burn center with major burn injuries followed at 1, 6, 12, and 24 months post discharge. The authors found that higher PTSD symptom severity soon after hospital discharge was prospectively related to greater psychosocial disability and poorer physical and social functioning. Deleterious effects of early PTSD were ameliorated by time and significant interaction terms indicated that the concurrent effect of PTSD on psychosocial disability, social functioning, and vitality attenuated during the 24-month recovery period.

Data collected from a prospective, multi-site and cohort study of major burn survivors showed that significant in-hospital psychological distress occurred in 34% of the patients. Clinically significant and reliable change in symptom severity by follow-up visits in 6, 12 and 24 months occurred infrequently. [29]

The psychological and physical consequences of sustaining a severe burn injury are well known and were previously discussed in this session. However, little attention is given to patients sustaining a small burns. [29] Several authors mention that the burn severity is not predictive of psychological health and small burns could also cause psychological distress. [30,31]

Table 1. DSM-IV Criteria for Post-traumatic Stress Disorder [26]

A. The person has been exposed to a traumatic event in which both of the following have been present: (1) The person experienced, witnessed, or was confronted with an event or events that involved actual or threatened death or serious injury, or a threat to the physical integrity of self or others (2) the person's response involved intense fear, helplessness, or horror. Note: In children, this may be expressed instead by disorganized or agitated behavior.
B. The traumatic event is persistently re-experienced in one (or more) of the following ways: (1) Recurrent and intrusive distressing recollections of the event, including images, thoughts, or perceptions. Note: In young children, repetitive play may occur in which themes or aspects of the traumatic incident are expressed. (2) Recurrent distressing dreams of the event. Note: In children, there may be frightening dreams without recognizable content. (3) Acting or feeling as if the traumatic event were recurring (includes a sense of reliving the experience, illusions, hallucinations, and dissociative flashback episodes, including those that occur upon awakening or when intoxicated). Note: In young children, trauma-specific reenactment may occur. (4) Intense psychological distress at exposure to internal or external cues that symbolize or resemble an aspect of the traumatic event. (5) Physiological reactivity on exposure to internal or external cues that symbolize or resemble an aspect of the traumatic event.
C. Persistent avoidance of stimuli associated with the trauma and numbing of general responsiveness (not present before the trauma), as indicated by three (or more) of the following: (1) Efforts to avoid thoughts, feelings, or conversations associated with the trauma (2) Efforts to avoid activities, places, or people that arouse recollections of the trauma (3) Inability to recall an important aspect of the trauma (4) Markedly diminished interest or participation in significant activities (5) Feelings of detachment or estrangement from others (6) Restricted range of affect (e.g., unable to have feelings of love) (7) Sense of a foreshortened future (e.g., does not expect to have a career, marriage, children, or a normal life span)
D. Persistent symptoms of increased arousal (not present before the trauma), as indicated by two (or more) of the following: (1) Difficulty falling or staying asleep (2) Irritability or outbursts of anger (3) Difficulty concentrating (4) Hypervigilance (5) Exaggerated startle response
F. The disturbance causes clinically significant distress or impairment in social, occupational, or other important areas of functioning.
Specify if: Acute: if duration of symptoms is less than 3 months; Chronic: if duration of symptoms is 3 months or more *Specify if*: With Delayed Onset: if onset of symptoms is at least 6 months after the stressor

In a prospective study, 45 patients with burn injuries ranging from less than 1% to 40% total body surface area were assessed using semi-structured interviews within two weeks of sustaining the burn, and followed-up at approximately three months post burn. Significant levels of anxiety, intrusions and avoidance were similar at two weeks and three months post burn for most of the patients and the prevalence of depression and Post Traumatic Stress Disorder (PTSD) increased 6- and 4-fold, respectively, over 3 months. Patients with small burn injuries of 1% or less experienced clinically significant levels of psychological difficulties post-burn. [30]

Another study that investigated the effect of smaller burn injuries on patient's physical and psychological health at 3-4 months after discharge from treatment showed that a minority of patients reported, at the follow-up point, that their physical and social function was still affected. [31]

Acne Scars

Acne is a disease caused by the blockage of sebaceous glands, increased sebum production and colonization by the *Propionibacterium acnes*. [32,33] It is one of the most prevalent skin conditions affecting teenagers and hormonal and genetic factors may also contribute to its occurrence. [33] Acne scar types include: ice-pick, rolling, and boxcar scars. [34, 35, 36] In order to minimize the risk of scarring and adverse psychological effects, the treatment of these patients should be started as early as possible. [32]

Several studies mention the occurrence of psychologic problems as a consequence of acne. [32,33,35,36] The psychologic change is not correlated with disease severity and patients with mild to moderate cases can present with suicidal ideation and depression. [33,37,38] A study involving 11 female patients presenting with mild to moderate acne showed a higher level of emotional and social impairment in terms of feelings of physical discomfort, anger, and the intermingling impact of these, among participants. [37]

Acne also has a negative effect on the way people are perceived by others. Adults and teenagers perceived other teens with acne as generally being less social, shy, more likely to be bullied and less successful in terms of finding a job. [39] The emotional and physical scars of acne can persist throughout the life of the affected individual and studies substantiate the psychological impact and support a causal, and at times reciprocal, link between acne and the emotional and functional status of the patient. [40]

Other psychological effects related to acne are body image alterations, depression, anxiety, poor self-esteem, altered social interactions, embarrassment and anger. Acne scars are also associated with lower academic performance, and are considered causes of unemployment. [41,42,43]

Having acne scars is also a risk factor for suicide. A study that investigated the causes of suicide in dermatological patients described that patients with long-standing and debilitating skin disease may become depressed enough to commit suicide. The authors also say that there is always an attendant risk of suicide in patients with established, severe psychiatric problems, who are referred to dermatologists with concurrent skin disorders. Patients, particularly women with facial complaints such as acne scars, may be extremely depressed and at greater risk for suicide. [44]

Acne is a harmful disease affecting mostly adolescents. Adolescence is a vulnerable time in life for an individual, during which a sense of identity and lifelong self-esteem is being developed. Providing early treatment and adequate psychological support is important to prevent physical scars and adverse psychological effects. [36]

Keloids and Hypertrophic Scars

Keloids and hypertrophic scars are benign fibrous growths that occur after wounding of the skin, usually caused by previous trauma. [45] These lesions are frequently painful, pruritic and may occasionally form strictures. They are not medically dangerous, but may result in significant cosmetic disfigurement. [46,47] Excessive scarring significantly affects the patient's quality of life, not only physically but also psychologically. [47]

Furtado and colleagues performed a study to evaluate factors that affect the quality of life of patients with keloids. Patients with keloids on non-visible areas of the body) and more than 10 years of disease reported higher scores on the physical domain of a quality of life questionnaire (QualiFibro questionnaire), which is specific for evaluation of the quality of life of patients with keloids and comprises the physical and psychological domains, and six visual numeric scales (VNS), of which three are related to psychological factors (satisfaction with appearance, shame of the disease, and suffering experienced), and the other three are related to physical factors (pruritus, pain and movement restriction). indicating increased severity compared with patients with keloids on visible areas of the body and disease duration of less than 10 years.

The authors also found a positive correlation between psychological (satisfaction with appearance, feelings of embarrassment about the disease and suffering experienced) and physical factors (pruritus, pain and movement restriction) evaluated using a visual numeric scale, and both domains of the QualiFibro questionnaire. [48]

The same authors performed another study to investigate the psychological stress on the prognosis of the postoperative recurrence of keloids. Twenty- five patients with keloids who were candidates for surgical resection and postoperative radiotherapy were evaluated for psychological stress on the day before the surgical procedure and during the 3rd, 6th, 9th and 12th months of postoperative care. During each return visit, two experts classified the lesions as non-recurrent and recurrent.

The parameters evaluated were pain and itching (Visual Numerical Scale), quality of life (Questionnaire QualiFibro/Cirurgia Plástica-UNIFESP), perceived stress (Perceived Stress Scale), depression and anxiety (Hospital Depression and Anxiety Scale), salivary cortisol and minimum and maximum galvanic skin responses (GSR) at rest and under stress (i.e., while the questionnaires were being filled out).

The authors found that the psychological stress influenced the recurrence of keloids in the post-operative period, which was demonstrated by the increase in the minimum and maximum galvanic skin responses during stress situations. [49]

Patients with hypertrophic scars and keloids may thus suffer from quality of life impairment similar to that of patients with other chronic skin diseases. [50] Psychological sequelae includes stigmatization, sleep disturbance, depression and disruption of daily activities, stress reactions and loss of self-esteem. [51, 52, 53]

Treatment of keloids and hypertrophic scars can be difficult, painful, long-lasting and sometimes unsatisfactory. [54] All these factors can cause anxiety and frustration for the patients. Physicians should be aware of the psychological impact that these lesions can cause to patients.

Medical Interventions

A medical intervention is an act performed to prevent harm to a patient or to improve the mental, emotional, or physical function of a patient. [55] Some medical interventions are surgical; others are based on pharmacological treatments, psychological treatments and minor procedures.

They all have in common the aim of reducing the discrepancy between an individual's ideal and actual state of health. [56] Many, but not all, disfiguring conditions are open to medical interventions. Some medical interventions for the conditions described in this chapter are described in table 02.

This chapter will address, in more detail, the psychological and psychopharmacological treatments.

Table 2. Medical Interventions for Post Burn Scars, Acne, Keloids and Hypertrophic Scars

POST BURN SCARS	Surgical Excision, Intralesional Injections, Compression, Physical Therapy, Lasers, Psychopharmacological Treatment Psychological Treatment.
ACNE SCARS	Surgery, Microneedling, Dermal Fillers, Dermabrasion, Lasers and Lights, Pharmacological Therapy, Psychopharmacological Treatment Psychological Treatment.
KELOIDS AND HYPERTROPIC SCARS	Surgery, Intralesional Injections, Dermabrasion, Lasers, Cryotherapy, Compression, Radiotherapy, Psychopharmacological Treatment Psychological Treatment.

Psychological Treatment

Burn Patients

Burn patients have often experienced a very frightening event and can be experiencing significant feelings of guilt, despair and anger. [57] Psychological support is necessary and should be provided, ideally, by clinicians specializing in human behavior, such as psychiatrists, psychiatric nurses, psychologists or other health personnel with similar levels of expertise. The treatment should begin as soon as possible and continue throughout the rehabilitation process. [58]

Several treatments have been used to treat depression symptoms. Cognitive behavioral therapy has shown positive effects for treatment of depression in burn patients.[6] This form of psychotherapy focuses on the examination of the relationships between thoughts, feelings and behaviors. Patients with mental illness can modify their patterns of thinking by exploring the thoughts that lead to self-destructive actions and beliefs that control and direct these thoughts. [59, 60] Patients presenting with post-traumatic stress disorder can be treated with eye movement reprocessing desensitization and exposure therapy, a type of cognitive behavioral therapy.[6] The eye movement reprocessing desensitization is a clinical treatment where the patients recalls the traumatic event while simultaneously undergoing bilateral stimulation that consist of moving the eyes form side to side. [61] Relaxation techniques, such as hypnosis, may be useful to reduce pain and anxiety. [62, 63] Problems in the social area can be mitigated by social skills training and community interventions. [6]

Acne Scars

Severe Acne and Acne Scars Can Ignite a Number of Different Emotional Reactions

Psychological treatments may vary based on each patient's unique needs and physician assessments. [37,38] Psychotherapy is indicated in depressive disorders, body dysmorphic disorder and social phobia. [64] Depression and anxiety may respond to cognitive-behavioral methods, relaxation techniques, such as hypnosis, self-hypnosis and psychodynamic psychotherapy. [65,66,67,68]

Keloids and Hypertrophic Scars

Patients with disfiguring keloids and hypertrophic scars often experience some psychological effects. Studies previously presented in this chapter show that they may experience a lower quality of life because of this. Psychotherapeutic approaches include cognitive behavioral therapy, psychodynamic therapy, interpersonal therapy and relaxation techniques. [66,69.70,71] Patients with disfigurement should be prepared to change how they respond to social attitudes. Social skills training may help the person to be more resilient and more able to deal with the minor stressors of life. [72] Other benefits of social support include the development of adaptive cognitions, reassurance of acceptance regardless of appearance, and encouragement to enter anxiety-provoking settings. [73]

Pyschopharmacological Treatment

A wide variety of medications with different pharmacological mechanisms of action are available for treatment of depression, anxiety and post-traumatic stress disorders. Many patients presenting psychological effects caused by scars may benefit from use of psychopharmacological agents. Thorough diagnostic information about the advantage, disadvantage and mechanism of action of these drugs are essential for treatment success. [74]

Some of the most common psychopharmacological agents prescribed are:

- SELECTIVE SEROTONIN REUPTAKE INHIBITORS (SSRIs): Commonly used as the first-line treatment for depression. They have a favorable side effect profile and low toxicity. Examples include: Fluoxetine, Fluvoxamine, Paroxetine, Sertraline, Citalopram, Escitalopram, Vilazodone [75,76]

- **TRICYCLIC ANTIDEPRESSANTS:** Acts by blocking the reuptake of neurotransmitters such as serotonin and norepinephrine. Examples include: Amitriptyline, Doxepin, Clomipramine, Imipramine, Trimipramine, Desipramine, Nortriptyline, Protriptlyne [77,78]
- **MONOAMINE OXIDASE INHIBITORS:** Acts by blocking the enzyme monoamine oxidase, which breaks down the neurotransmitters serotonin, dopamine, and norepinephrine. Examples include: Moclobemide, Isocarboxazid, Phenelzine, Selegiline and Tranylcypromine. [79]
- **SEROTONIN-NOREPINEPHRINE REUPTAKE INHIBITORS:** Acts upon, and increase the levels of serotonin and norepinephrine. Examples include: Venlafaxine [80]
- **NORADRENEGIC AND SPECIFIC SEROTONERGIC ANTIDEPRESSANTS:** Acts by blocking the presynaptic alpha-2 adrenergic receptors and certain serotonin receptors, increasing norepinephrine and serotonin neurotransmission. Examples include: Mirtazapine and Mianserin. [81]
- **NOREPINEPHRINE REUPTAKE INHIBITORS:** Acts via norepinephrine Examples include: Viloxazine, Reboxetine, Atomoxetine [82]
- **NOREPINEPHRINE-DOPAMINE REUPTAKE INHIBITORS:** Inhibit the neuronal reuptake of norepinephrine and dopamine. Examples include: Bupropion [83]
- **SELECTIVE SEROTONIN REUPTAKE ENHANCERS:** Enhances the plasmalemmal reuptake of serotonin. Examples include: Tianeptine

Conclusion

Psychological and physical effects caused by different types of scars can be long lasting and cause severe distress and discomfort. Patients experiencing disfigurement by scars, often present problems in their social interaction and behavior. The most common types of scars that may affect the psychological aspect of an individual are those caused by burns, acne and other traumas that can leave a disfiguring keloid or hypertrophic scar. Depression, anxiety, and low self-esteem are some examples of the psychological effects that scars can cause. Physicians and other health personnel involved in the treatment of these patients must provide good psychological support. Taking time to listen to the patient's concerns, providing good information and listening carefully to their questions can help the treatment process and improve outcomes.

References

[1] Vercelli S, Ferriero G, Sartorio F, Stissi V, Franchignoni F. How to assess postsurgical scars: a review of outcome measures. *Disabil. Rehabil.* 2009;31(25):2055-63.

[2] Brown BC, McKenna SP, Siddhi K, McGrouther DA, Bayat A. The hidden cost of skin scars: quality of life after skin scarring. *J. Plast. Reconstr. Aesthet. Surg.* 2008 Sep;61(9):1049-58. Epub 2008 Jul 9.

[3] Bock O, Schmid-Ott G, Malewski P, Mrowietz U.Quality of life of patients with keloid and hypertrophic scarring. *Arch. Dermatol. Res*. 2006 Apr;297(10):433-8. Epub 2006 Mar 10.

[4] Nițescu C, Calotă DR, Stăncioiu TA, Marinescu SA, Florescu IP, Lascăr I. Psychological impact of burn scars on quality of life in patients with extensive burns who received allotransplant. *Rom. J. Morphol. Embryol*. 2012;53(3):577-83.

[5] Dunker MS, Bemelman WA, Slors JF, van Duijvendijk P, Gouma DJ. Functional outcome, quality of life, body image, and cosmesis in patients after laparoscopic-assisted and conventional restorative proctocolectomy: a comparative study. *Dis. Colon. Rectum*. 2001 Dec;44(12):1800-7.

[6] Van Loey NE, Van Son MJ. Psychopathology and psychological problems in patients with burn scars: epidemiology and management. *Am. J. Clin. Dermatol*. 2003;4(4):245-72.

[7] Robert R, Meyer W, Bishop S, Rosenberg L, Murphy L, Blakeney P. Disfiguring burn scars and adolescent self-esteem. *Burns*. 1999 Nov;25(7):581-5.

[8] Thompson A, Kent G. Adjusting to disfigurement: processes involved in dealing with being visibly different. *Clin. Psychol. Rev*. 2001 Jul;21(5):663-82.

[9] Versnel SL, Plomp RG, Passchier J, Duivenvoorden HJ, Mathijssen IM. Long-term psychological functioning of adults with severe congenital facial disfigurement. *Plast. Reconstr. Surg*. 2012 Jan;129(1):110-7.

[10] Bradbury E. The psychological and social impact of disfigurement to the hand in children and adolescents. *Dev. Neurorehabil*. 2007 Apr-Jun;10(2):143-8.

[11] Tebble NJ, Thomas DW, Price P. Anxiety and self-consciousness in patients with minor facial lacerations. *J. Adv. Nurs*. 2004 Aug;47(4):417-26.

[12] Callahan C. Facial disfigurement and sense of self in head and neck cancer. *Soc. Work Health Care*. 2004;40(2):73-87.

[13] Shepherd JP. Strategies for the study of long-term sequelae of oral and facial injuries. *J. Oral Maxillofac. Surg*. 1992 Apr;50(4):390-9.

[14] Sen P, Ross N, Rogers S. Recovering maxillofacial trauma patients: the hidden problems. *J. Wound Care*. 2001 Mar;10(3):53-7.

[15] Roccia F, Dell'Acqua A, Angelini G, Berrone S. Maxillofacial trauma and psychiatric sequelae: post-traumatic stress disorder. *J. Craniofac. Surg*. 2005 May;16(3):355-60.

[16] Millstone,S. Coping With Disfigurement 1: Causes and effects. Available: http://www.nursingtimes.net/nursing-practice/clinical-zones/public-health/coping-with-disfigurement-1-causes-and-effects/993378.article. Access: October, 8,2012.

[17] Shetty V, Dent DM, Glynn S, Brown KE. Psychosocial sequelae and correlates of orofacial injury. *Dent. Clin. North Am*. 2003 Jan;47(1):141-57, xi.

[18] The free dictionary. Available: http://medical-dictionary.thefreedictionary.com/burn. Access 08, October 2012.

[19] Goel A, Shrivastava P. Post-burn scars and scar contractures. *Indian J. Plast. Surg*. 2010 September; 43(Suppl): S63–S71. doi: 10.4103/0970-0358.70724.

[20] Van Loey NE, Van Son MJ. Psychopathology and psychological problems in patients with burn scars: epidemiology and management. *Am. J. Clin. Dermatol*. 2003;4(4):245-72.

[21] Charlton JE, Klein R, Gagliardi G, Heimbach DM. Factors affecting pain in burned patients a preliminary report. *Postgrad. Med. J,* 59 (695) (1983), pp. 604–607.

[22] Roh YS, Chung HS, Kwon B, Kim G. Association between depression, patient scar assessment and burn-specific health in hospitalized burn patients, Burns, Volume 38, Issue 4, June 2012, Pages 506-512, ISSN 0305-4179, 10.1016/j.burns.2011.12.027.

[23] Wiechman S, Ptacek, J, Patterson D, Gibran N, Engrav L, Heimbach DM. Rates, trends, and severity of depression after burn injuries. *J. Burn Care Rehabil*, 22 (6) (2001), pp. 417–424

[24] Thombs B.D, Bresnick MG, Magyar-Russell G, Lawrence J, McCann, U.D, Fauerbach JA. Symptoms of depression predict change in physical health after burn injury. *Burns*, 33 (3) (2007), pp. 292–298.

[25] Bovin MJ, Marx BP. The importance of the peritraumatic experience in defining traumatic stress. *Psychol. Bull*. 2011 Jan;137(1):47-67.

[26] American Psychiatric Association. (2000). *Diagnostic and statistical manual of mental disorders* (Revised 4th ed.). Washington, DC: Author.

[27] Perry S, Difede J, Musngi G, Frances AJ, Jacobsberg L. Predictors of posttraumatic stress disorder after burn injury. *Am. J. Psychiatry*. 1992 Jul;149(7):931-5.

[28] Corry NH, Klick B, Fauerbach JA. Posttraumatic stress disorder and pain impact functioning and disability after major burn injury. *J. Burn. Care Res.* 2010 Jan-Feb;31(1):13-25.

[29] Fauerbach JA, McKibben J, Bienvenu OJ, Magyar-Russell G, Smith MT, Holavanahalli R, Patterson DR, Wiechman SA, Blakeney P, Lezotte D. Psychological distress after major burn injury. *Psychosom. Med.* 2007 Jun;69(5):473-82.

[30] Tedstone JE, Tarrier N. An investigation of the prevalence of psychological morbidity in burn-injured patients. *Burns*. 1997 Nov-Dec;23(7-8):550-4.

[31] Shakespeare V. Effect of small burn injury on physical, social and psychological health at 3-4 months after discharge. *Burns*. 1998 Dec;24(8):739-44.

[32] Ayer J, Burrows N. Acne: more than skin deep. *Postgrad. Med. J.* 2006 August; 82(970): 500–506. doi: 10.1136/pgmj.2006.045377.

[33] Layton AM. Optimal management of acne to prevent scarring and psychological sequelae. *Am. J. Clin. Dermatol.* 2001;2(3):135-41.

[34] Jacob CI, Dover JS, Kaminer MS. Acne scarring: a classification system and review of treatment options. *J. Am. Acad. Dermatol.* 2001 Jul;45(1):109-17.

[35] Basta-Juzbašić A. Current therapeutic approach to acne scars. *Acta Dermatovenerol. Croat.* 2010;18(3):171-5.

[36] Goodman G. Acne and acne scarring - the case for active and early intervention. *Aust. Fam. Physician.* 2006 Jul;35(7):503-4.

[37] Pruthi G, Babu N. *Physical and Psychosocial Impact of Acne in Adult Females Indian J. Dermatol.* 2012 Jan-Feb; 57(1): 26–29. doi: 10.4103/0019-5154.92672.

[38] Levy LL, Zeichner JA. Management of acne scarring, part II: a comparative review of non-laser-based, minimally invasive approaches. *Am. J. Clin. Dermatol.* 2012 Oct 1;13(5):331-40. doi: 10.2165/11631410-000000000-00000.

[39] Ritvo E, Del Rosso J, Stilman M, La Riche C. Psychosocial judgements and perceptions of adolescents with acne vulgaris: A blinded, controlled comparison of adult and peer evaluations. *Biopsychosoc. Med.* 2011; 5: 11. Published online 2011 August 13. doi: 10.1186/1751-0759-5-11.

[40] Fried RG, Wechsler A. Psychological problems in the acne patient. *Dermatol. Ther.* 2006 Jul-Aug;19(4):237-40.

[41] Koo JY, Smith LL. Psychologic aspects of acne. *Pediatr. Dermatol.* 1991 Sep;8(3):185-8.
[42] Rivera AE. Acne scarring: a review and current treatment modalities. *J. Am. Acad. Dermatol.* 2008 Oct;59(4):659-76. Epub 2008 Jul 26.
[43] Fife D. Practical Evaluation and Management of Atrophic Acne Scars: Tips for the General Dermatologist. *J. Clin. Aesthet. Dermatol.* 2011 August; 4(8): 50–57.
[44] Cotterill JA, Cunliffe WJ. Suicide in dermatological patients. *Br. J. Dermatol.* 1997 Aug;137(2):246-50.
[45] English RS, Shenefelt PD. Keloids and hypertrophic scars. *Dermatol. Surg.* 1999 Aug;25(8):631-8.
[46] Urioste SS, Arndt KA, Dover JS. Keloids and hypertrophic scars: review and treatment strategies. *Semin Cutan Med. Surg.* 1999 Jun;18(2):159-71.
[47] Gauglitz GG, Korting HC, Pavicic T, Ruzicka T, Jeschke MG. Hypertrophic scarring and keloids: pathomechanisms and current and emerging treatment strategies. *Mol. Med.* 2011 Jan-Feb;17(1-2):113-25. Epub 2010 Oct 5.
[48] Furtado F, Hochman B, Ferrara SF, Dini GM, Nunes JM, Juliano Y, Ferreira LM. What factors affect the quality of life of patients with keloids? *Rev. Assoc. Med. Bras.* 2009 Nov-Dec;55(6):700-4.
[49] Furtado F, Hochman B, Farber PL, Muller MC, Hayashi LF, Ferreira LM. Psychological stress as a risk factor for postoperative keloid recurrence. *J. Psychosom. Res.* 2012 Apr;72(4):282-7. Epub 2012 Jan 26.
[50] Bock O, Schmid-Ott G, Malewski P, Mrowietz U. Quality of life of patients with keloid and hypertrophic scarring. *Arch. Dermatol. Res.* 2006 Apr;297(10):433-8. Epub 2006 Mar 10.
[51] Puri N, Taiwar A. The Efficacy of Silicone Gel for the Treatment of Hypertrophic Scars and Keloids. *J. Cutan Aesthet. Surg.* 2009 Jul-Dec; 2(2): 104–106. doi: 10.4103/0974-2077.58527
[52] Ahn ST. Topical silicone gel: A new treatment for hypertrophic scars. *Surgery.* 1989;106:781–7.
[53] Ahn ST. Topical silicone gel for the prevention and treatment of hypertrophic scar. *Arch. Surg.* 1991;126:499–504.
[54] Shaffer JJ, Taylor SC, Cook-Bolden F. Keloidal scars: a review with a critical look at therapeutic options. J Am Acad Dermatol 46:S63–S97
[55] The free dictionary. Available: http://medical-dictionary.thefreedictionary.com/intervention. Access: 15 October, 2012.
[56] Andrew Thompson, Gerry Kent, Adjusting to disfigurement: processes involved in dealing with being visibly different, *Clinical Psychology Review*, Volume 21, Issue 5, July 2001, Pages 663-682, ISSN 0272-7358, 10.1016/S0272-7358(00)00056-8.
[57] Procter F. Rehabilitation of the burn patient *Indian J. Plast. Surg.* 2010 September; 43(Suppl): S101–S113. doi: 10.4103/0970-0358.70730.
[58] Morris, J. and Mcfadd, A. Mental-Health Team on A Burn Unit Multidisciplinary Approach. *Journal of Trauma-Injury Infection and Critical Care* 1978;18(9):658-64.
[59] Embling S. The effectiveness of cognitive behavioural therapy in depression. *Nurs Stand.* 2002 Dec 18-31;17(14-15):33-41.

[60] Burns DD, Nolen-Hoeksema S. Therapeutic empathy and recovery from depression in cognitive-behavioral therapy: a structural equation model. *J. Consult. Clin. Psychol.* 1992 Jun;60(3):441-9.

[61] Van der Kolk BA, Spinazzola J, Blaustein ME, Hopper JW, Hopper EK, Korn DL, Simpson WB. A randomized clinical trial of eye movement desensitization and reprocessing (EMDR), fluoxetine, and pill placebo in the treatment of posttraumatic stress disorder: treatment effects and long-term maintenance. *J. Clin. Psychiatry.* 2007 Jan;68(1):37-46.

[62] Frenay MC, Faymonville ME, Devlieger S, Albert A, Vanderkelen A. Psychological approaches during dressing changes of burned patients: a prospective randomised study comparing hypnosis against stress reducing strategy. *Burns.* 2001 Dec;27(8):793-9.

[63] Vickers A, Zollman C. Hypnosis and relaxation therapies. *BMJ.* 1999 November 20; 319(7221): 1346–1349.

[64] Uzun O, Başoğlu C, Akar A, Cansever A, Ozşahin A, Cetin M, Ebrinç S. Body dysmorphic disorder in patients with acne. *Compr. Psychiatry.* 2003 Sep-Oct;44(5):415-9.

[65] Shenefelt PD. Biofeedback, cognitive-behavioral methods, and hypnosis in dermatology: is it all in your mind? *Dermatol. Ther.* 2003;16(2):114-22.

[66] Shenefelt PD. Hypnosis in dermatology. *Arch. Dermatol.* 2000 Mar;136(3):393-9.

[67] Panconesi E, Hautmann G. Psychotherapeutic approach in acne treatment. *Dermatology.* 1998;196(1):116-8.

[68] Bowes LE, Alster TS. Treatment of facial scarring and ulceration resulting from acne excoriée with 585-nm pulsed dye laser irradiation and cognitive psychotherapy. *Dermatol. Surg.* 2004 Jun;30(6):934-8.

[69] Bolton, M. Lobben I, Stern T. The Impact of Body Image on Patient Care. *Prim. Care Companion J. Clin. Psychiatry.* 2010; 12(2): PCC.10r00947. doi: 10.4088/PCC. 10r00947blu.

[70] Valente SM. Visual disfigurement and depression. *Plast. Surg. Nurs.* 2004 Oct-Dec;24(4):140-6; quiz 147-8.

[71] Miliora MT. Facial disfigurement: a self-psychological perspective on the "hide-and-seek" fantasy of an avoidant personality. *Bull. Menninger Clin.* 1998 Summer;62(3):378-94.

[72] Bradbury E. Meeting the psychological needs of patients with facial Disfigurement. *British Journal of Oral and Maxillofacial Surgery* 50 (2012) 193–196.

[73] Carver, C. and Scheier, M., 1981. *Attention and self-regulation: A control theory approach to human behaviour.* New York: Springer-Verlag.

[74] Bourin, M. Psychopharmacological Treatment of Depression. Klinik Psikofarmakoloji Bu☐lteni, Cilt: 11, Say›: 1, 2001 / *Bulletin of Clinical Psychopharmacology*, Vol: 11, N.: 1, 2001

[75] Eckert A, Reiff J, Müller WE. [Medical interactions with antidepressives. Benefits of the specific serotonin reuptake inhibitor citalopram]. *Med. Monatsschr. Pharm.* 1998 May;21(5):138-50.

[76] Vaswani M, Linda FK, Ramesh S. Role of selective serotonin reuptake inhibitors in psychiatric disorders: a comprehensive review. *Prog. Neuropsychopharmacol. Biol. Psychiatry.* 2003 Feb;27(1):85-102.

[77] Jeffreys M, Capehart B, Friedman MJ. Pharmacotherapy for posttraumatic stress disorder: Review with clinical applications. *J. Rehabil. Res. Dev*. 2012 Jul;49(5):703-16.

[78] Hirschfeld RM. The epidemiology of depression and the evolution of treatment. *J. Clin. Psychiatry*. 2012;73 Suppl 1:5-9.

[79] Remick R, Froese C. Monoamine Oxidase Inhibitors: Clinical Review. *Can. Fam. Physician*. 1990 June; 36: 1151–1155.

[80] Montgomery SA. Tolerability of serotonin norepinephrine reuptake inhibitor antidepressants. *CNS Spectr*. 2008 Jul;13(7 Suppl 11):27-33.

[81] Stimmel GL, Dopheide JA, Stahl SM. Mirtazapine: an antidepressant with noradrenergic and specific serotonergic effects. *Pharmacotherapy*. 1997 Jan-Feb;17(1):10-21.

[82] Hajós M, Fleishaker JC, Filipiak-Reisner JK, Brown MT, Wong EH. The selective norepinephrine reuptake inhibitor antidepressant reboxetine: pharmacological and clinical profile. *CNS Drug Rev*. 2004 Spring;10(1):23-44.

[83] Koenig AM, Thase ME. First-line pharmacotherapies for depression - what is the best choice? *Pol. Arch. Med. Wewn*. 2009 Jul-Aug;119(7-8):478-86.

[84] Gada M. Treatment of depression with the serotonin reuptake enhancer tianeptine in the primary care setting of India. *J. Indian Med. Assoc*. 2005 Feb;103(2):105-6.

Pathogenesis of Scarring

In: Scars and Scarring
Editor: Yongsoo Lee

ISBN: 978-1-62808-005-6
© 2013 Nova Science Publishers, Inc.

Chapter 3

Pathogenesis of Scars: An Overview

Chao-Kai Hsu[1,*2], Julia Yu-Yun Lee[2] and Ming-Jer Tang[3]

[1]Institute of Clinical Medicine,
[2]Department of Dermatology,
[3]Department of Physiology,
National Cheng-Kung University, College of Medicine and Hospital,
Tainan, Taiwan

Abstract

Scars are areas of fibrous tissue that replace the normal skin tissue following injury or disease. The processes of wound healing are dynamic and quite complex. Various factors, including growth factors, turnover of extracellular matrix and genetic susceptibility, contribute to the formation of various types of scars that can be normotrophic, atrophic, hypertrophic, keloid, or mixed. Clinically, keloids and hypertrophic scars are more common in the body areas subjected to increased skin tension, such as the anterior chest, shoulder and upper arm. Recent clinical and basic studies have provided evidence that local mechanical stimulation influences significantly the formation and degree of abnormal scar. The pathogenic role of mechanical force is supported by the preferential growth of the keloid scar along the direction of the skin tension with the characteristic butterfly or crab's claw shape of keloids on the anterior chest being the best example. There has been substantial growth in the basic research regarding the changes in both biomechanical and biophysical properties of cells and their effects on the progression of some human diseases. The interaction between cell and extracellular matrix can not only determine the shape and orientation of cells but also regulate important cellular functions, including migration, differentiation, and proliferation. Identification of the specific signal transduction pathways involved in abnormal wound healing will propel the development of novel methods for scar prevention and treatment. In this Chapter, we will review the orchestrated phases of wound healing process, and the pathogenesis of abnormal scars.

---

[*] kylehsu@mail.ncku.edu.tw

Introduction

Scars are areas of fibrous tissue that replace the normal skin tissue following injury or disease. Wound healing is a complex process that can be roughly divided into 3 overlapping phases, including inflammation, tissue formation, and tissue remodeling. Various factors responsible for wound healing, including growth factors, turnover of extracellular matrix and genetic susceptibility, contribute to the formation of various types of scars. Recent clinical and basic studies have shown that mechanobiology plays a vital role in the pathogenesis of abnormal scarring. In this chapter, we give a review of the cutaneous wound healing process, the most significant molecular or cellular factors that affect wound healing, and the potential mechanisms involved.

Cutaneous Wound Healing

Cutaneous wound healing is a dynamic and complex interaction between keratinocytes of the epidermis, stromal cells and hematocytes of the dermis, extracellular matrix and various soluble mediators. The complex process of wound healing can be temporally grouped into three phases—"inflammation", "tissue formation (cell proliferation)" and "matrix remodeling" (Figure 1) [1]. These three phases of wound healing are not straight subsequent events but rather overlapping in time.

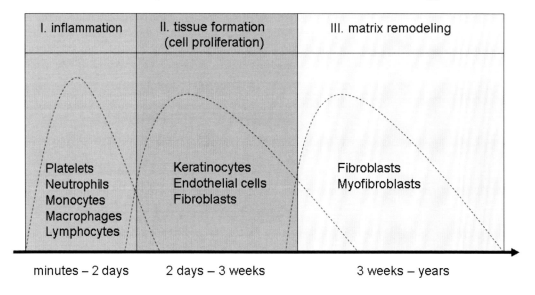

Figure 1. Three phases of cutaneous wound healing.

Table 1. The source and function of growth factors and cytokines involved in wound healing

Growth factors and cytokines	Major Source	Properties/effects
Transforming growth factor-β1 (TGF-β1)	Platelets, macrophages, fibroblasts	Chemotaxis of neutrophils, macrophages and fibroblasts; extracellular-matrix synthesis and remodeling; Epidermal-cell motility
Platelet-derived growth factor (PDGF)	Platelets, macrophages, epidermal cells	Chemotaxis of neutrophils, macrophages and fibroblasts; Fibroblast proliferation; macrophage activation; extracellular-matrix synthesis
Fibroblast growth factor (FGF)	Macrophages, fibroblasts	Angiogenesis
Keratinocyte growth factor (KGF) (A member of FGF family)	Fibroblasts	Proliferation and migration of epidermal cells
Vascular endothelial growth factor (VEGF)	Macrophages, fibroblasts	Angiogenesis and inducer of vascular permeability

1. Inflammation Phase

The first phase of wound healing is characterized by "hemostasis" and "inflammation". Some authors divide wound healing process into 4 stages, and nominate "hemostasis" as the first stage [2]. Skin injury causes the disruption of blood vessels in the dermis, which subsequently causes the extravasation of blood cells and other blood constituents (Figure 2). Platelets adhere, aggregate, and release several clotting factors to facilitate coagulation of blood clots. The blood clots serve as scaffolding for arriving cells, such as neutrophils, monocytes and fibroblasts. Platelets not only facilitate the formation of hemostatic clots, but they also secrete several mediators for wound healing. The two most important signals are platelet-derived growth factor (PDGF) and transforming growth factor-beta 1 (TGF-β1). The PDGF initiates the chemotaxis of neutrophils, macrophages and fibroblasts. Neutrophils are the earliest to arrive among the infiltrating cells, and are responsible for cleansing foreign particles and bacteria. The infiltrating monocytes further differentiate into activated macrophages, which function as phagocytosis as well as produce multiple inflammatory cytokines and growth factors, such as PDGF, TGF-β1, vascular endothelial growth factor (VEGF) and fibroblast growth factor (FGF), to facilitate the wound healing [3]. Latent TGF-β1, released by degranulating platelets, is activated from its latent complex via proteolytic and non-proteolytic mechanisms [4]. Active TGF-β1 elicits rapid chemotaxis of neutrophils and monocytes to the wound site [5]. In concert with the extracellular-matrix molecules, PDGF and TGF-β1 stimulate fibroblasts of the tissue around the wound to migrate, proliferate and express appropriate integrin receptors [6]. The paracrine and autocrine TGF-â1 dermal signaling mechanisms further mediate macrophage recruitment, re-epithelization, and wound contraction [7]. VEGF, primarily produced by fibroblasts and macrophages, functions as inducer for angiogenesis and vascular permeability [8]. In contrast to VEGF, which is an endothelial cell-specific mitogen, FGF acts on a variety of different cell types. It has a direct and an indirect stimulation effects on angiogenesis. Keratinocyte growth factor (KGF) is a member of FGF family. KGF is weakly expressed in the human skin, but is strongly upregulated in dermal fibroblasts after skin injury [9]. KGF binds to a transmembrane receptor on keratinocytes, and induces proliferation and migration of keratinocytes. Lymphocytes come into the wound area at the later stage of the inflammation phase. They are not considered to be the major inflammatory cells involved in the wound healing process, and their precise role remains unclear [2]. The detailed functions and sources of major growth factors and cytokines involved in wound healing are listed in Table 1.

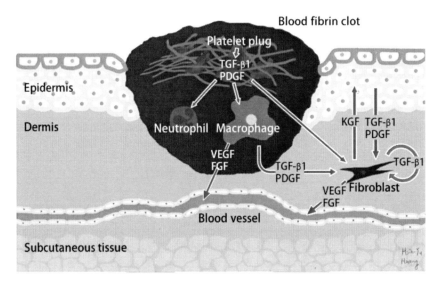

Figure 2. Inflammation phase (minutes to 2 days). Platelets release clotting factors to initiate coagulation, and several mediators that attract neutrophils, monocytes, macrophages and fibroblasts. The formation of a blood clot re-establishes hemostasis and provides a provisional matrix for cell migration. The infiltrating neutrophils are responsible for cleansing foreign particles and bacteria, and the activated macrophages function as scavengers to remove foreign materials, cell debris and dead cells. Cytokines and growth factors released by macrophages, including PDGF, fibroblast growth factor (FGF) and tumor necrosis factor-alpha (TNF-α), facilitate the wound healing process. Vascular endothelial growth factor (VEGF), which is primarily produced by fibroblasts and macrophages functions as chemotactic agent and inducer of angiogenesis vascular permeability. Keratinocyte growth factor (KGF) mainly from dermal fibroblasts induces proliferation and migration of keratinocytes. [Note: Figure 2 and Figure 3 are adapted from Reference 1].

2. Tissue Formation (Cell Proliferation) Phase

The tissue formation phase, also called cell proliferation phase, is characterized by angiogenesis, re-epithelialization (epidermal regeneration), collagen deposition and wound contraction (Figure 3). This phase begins with the infiltration of fibroblasts and the sprouting of new blood vessels (angiogenesis or neovascularization). Fibroblasts proliferate and produce extracellular matrix, including various types of collagen and fibronectin. When the wound bed is more or less filled with the granulation tissue, re-epitheliazation process takes place in which keratinocytes proliferate and migrate in sheets to cover the wound bed. With the deposition of collagen and fibronectin in the granulation tissue, actin-rich fibroblasts (myofibroblasts) express fibronectin receptors, and exert a contractile force to make the wound smaller [10]. The production of extracellular matrix is counterbalanced by its turnover and catabolism principally mediated by several proteolytic enzymes termed matrix metalloproteinases (MMPs) [11]. MMPs comprise a family of 24 distinct but structurally related enzymes, which can be further divided into four subgroups, specifically, collagenases, stromelysins, gelatinases and membrane type-MMPs, based on substrate specificity [12, 13]. Among these MMPs, collagenase (MMP-1) cuts intact collagen at a single site; gelatinases (MMP-2 and MMP-9) degrade partially denatured collagen (gelatin); and stromelysin (MMP-3) degrades multiple protein substrates in the extracellular matrix. MMPs not only metabolize collagen or other extracellular matrix components, recent studies suggests that they also influence inflammation and re-epithelialization [12, 14]. MMPs are produced by several cell types involved in wound healing, including keratinocytes, fibroblasts, endothelial cells and inflammatory cells. The expression of MMPs is modulated in response to signals from cytokines or growth factors as well as cell–matrix interactions [12].

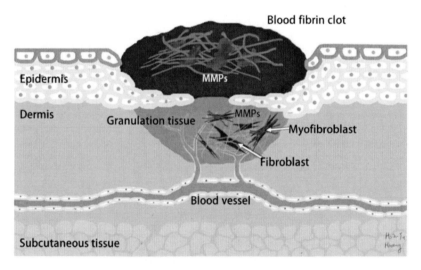

Figure 3. Tissue formation (cell proliferation) (2 days to 3 weeks). Blood vessels sprout into the granulation tissue as re-epithelialization occurs. Matrix metalloproteinases (MMPs) are produced by keratinocytes, fibroblasts, endothelial cells and inflammatory cells. MMPs not only metabolize collagen or other extracellular matrix components, but they also influence inflammation and re-epithelialization.

3. Matrix Remodeling Phase

The matrix remodeling phase, also named as maturation phase, typically begins about 3 weeks after the injury, and may last from 3 weeks to 2 years, depending on the size of the wound. The disorganized collagen fibers are remodeled and gradually aligned themselves along tensile forces (Figure 4). The process continues until the scar tissue has regained about 80 % of the skin's original strength. Type III collagen deposited during the proliferation phase is gradually replaced by type I collagen, which is more tightly crosslinked and provides more tensile strength to the matrix than type III collagen. Collagen remodeling during matrix remodeling phase is dependent on the continued synthesis and catabolism of collagen. The activities of MMPs are negatively regulated by specific endogenous tissue inhibitors of metalloproteinases (TIMPs), which bind to the active MMP enzyme with high affinity [1, 15]. Four TIMPs (TIMP 1-4) have been identified, and each has the ability to bind and inhibit MMP activities in a varying degree [16]. During the matrix remodeling phase, the role of myofibroblasts is close to completion, the unneeded cells undergo apoptosis, leaving a collagen-rich scar tissue that is slowly re-modeled over several months (Figure 4A) [17]. In pathological conditions, such as hypertrophic scar or keloid, myofibroblasts persist and continue to produce excessive extracellular matrix (Figure 4B). In addition, higher number of vessels and distinct pattern of vascularization can be seen in hypertrophic scars and keloids [18].

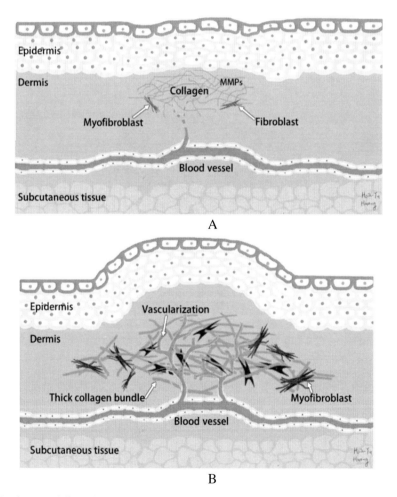

Figure 4. Matrix remodeling phase (3 weeks to 2 years). A, Normal scar B, Pathological scar. Fibroblasts produce new collagen, which increases tensile strength to the wound. When a normal healing wound closes, myofibroblasts disappear by apoptosis. In pathological situations, such as hypertrophic scar or keloid, myofibroblasts persist and continue to produce excessive extracellular matrix. Greater number of blood vessels and distinct pattern of vascularization can be seen in pathological scars.

Cutaneous wound healing is a complex process involving blood clotting, inflammation, new tissue formation, and finally tissue remodeling. Although the details of the wound healing process seem to be elucidated, the exact mechanism of wound healing regulation remains to be fully understood.

Overview of Scars

An ideal scar is a fine line or an area of smooth skin surface with minimal pigmentation and without any irregular texture or contractures distorting the adjacent skin. Abnormal scar formation is influenced by variable factors such as type of wounding, (trauma, burn, and surgery), location, treatment (operative techniques or radiation), relevant underlying chronic illnesses (diabetes, arterial insufficiency), gender, gravidity, age, race, skin type or even lifestyle (sun exposure, smoking). According to the scar classification schemes proposed by Mustoe *et al.* in 2002, scars are classified as 6 types: mature scar, immature scar, linear hypertrophic scar, widespread scar, minor keloid and major keloid [19]. Among these, hypertrophic scar and keloid are common forms of abnormal scar resulting from abnormal responses to wounding. Keloids are defined as scars growing beyond the confines of the original wounds, and rarely regress over time. Hypertrophic scars, on the other hand, are elevated scars that remain within the boundaries of the wound and frequently regress spontaneously [20].

Pathological Findings of Hypertrophic Scars and Keloid

Histopathologically, a keloid is characterized by a cellular fibrous tissue with thick hyalinized eosinophilic collagen fibers (keloidal collagen) and a horizontal, tongue-like advancing edge in the dermis [21]. Conversely, little or no keloidal collagen is found in hypertrophic scar [21, 22]. Recent studies found that α-smooth muscle actin (α-SMA) is commonly expressed in a healing wound and hypertrophic scar. Ehrlich *et al.* found diffuse expression of α-SMA in 18 of 22 hypertrophic scars but only minimal or focal expression of this marker in 2 of 17 keloids [23]. However, Lee *et al.* found that common α-SMA expression in both hypertrophic scar (70%) and keloid (45%) [21]. Therefore, the extent of α-SMA expression may not be a differentiating marker between hypertrophic scar and keloid, as suggested earlier by Ehrlich *et al.* Other pathological features of keloids include a non-flattened epidermis, non-fibrotic papillary dermis, horizontal cellular fibrous band in the upper reticular dermis, and prominent fascia-like dense collagenous band near the base of the scar [21].

Pathogenesis of Keloid

The pathogenesis of keloids is fairly complex, and involves both genetic and environmental factors. Keloids develop subsequent to injury or inflammation in certain skin disorders, such as acne vulgaris, folliculitis, chikenpox, or vaccinations (mostly BCG vaccination). Keloids often begin months after skin injury or inflammatory process, but may develop as far out as a year later [24, 25]. The proposed mechanisms of keloid formation include (1) dysregulation of various cytokines/growth factors (2) aberrant collagen turnover (3) genetic susceptibility (4) mechanical force [25-30]. Still, there is no single unifying hypothesis that can adequately explain the formation of keloid.

(1) *Cytokines/growth factors dysregulation:* A great number of cytokines and growth factors are linked to all phases of wound healing. Therefore, the majority of keloid studies are focused on the evaluation of protein factors and the involved upstream and downstream signaling pathways. Keloid fibroblasts show an increased amount of growth factors and their receptors. Furthermore, keloid fibroblasts also respond more briskly to growth factor-induced signals [3]. TGF-β1, PDGF, and other cytokines/growth factors have been implicated as important factors involved in the formation of keloid and hypertrophic scar [20, 31], and TGF-β1/Smad pathway plays a key role in keloid pathogenesis [32, 33]. He *et al.* showed that the ERK, JNK and p38 pathways mediate TGF-β1/Smad signal transduction and might be considered as specific targets of drug therapy for keloids [34]. PDGF is a strong inducer of fibroblastic production of collagen, and it has been observed that both PDGF and its receptor are markedly overexpressed in hypertrophic scar and keloids [35]. Recent studies showed that PDGF, which is secreted by macrophages during the proliferative phase of wound healing stimulates fibroblasts to produce and secrete osteopontin, an extracellular glycoprotein that enhances fibroplasia [36].

(2) *Aberrant extracellular matrix turnover:* The synthesis of extracellular matrix is counterbalanced by its degradation principally mediated by MMPs [11]. The catalytic activity of MMPs is generally low in normal tissue, but is increased during inflammation and wound repair [37]. While the transcription of MMPs can be regulated by cytokines and growth factors, the catalytic activity of MMPs is regulated by TIMP [38]. Therefore, the balance between MMP and TIMP expression is essential for tissue homeostasis and is linked to various pathogenic conditions. Fujiwara *et al.* found that the production of type 1 collagen, MMP-1, MMP-2, and TIMP-1 by keloid fibroblasts was 3-fold, 6-fold, 2.4-fold, and 2-fold greater than that of normal dermal fibroblasts, respectively [32]. Furthermore, the TGF-β1 played a role in this regulation of collagen and MMPs production. Imaizumi *et al.* demonstrated significantly increased expressions of MMP-2, TIMP-2 and TIMP-3 in keloids compared with mature scars. MMP-2 activity can be enhanced in keloid fibroblasts between collagen bundles in cooperation with TIMP-2 and membrane-type 1 MMP. This could contribute to remodeling of collagen in keloid tissue and invasion of fibroblasts into the peripheral normal regions through increased degradation of extracellular matrix [39]. Russell *et al.* observed that decreased expression of MMP3 in cultured keloid fibroblasts were maintained for many cell generations [40].

(3) *Genetic susceptibility:* The findings of familial predisposition, high prevalence in certain populations and occurrence in twins suggest a significant genetic factor in the pathogenesis of keloid. However, to date no single causative gene responsible has been identified for the development of keloid. Recent data suggests that carriers of

certain specific major histocompatibility complex alleles, HLADRB1*15, HLA-DQA1*0104, DQB1*0501 and DQB1*0503 in particular, are at increased risks of developing keloid scarring [41]. Smith JC et al. observed that keloid expressed differential regulation of approximately 500 of 38,000 genes by microarray study [42]. Of particular interest was the increased expression of several insulin-like growth factor (IGF)-binding and related proteins, and decreased expression of a subset of Wnt pathway inhibitors and multiple IL-1-inducible genes. These findings suggest that multiple fibrosis-related pathways are involved in the pathogenesis of keloids. In 2010, Nakashima et al. reported a genome-wide association study among 824 individual cases with keloid and 3,205 unaffected controls in a Japanese population [43]. They identified 4 susceptibility loci. Further fine mapping by SNPs revealed that a 185-kb region containing E3 ubiquitin ligase, NEDD4, was strongly associated with keloid ($P = 4.8 \times 10^{-11}$). NEDD4 was previously suggested to negatively regulate TGF-β signaling with ubiquitin-mediated degradation of SMAD4 [44].

(4) *Mechanical force:* Clinically, the recognition of the tension line (Langer's lines) is important for surgical operations, particularly cosmetic surgery. The incisions created parallel to skin tension lines rarely form abnormal scars, whereas those placed at sites of joint motion frequently do [45]. Keloids are more likely to form in the body sites subjected to an increased skin tension or stiffness, such as presternal region, shoulder (especially the scapular area), and ear lobe (Delete the below sensence readers may question about the inclusion of ear lobe here) [28, 46]. These sites all have in common that they are constantly or frequently subjected to skin stretching due to the cyclic body movements in daily life, such as breathing and upper limbs movement [47, 48]. Another clinical observation shows that abnormal scarring rarely develops in elderly patients whose skin characteristically has low tension [49]. Interestingly, it has been reported that keloids transplanted to areas of low tension resolved subsequently [50]. These clinical phenomena imply that mechanical stimulation may play a role in keloid formation. Ogawa et al. analyzed the relationship between keloid growth patterns and stretching tension using a visualized finite element study. The results suggest that stretching tension is an important local factor associated with keloid growth [51]. Furthermore, Ogawa et al. hypothesized that keloid may be a mechanoreceptor or mechanosensitive nociceptor disorder [28, 47, 48].

There has been substantial growth in the research related to the changes in both biomechanical and biophysical properties of cells and their effect on the progression of human diseases, especially cancer metastasis [52-54]. Cell- extracellular matrix interactions not only determine the shape and orientation of cells within the extracellular matrix but also regulate important cellular functions, including migration, differentiation, and proliferation [55, 56]. The pioneering study of exploring the effect of mechanical tension on fibroblast phenotype is from Pelham and Wang [57]. They have demonstrated that NIH-3T3 fibroblasts seeded on a soft surface were less well spread with fewer actin stress fibers than cells seeded on stiff surfaces. Arora et al. have reported that TGF-β1-induced gingival fibroblasts differentiation and expression of α-SMA are dependent on matrix stiffness [58]. Li et al. have shown that both TGF-β1 and matrix stiffness play a role in the pathogenesis of liver cirrhosis, which is characterized by portal fibroblast activation and excessive accumulation of extracellular matrix proteins [59]. The above studies demonstrated that fibroblasts are sensitive to changes in extracellular matrix composition and structure.

Wang Z *et al.* hypothesized that a difference exists in the transcriptional response of keloid fibroblasts to mechanical strain compared with normal fibroblasts [60]. They seeded normal and keloid fibroblasts in a device delivering equibiaxial strain, and found that keloid fibroblasts formed more focal adhesion complexes as measured by immunofluorescence for focal adhesion kinase (FAK), integrin β1, and vinculin. Keloid fibroblasts produced more mRNA for TGF-β1, TGF-β2, and collagen Iα after mechanical strain compared to normals, and this was correlated with protein production. This was the pilot study showing that keloid fibroblasts have an exaggerated response to mechanical strain compared to normal fibroblasts. Gurtner's group first demonstrated that mechanical stress applied to a healing wound is sufficient to produce hypertrophic scars in mice [61]. They found that mechanical loading early in the proliferative phase of wound healing produces hypertrophic scars by inhibiting cellular apoptosis. Furthermore, they found that mechanical force regulates fibrosis through inflammatory FAK-ERK-MCP-1 pathways [62]. They demonstrated the important role of focal adhesion kinase (FAK) and monocyte chemoattractant protein-1 (MCP-1) in the mechanical force-induced skin fibrosis, and the crosstalk between the mechanotransduction pathway and inflammatory signaling.

Conclusion and Perspectives

Excessive scarring is a fibrotic disorder resulting from an abnormal wound-healing process. The pathogenesis of excessive scarring is complex and involves both genetic and environmental factors. Although mechanobiology research has recently revealed promising signaling pathways participating in scarring, much remains to be elucidated in terms of the mechanotransduction pathways that lead to the development and progression of scars. Further research into these scar-related mechanisms, especially the mechanotransduction pathway, is likely to reveal promising molecules that could be used for targeted pharmaceutical or clinical treatment in the near future.

Acknowledgments

This work was supported in part by grants from National Cheng Kung University Hosptial (NCKUH-101-5017 & 100-5011) and National Science Council (NSC99-2314-B-006-008-MY3). We thank to Hsin-Yu Huang for his assistance in the drawing of figures.

References

[1] Singer AJ, Clark RA. Cutaneous wound healing. *N Engl J Med.* 1999 Sep 2;341(10):738-46. PubMed PMID: 10471461. Epub 1999/09/02. eng.

[2] Diegelmann RF, Evans MC. Wound healing: an overview of acute, fibrotic and delayed healing. *Front Biosci.* 2004 Jan 1;9:283-9. PubMed PMID: 14766366.

[3] Mahdavian Delavary B, van der Veer WM, van Egmond M, Niessen FB, Beelen RH. Macrophages in skin injury and repair. *Immunobiology.* 2011 Jul;216(7):753-62. PubMed PMID: 21281986. Epub 2011/02/02. eng.

[4] Khalil N. TGF-beta: from latent to active. *Microbes Infect.* 1999 Dec;1(15):1255-63. PubMed PMID: 10611753.

[5] Wahl SM, Hunt DA, Wakefield LM, McCartney-Francis N, Wahl LM, Roberts AB, et al. Transforming growth factor type beta induces monocyte chemotaxis and growth factor production. *Proc Natl Acad Sci U S A.* 1987 Aug;84(16):5788-92. PubMed PMID: 2886992. Pubmed Central PMCID: 298948.

[6] Xu J, Clark RA. Extracellular matrix alters PDGF regulation of fibroblast integrins. *J Cell Biol.* 1996 Jan;132(1-2):239-49. PubMed PMID: 8567727. Pubmed Central PMCID: 2120701.

[7] Martinez-Ferrer M, Afshar-Sherif AR, Uwamariya C, de Crombrugghe B, Davidson JM, Bhowmick NA. Dermal transforming growth factor-beta responsiveness mediates wound contraction and epithelial closure. *Am J Pathol.* 2010 Jan;176(1):98-107. PubMed PMID: 19959810. Pubmed Central PMCID: 2797873.

[8] Bao P, Kodra A, Tomic-Canic M, Golinko MS, Ehrlich HP, Brem H. The role of vascular endothelial growth factor in wound healing. *J Surg Res.* 2009 May 15;153(2):347-58. PubMed PMID: 19027922. Pubmed Central PMCID: 2728016.

[9] Beer HD, Gassmann MG, Munz B, Steiling H, Engelhardt F, Bleuel K, et al. Expression and function of keratinocyte growth factor and activin in skin morphogenesis and cutaneous wound repair. *J Investig Dermatol Symp Proc.* 2000 Dec;5(1):34-9. PubMed PMID: 11147673.

[10] Clark RA. Fibronectin matrix deposition and fibronectin receptor expression in healing and normal skin. *J Invest Dermatol.* 1990 Jun;94(6 Suppl):128S-34S. PubMed PMID: 2161886. Epub 1990/06/01. eng.

[11] Mirastschijski U, Schnabel R, Claes J, Schneider W, Agren MS, Haaksma C, et al. Matrix metalloproteinase inhibition delays wound healing and blocks the latent transforming growth factor-beta1-promoted myofibroblast formation and function. *Wound Repair Regen.* 2010 Mar-Apr;18(2):223-34. PubMed PMID: 20409148. Pubmed Central PMCID: 2859473.

[12] Gill SE, Parks WC. Metalloproteinases and their inhibitors: regulators of wound healing. *Int J Biochem Cell Biol.* 2008;40(6-7):1334-47. PubMed PMID: 18083622. Pubmed Central PMCID: 2746915.

[13] Parks WC. Matrix metalloproteinases in repair. *Wound Repair Regen.* 1999 Nov-Dec;7(6):423-32. PubMed PMID: 10633001.

[14] Parks WC, Wilson CL, Lopez-Boado YS. Matrix metalloproteinases as modulators of inflammation and innate immunity. *Nature reviews Immunology.* 2004 Aug;4(8):617-29. PubMed PMID: 15286728.

[15] Madlener M, Parks WC, Werner S. Matrix metalloproteinases (MMPs) and their physiological inhibitors (TIMPs) are differentially expressed during excisional skin wound repair. *Exp Cell Res.* 1998 Jul 10;242(1):201-10. PubMed PMID: 9665817.

[16] Kugler A. Matrix metalloproteinases and their inhibitors. *Anticancer Res.* 1999 Mar-Apr;19(2C):1589-92. PubMed PMID: 10365151.

[17] Midwood KS, Williams LV, Schwarzbauer JE. Tissue repair and the dynamics of the extracellular matrix. *Int J Biochem Cell Biol.* 2004 Jun;36(6):1031-7. PubMed PMID: 15094118. Epub 2004/04/20. eng.

[18] Amadeu T, Braune A, Mandarim-de-Lacerda C, Porto LC, Desmouliere A, Costa A. Vascularization pattern in hypertrophic scars and keloids: a stereological analysis. *Pathology, research and practice.* 2003;199(7):469-73. PubMed PMID: 14521263.

[19] Mustoe TA, Cooter RD, Gold MH, Hobbs FD, Ramelet AA, Shakespeare PG, et al. International clinical recommendations on scar management. *Plast Reconstr Surg.* 2002 Aug;110(2):560-71. PubMed PMID: 12142678. Epub 2002/07/27. eng.

[20] Tuan TL, Nichter LS. The molecular basis of keloid and hypertrophic scar formation. *Mol Med Today.* 1998 Jan;4(1):19-24. PubMed PMID: 9494966. Epub 1998/03/12. eng.

[21] Lee JY, Yang CC, Chao SC, Wong TW. Histopathological differential diagnosis of keloid and hypertrophic scar. *Am J Dermatopathol.* 2004 Oct;26(5):379-84. PubMed PMID: 15365369. Epub 2004/09/15. eng.

[22] Muir IF. On the nature of keloid and hypertrophic scars. *Br J Plast Surg.* 1990 Jan;43(1):61-9. PubMed PMID: 2310898.

[23] Ehrlich HP, Desmouliere A, Diegelmann RF, Cohen IK, Compton CC, Garner WL, et al. Morphological and immunochemical differences between keloid and hypertrophic scar. *Am J Pathol.* 1994 Jul;145(1):105-13. PubMed PMID: 8030742. Epub 1994/07/01. eng.

[24] Brissett AE, Sherris DA. Scar contractures, hypertrophic scars, and keloids. *Facial Plast Surg.* 2001 Nov;17(4):263-72. PubMed PMID: 11735059.

[25] Robles DT, Moore E, Draznin M, Berg D. Keloids: pathophysiology and management. *Dermatol Online J.* 2007;13(3):9. PubMed PMID: 18328203. Epub 2008/03/11. eng.

[26] Al-Attar A, Mess S, Thomassen JM, Kauffman CL, Davison SP. Keloid pathogenesis and treatment. *Plast Reconstr Surg.* 2006 Jan;117(1):286-300. PubMed PMID: 16404281. Epub 2006/01/13. eng.

[27] Butler PD, Longaker MT, Yang GP. Current progress in keloid research and treatment. *J Am Coll Surg.* 2008 Apr;206(4):731-41. PubMed PMID: 18387480. Epub 2008/04/05. eng.

[28] Ogawa R, Akaishi S, Huang C, Dohi T, Aoki M, Omori Y, et al. Clinical Applications of Basic Research that Shows Reducing Skin Tension Could Prevent and Treat Abnormal Scarring: The Importance of Fascial/Subcutaneous Tensile Reduction Sutures and Flap Surgery for Keloid and Hypertrophic Scar Reconstruction. *J Nippon Med Sch.* 2011;78(2):68-76. PubMed PMID: 21551963. Epub 2011/05/10. eng.

[29] Ogawa R. Mechanobiology of scarring. *Wound Repair Regen.* 2011 Sep;19 Suppl 1:s2-9. PubMed PMID: 21793962. Epub 2011/08/04. eng.

[30] Agha R, Ogawa R, Pietramaggiori G, Orgill DP. A review of the role of mechanical forces in cutaneous wound healing. *J Surg Res.* 2011 Dec;171(2):700-8. PubMed PMID: 22005503. Epub 2011/10/19. eng.

[31] Niessen FB, Spauwen PH, Schalkwijk J, Kon M. On the nature of hypertrophic scars and keloids: a review. *Plast Reconstr Surg.* 1999 Oct;104(5):1435-58. PubMed PMID: 10513931. eng.

[32] Fujiwara M, Muragaki Y, Ooshima A. Keloid-derived fibroblasts show increased secretion of factors involved in collagen turnover and depend on matrix

metalloproteinase for migration. *Br J Dermatol.* 2005 Aug;153(2):295-300. PubMed PMID: 16086739. Epub 2005/08/10. eng.

[33] Leask A, Abraham DJ. TGF-beta signaling and the fibrotic response. *FASEB J.* 2004 May;18(7):816-27. PubMed PMID: 15117886. Epub 2004/05/01. eng.

[34] He S, Liu X, Yang Y, Huang W, Xu S, Yang S, et al. Mechanisms of transforming growth factor beta(1)/Smad signalling mediated by mitogen-activated protein kinase pathways in keloid fibroblasts. *Br J Dermatol.* 2010 Mar;162(3):538-46. PubMed PMID: 19772524.

[35] Haisa M, Okochi H, Grotendorst GR. Elevated levels of PDGF alpha receptors in keloid fibroblasts contribute to an enhanced response to PDGF. *J Invest Dermatol.* 1994 Oct;103(4):560-3. PubMed PMID: 7930682.

[36] Mori R, Shaw TJ, Martin P. Molecular mechanisms linking wound inflammation and fibrosis: knockdown of osteopontin leads to rapid repair and reduced scarring. *J Exp Med.* 2008 Jan 21;205(1):43-51. PubMed PMID: 18180311. Pubmed Central PMCID: 2234383.

[37] Overall CM, Lopez-Otin C. Strategies for MMP inhibition in cancer: innovations for the post-trial era. *Nat Rev Cancer.* 2002 Sep;2(9):657-72. PubMed PMID: 12209155.

[38] Brew K, Dinakarpandian D, Nagase H. Tissue inhibitors of metalloproteinases: evolution, structure and function. *Biochim Biophys Acta.* 2000 Mar 7;1477(1-2):267-83. PubMed PMID: 10708863.

[39] Imaizumi R, Akasaka Y, Inomata N, Okada E, Ito K, Ishikawa Y, et al. Promoted activation of matrix metalloproteinase (MMP)-2 in keloid fibroblasts and increased expression of MMP-2 in collagen bundle regions: implications for mechanisms of keloid progression. *Histopathology.* 2009 May;54(6):722-30. PubMed PMID: 19438747.

[40] Russell SB, Russell JD, Trupin KM, Gayden AE, Opalenik SR, Nanney LB, et al. Epigenetically altered wound healing in keloid fibroblasts. *J Invest Dermatol.* 2010 Oct;130(10):2489-96. PubMed PMID: 20555348. Pubmed Central PMCID: 2939920.

[41] Brown JJ, Bayat A. Genetic susceptibility to raised dermal scarring. *Br J Dermatol.* 2009 Jul;161(1):8-18. PubMed PMID: 19508304.

[42] Smith JC, Boone BE, Opalenik SR, Williams SM, Russell SB. Gene profiling of keloid fibroblasts shows altered expression in multiple fibrosis-associated pathways. *J Invest Dermatol.* 2008 May;128(5):1298-310. PubMed PMID: 17989729. Epub 2007/11/09. eng.

[43] Nakashima M, Chung S, Takahashi A, Kamatani N, Kawaguchi T, Tsunoda T, et al. A genome-wide association study identifies four susceptibility loci for keloid in the Japanese population. *Nat Genet.* 2010 Sep;42(9):768-71. PubMed PMID: 20711176. Epub 2010/08/17. eng.

[44] Izzi L, Attisano L. *Ubiquitin-dependent regulation of TGFbeta signaling in cancer.* Neoplasia. 2006 Aug;8(8):677-88. PubMed PMID: 16925950. Pubmed Central PMCID: 1601946. Epub 2006/08/24. eng.

[45] Wilhelmi BJ, Blackwell SJ, Phillips LG. Langer's lines: to use or not to use. *Plast Reconstr Surg.* 1999 Jul;104(1):208-14. PubMed PMID: 10597698. Epub 1999/12/22. eng.

[46] Conejo-Mir JS, Corbi R, Linares M. Carbon dioxide laser ablation associated with interferon alfa-2b injections reduces the recurrence of keloids. *J Am Acad Dermatol.* 1998 Dec;39(6):1039-40. PubMed PMID: 9843032. Epub 1998/12/08. eng.

[47] Ogawa R. Keloid and hypertrophic scarring may result from a mechanoreceptor or mechanosensitive nociceptor disorder. *Med Hypotheses.* 2008 Oct;71(4):493-500. PubMed PMID: 18614294. Epub 2008/07/11. eng.

[48] Akaishi S, Ogawa R, Hyakusoku H. Keloid and hypertrophic scar: neurogenic inflammation hypotheses. *Med Hypotheses.* 2008;71(1):32-8. PubMed PMID: 18406540. Epub 2008/04/15. eng.

[49] Peacock EE, Jr., Madden JW, Trier WC. Biologic basis for the treatment of keloids and hypertrophic scars. *South Med J.* 1970 Jul;63(7):755-60. PubMed PMID: 5427162. Epub 1970/07/01. eng.

[50] Diegelmann RF, Cohen IK, McCoy BJ. Growth kinetics and collagen synthesis of normal skin, normal scar and keloid fibroblasts in vitro. *J Cell Physiol.* 1979 Feb;98(2):341-6. PubMed PMID: 422662. Epub 1979/02/01. eng.

[51] Akaishi S, Akimoto M, Ogawa R, Hyakusoku H. The relationship between keloid growth pattern and stretching tension: visual analysis using the finite element method. *Ann Plast Surg.* 2008 Apr;60(4):445-51. PubMed PMID: 18362577. Epub 2008/03/26. eng.

[52] Levental KR, Yu H, Kass L, Lakins JN, Egeblad M, Erler JT, et al. Matrix crosslinking forces tumor progression by enhancing integrin signaling. *Cell.* 2009 Nov 25;139(5):891-906. PubMed PMID: 19931152. Pubmed Central PMCID: 2788004. Epub 2009/11/26. eng.

[53] Fletcher DA, Mullins RD. Cell mechanics and the cytoskeleton. *Nature.* 2010 Jan 28;463(7280):485-92. PubMed PMID: 20110992. Pubmed Central PMCID: 2851742. Epub 2010/01/30. eng.

[54] Wirtz D, Konstantopoulos K, Searson PC. The physics of cancer: the role of physical interactions and mechanical forces in metastasis. *Nat Rev Cancer.* 2011;11(7):512-22. PubMed PMID: 21701513. Epub 2011/06/28. eng.

[55] Eckes B, Kessler D, Aumailley M, Krieg T. Interactions of fibroblasts with the extracellular matrix: implications for the understanding of fibrosis. *Springer Semin Immunopathol.* 1999;21(4):415-29. PubMed PMID: 10945034. Epub 2000/08/17. eng.

[56] Zaman MH, Trapani LM, Sieminski AL, Mackellar D, Gong H, Kamm RD, et al. Migration of tumor cells in 3D matrices is governed by matrix stiffness along with cell-matrix adhesion and proteolysis. *Proc Natl Acad Sci U S A.* 2006 Jul 18;103(29):10889-94. PubMed PMID: 16832052. Pubmed Central PMCID: 1544144. Epub 2006/07/13. eng.

[57] Pelham RJ, Jr., Wang Y. Cell locomotion and focal adhesions are regulated by substrate flexibility. *Proc Natl Acad Sci U S A.* 1997 Dec 9;94(25):13661-5. PubMed PMID: 9391082. Pubmed Central PMCID: 28362. Epub 1998/02/12. eng.

[58] Arora PD, Narani N, McCulloch CA. The compliance of collagen gels regulates transforming growth factor-beta induction of alpha-smooth muscle actin in fibroblasts. *Am J Pathol.* 1999 Mar;154(3):871-82. PubMed PMID: 10079265. Epub 1999/03/18. eng.

[59] Li Z, Dranoff JA, Chan EP, Uemura M, Sevigny J, Wells RG. Transforming growth factor-beta and substrate stiffness regulate portal fibroblast activation in culture.

Hepatology. 2007 Oct;46(4):1246-56. PubMed PMID: 17625791. Epub 2007/07/13. eng.

[60] Wang Z, Fong KD, Phan TT, Lim IJ, Longaker MT, Yang GP. Increased transcriptional response to mechanical strain in keloid fibroblasts due to increased focal adhesion complex formation. *J Cell Physiol.* 2006 Feb;206(2):510-7. PubMed PMID: 16155910. Epub 2005/09/13. eng.

[61] Aarabi S, Bhatt KA, Shi Y, Paterno J, Chang EI, Loh SA, et al. Mechanical load initiates hypertrophic scar formation through decreased cellular apoptosis. *FASEB J.* 2007 Oct;21(12):3250-61. PubMed PMID: 17504973. Epub 2007/05/17. eng.

[62] Wong VW, Rustad KC, Akaishi S, Sorkin M, Glotzbach JP, Januszyk M, et al. Focal adhesion kinase links mechanical force to skin fibrosis via inflammatory signaling. *Nat Med.* 2012 Jan;18(1):148-52. PubMed PMID: 22157678.

In: Scars and Scarring
Editor: Yongsoo Lee

ISBN: 978-1-62808-005-6
© 2013 Nova Science Publishers, Inc.

Chapter 4

Redox-Signaling during Wound Healing: A Role for Cytoprotective Enzymes in Scar Prevention?

Ditte M. S. Lundvig and Frank A. D. T. G. Wagener[*]

Department of Orthodontics and Craniofacial Biology, Nijmegen Centre for Molecular Life Sciences, Radboud University Nijmegen Medical Centre, Nijmegen, The Netherlands

Abstract

Wound healing is an intricate process involving the concerted action of various growth factors, chemokines, and cell types. Normally, tissue restoration occurs non-problematically, however, when wound healing is impaired it may lead to chronic non-healing wounds or excessive scar formation, accompanied by functional and esthetical problems. The mechanisms underlying impaired wound healing are still scarcely understood.

Generation of reactive oxygen species (ROS) is part of the normal wound healing process to prevent pathogen invasion, and low levels of ROS are required for cellular signaling. However, insufficient ROS detoxification or overproduction of excessive amounts of ROS generates oxidative and inflammatory stress, resulting in oxidative modification of proteins and cellular damage, contributing to impaired wound healing and excessive scarring.

Wounding and cell injury lead to a local accumulation of hemoproteins and free heme. Heme is a crucial molecule for the functioning of heme proteins, however, when free heme is released from proteins it acts as a pro-inflammatory and pro-oxidative molecule. Heme exposure promotes vasoconstriction, complement system activation, and inflammatory cell infiltration, which are important responses in the early phase of wound healing. However, high levels of free heme promotes ROS generation via the Fenton reaction and thereby increases oxidative stress in the wound. Thus, a tight control on the

---

[*] F.Wagener@dent.umcn.nl (Frank Wagener).

level of free heme and the overall redox balance in the wound is crucial in preventing impaired wound healing and scar formation.

The cellular redox balance is regulated by several antioxidant and pro-oxidant enzymes as well as a variety of extracellular and intracellular (anti)oxidants. In this review, we address the role of these enzymes with emphasis on the cytoprotective heme oxygenase (HO) system in regulating the cellular redox balance to prevent excessive scar formation.

Abbreviations

AGE,	advanced glucation end-products;
AngII,	angiotensin II;
AP-1,	activator protein-1;
APE/Ref-1,	apurinic/apyrimidinic endonuclease/redox effector factor-1;
ARE,	antioxidant responsive element;
BVR,	biliverdin reductase;
Cat,	catalase;
CGD,	chronic granulomatous disease;
CO,	carbon monoxide;
COHb,	carboxyhemoglobin;
CO-RM,	carbon monoxide-releasing molecule;
ECM,	extracellular matrix;
ETC,	electron transport chain;
EMMPRIN,	extracellular matrix metalloproteinase inducer;
ERK,	extracellular signal-regulated protein kinases;
G6PD,	glucose 6-phosphate dehydrogenase;
GC,	guanylyl cyclase;
GPx,	glutathione peroxidase;
GR,	glutathione reductase;
GSH,	reduced glutathione;
GSSG,	glutathione disulfide;
GST,	transcription factor p65 protein;
H_2O_2,	hydrogen peroxide;
Hb,	hemoglobin;
HSCs	hepatic stellate cells
HDAC,	histone deacetylase;
HO•,	hydroxyl radical;
HO,	heme oxygenase;
HIF-1,	hypoxia inducible factor-1;
HSC,	hepatic stellate cells;
IL-1,	interleukin-1;
INFγ,	interferon-γ;
IRP,	iron regulatory protein;
JNK,	c-Jun N-terminal kinases;
KO,	knockout;

LDL,	low density lipoprotein;
LPS,	lipopolysaccharide;
MAPK,	mitogen-activated protein kinase;
MMP,	matrix metalloproteinase;
NF-κB,	nuclear factor-κB;
NO,	nitric oxide;
Nox,	NADPH oxidase;
Nrf2,	NF-E2-related factor 2;
$O_2^{\cdot-}$,	superoxide anion;
PKC,	protein kinase C;
Prdx,	peroxiredoxin;
RNS,	reactive nitrogen species;
ROS,	reactive oxygen species;
SOD,	superoxide dismutase;
TGF,	transforming growth factor;
TNFα,	tumor necrosis factor-α

I. Introduction

Normal Wound Healing

Following wounding, a series of events takes place to prevent blood loss, to eliminate pathogen invasion, and ultimately, to promote tissue integrity and homeostasis. Wound healing occurs in three distinct, but overlapping, phases: inflammation, proliferation, and remodeling.

The inflammatory phase is preceded by the formation of a fibrin clot that serves as a provisional matrix for infiltrating and proliferating cells and acts as a reservoir for growth factors and cytokines [1]. These factors orchestrate and fine-tune the different wound healing processes, including angiogenesis and recruitment of neutrophils and monocytes /macrophages to the wound area [2]. Neutrophils are important in eliminating invading pathogens by their respiratory burst activity and in activating fibroblasts and keratinocytes [3]. Monocytes can differentiate into macrophages that clean up the wound area by engulfing damaged cells, microorganisms and damaged tissue. Furthermore, macrophages secrete various cytokines and growth factors that control the inflammatory response and initiate the proliferative phase [1].

This proliferative phase is characterized by the infiltration and proliferation of keratinocytes and activated fibroblasts into the wound area replacing damaged cells and synthesizing and depositing extracellular matrix (ECM) components, predominantly collagen I and III [4]. Simultaneously, a fraction of these fibroblasts transform into myofibroblasts that close the wound by contraction. During this phase endothelial cells restore tissue blood and oxygen supply by making new blood vessels, a process known as angiogenesis.

The wound healing process ends with a long-lasting remodeling phase, involving apoptosis of endothelial cells, myofibroblasts, and inflammatory cells. Moreover, remodeling of the ECM proteins occurs, leading to maturation and cross-linking of collagen and subsequently tissue restoration and scar formation [5, 6].

Fibrosis and Scarring

Wound healing is a protective mechanism aimed at restoring tissue integrity after injury. However, dysregulation of this delicate process and chronic injury may lead to tissue fibrosis characterized by excessive deposition of ECM components, scarring and organ dysfunction/failure. Fibrosis can occur in almost any organ or tissue, and examples of fibrotic diseases are liver cirrhosis, chronic pancreatitis, renal fibrosis, idiopathic pulmonary fibrosis, and hypertrophic scarring. Despite the demanding medical needs of this group of patients no effective anti-fibrotic therapies exist due to limited knowledge about the etiology of fibrogenesis.

Tissue fibrosis is considered to be caused by failed termination of the wound healing response. During normal wound healing activated (myo)fibroblasts proliferate and migrate into the wound area, where they produce and deposit ECM proteins after which they normally will disappear by apoptosis, leaving a rather acellular scar. In contrast, fibrosis in different organs is associated with the persistent presence of activated ECM-producing cells in injured tissues. Different activated cells are responsible for this in different organs They are known as stellate cells in the liver and pancreas, mesangial cells in the kidney, and (myo)fibroblasts in the lung and skin.

Albeit from different origins, several common biological and molecular events occur during fibrogenesis and a number of fibrogenic factors have been identified, like chronic injury (e.g. ischemia, toxins), (viral) infections, and physical injury, resulting in prolonged inflammation [7]. Also, a number of fibrogenic growth factors and cytokines involved in fibroblast recruitment, activation and proliferation are known [8]. The cytokine transforming growth factor (TGF)β-1 is considered the most potent pro-fibrotic factor [9] and transgenic mice over-expressing TGFβ-1 suffer from fibrosis in multiple organs [10]. TGFβ-1 release from damaged cells and inflammatory cells is central to the activation of ECM-producing cells, e.g. myofibroblasts. Once activated, myofibroblasts themselves secrete TGFβ-1, sustaining their own activation [11, 12]. The detrimental role of TGFβ-1 in fibrogenesis is further supported by the findings that increased levels of TGFβ-1 are found in fibrotic kidney [13, 14], lung [15], and liver [16]. Besides these factors also oxidative stress and inflammation are thought to contribute to fibrosis and scarring.

Redox Balance

Reactive oxygen species (ROS) are free radicals generated from molecular oxygen, such as superoxide anion ($O_2^{\cdot-}$), hydroxyl radical (HO•), and non-radical species including hydrogen peroxide (H_2O_2). Today, it is well accepted that ROS play an important role as regulatory mediators in signaling processes [17, 18]. In moderate concentrations, ROS act as important regulatory mediators in different signaling processes [19, 20]. Redox-regulated proteins sense the cellular redox state by different mechanisms, and can modify biological activity though affecting signaling pathways and through direct modifications of biomolecules, especially proteins [20].

The redox system can alter protein function by affecting protein levels via transcriptional regulation and protein stability, or by directly affecting protein function through posttranslational modifications [20]. Several transcription factors, including activator protein-1 (AP-1), nuclear factor κB (NF-κB), hypoxia inducible factor-1 (HIF-1), and p53, contain redox-sensitive cysteine residues in their DNA binding sites [21]. Thiol oxidation of these reactive cysteine residues upon ROS exposure affect the DNA binding function and thus regulates the gene transcription of redox sensitive genes [20, 22, 23]. Also, apurinic/apyrimidinic endonuclease/redox effector factor-1 (APE/Ref-1) protein affects the redox state of reactive cysteines in several redox-sensitive transcription factors, like AP-1, HIF-1, NF-κB, and p53, and is thus an indirect regulator of gene transcription mediated by these transcriptional regulators [24]. Additionally, ROS-mediated regulation of gene transcription occurs through redox-sensitive histone deacetylases (HDACs), which regulate transcription factor interactions with DNA binding sites [25].

Oxidative posttranslational modifications form a major mechanism of redox regulation of protein function [26] targeting multiple types of amino acids with various susceptibilities and subsequent structural and functional consequences [27]. The functional effect of the oxidative modification is dependent on the type and the importance of the modified amino acid in the function of the protein. For instance, reversible oxidation of cysteines and oxidative nitration of tyrosines regulate the activity of various kinases involved in signaling pathways, including c-Jun N-terminal kinases (JNK), mitogen-activated protein kinase (MAPK), and protein kinase C (PKC) [20]. Altered kinase activities due to oxidative modifications affect downstream signaling pathways, transcription factor activation, and contribute to additional redox-regulated gene transcription [28]. However, dependent on the level of ROS and the subsequent degree of oxidative protein modification different cellular outcomes are observed. Oxidative modifications may besides directly affecting protein function also modulate protein-protein interactions and thereby affect the stability of protein complexes and activity of the protein partners involved [29]. For instance, NF-κB is sequestered by IκB in the cytosol. ROS activate IκB kinases that phosphorylate IκB leading to its degradation and activation of NF-κB. Next, NF-κB translocates to the nucleus, and activates transcription of various target genes [30]. Moderate ROS levels promotes NF-κB activation and cell survival, whereas high levels of ROS inactivates NF-κB, leading to cell death [20, 28]. Similarly, activation of the master regulator of several antioxidant genes, NF-E2-related factor 2 (Nrf2), is controlled by binding partner Keap1 [20, 31]. Oxidative modification of Keap1 leads to dissociation of the Nrf2-Keap1 complex, allowing Nrf2 to translocate to the nucleus to activate transcriptional expression of target genes [32].

Paradoxically, ROS-signaling also promotes pathways protecting against oxidative stress, restoring a balanced ratio between cellular oxidants and antioxidants [33, 34]. However, it is beyond the scope of this chapter to describe all pathways affected by ROS in detail, and we refer to comprehensive reviews on pathways and redox-sensitive master regulators of gene expression [22, 31].

Redox Balance in Wound Healing

ROS are important for diverse processes during wound healing [35], as host phagocytic cells use self-generated ROS as microbicidal defense [36]. ROS produced by inflammatory cells during wound healing induce a cascade of cell signaling networks and generate a ROS wave propagating throughout tissues and carry signals across large distances [37]. For example, low levels of ROS mediate intra- en intercellular signaling [38, 39] during wound healing associated processes like angiogenesis [40].

When in excess, ROS exert their damaging effects in mainly two ways: 1) by oxidatively modifying and damaging macromolecules, which alters protein/DNA function and subsequently leads to pathological effects, and (2) by affecting the redox state of factors involved in signal transduction, leading to hyper- or hypo-activation of signaling pathways [41]. Paradoxically, both hypoxia and hyperoxia increase ROS production, but increased ROS levels overrule the beneficial effect of oxygen treatment either by direct tissue and molecular damage [42] or by activating transcription factors like NF-κB [reviewed in 43] that trigger downstream signaling cascades leading to cytokine release and inflammation [44].

Thus, under physiological conditions low concentrations of intracellular ROS are important in cellular signaling and maintaining physiological functions. However, under pathological conditions, increased ROS levels contribute to tissue dysfunction and oxidative damage due to chronic oxidative stress. Indeed, oxidative stress is closely linked to fibrosis [10]. Fetal wound healing, which normally occurs in the absence of scar formation, is affected by ROS and inflammation leading to increased fibroblast proliferation and fibrosis [45, 46]. Although substantial research has been performed during the years on increasing the understanding of wound healing and pathological scarring, the decisive and controlling mechanisms still remain to be elucidated.

For instance, hypertension has been linked to increased ROS concentrations, and impaired endogenous antioxidant systems [47-49]. During the development of hypertension, ROS buildup is predominantly due to NADPH oxidase (Nox) activity, and a mutual reinforcement between ROS and angiotensin II (AngII) exists [49]. Increased ROS levels accompanied by increased Nox activity have been detected *in vivo* and *in vitro* after AngII exposure [reviewed in 50]. Importantly, both oxidative stress and AngII induce collagen I and III expression and remodeling *in vivo* and *in vitro* [50], and both have been linked to the development of cardiac fibrosis [51]. AngII also induces different fibrogenic cascades in hepatic stellate cells (HSCs) including pro-inflammatory cytokine production, cell activation, TGFβ-1 synthesis and collagen production [52, 53]. Furthermore, AngII induction has recently been demonstrated to promote hepatic myofibroblast survival and liver fibrosis by regulating transcription factor phosphorylation [54].

A major determinant of excessive scar formation is time; if wound healing exceeds more than 3 weeks, 78% of the wounds develop excessive or hypertrophic scars [55]. In cutaneous wound healing, the prolongation of healing time as a result of overproduction of ROS and inflammatory mediators leads to an extension of the repair phase due to increased growth factor concentrations that stimulate fibroblast proliferation [56]. Moreover, excessive production and deposition of ECM occurs in skin leading to formation of hypertrophic scarring [57]. Also, activation of HSCs is stimulated by ROS secreted by damaged hepatocytes, liver tissue macrophages (Kupffer cells), and neutrophils [10, 58]. Moreover, neutrophils, alveolar macrophages, and epithelial cells contribute to ROS production in the lungs [59], whereas antioxidant compounds counteract bleomycin-induced pulmonary fibrosis and tissue damage [60]. Importantly, Nox has been directly linked to pulmonary fibrosis, as mice devoid of Nox activity are protected against bleomycin-induced fibrosis [61]. Furthermore, increased oxidative stress has been demonstrated after unilateral ureteral obstruction, a well-established experimental model of renal interstitial fibrosis [62], and ROS scavenging reduced post-ischemic damage including fibrosis progression after kidney transplantation [63].

Thus, a tight control of the cellular redox balance is crucial, as excessive ROS production or decreased activity of ROS detoxifying enzymes results in aberrant wound healing [46, 64] caused by exacerbated tissue damage due to macromolecular damage or by fibrogenic responses via stress-induced pathways affecting cell hypertrophy, migration, proliferation, apoptosis and ECM regulation [65-69](Figure 1). Here, we review the role of different oxidant and antioxidant systems during wound healing and their influence on fibrotic processes.

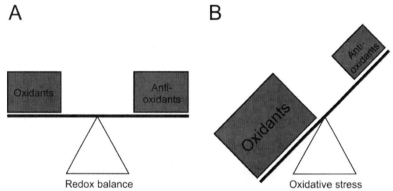

(A) The generation of ROS by oxidants is regulated by antioxidant systems. Non-enzymatic antioxidants, antioxidant enzymes, and metal-binding proteins scavenge ROS or reduce their production, thereby maintaining the redox balance in healthy cells and tissues. (B) Oxidative stress occurs when antioxidant systems are being overwhelmed due to either increased oxidant levels or reduced antioxidant capacity.

Figure 1. Redox balance and oxidative stress.

II. Cellular Oxidant and Antioxidant Systems

ROS production occurs naturally in all cells during normal metabolic processes, and mitochondrial respiration is the major ROS source [recently reviewed by 70].

Under physiological conditions ROS buildup is limited by numerous endogenous antioxidant defense systems, including both enzymatic and non-enzymatic mechanisms that either scavenge generated ROS before it can cause damage or prevent its formation (Figure 2). To keep the redox balance under control a complex network of pro- and anti-oxidant enzymes exists. However, it can be envisioned that in case the cytoprotective antioxidant factors get overwhelmed as may occur following hyperglycemia, the balance gets skewed towards oxidative stress and may lead to abnormal wound healing and scar formation.

IIa. Oxidant Systems

Various enzyme systems produce ROS secondary to their main enzymatic function, including xanthine oxidoreductase [71], mitochondrial respiratory chain [70], lipid peroxidases [72], cytochrome P450 enzymes [73], and endothelial nitric oxide synthase [74]. Nitric oxide synthase produces the free radical nitric oxide, which under normal conditions acts protective, but which under oxidative circumstances can be converted into other reactive nitrogen species (RNS) like peroxynitrite [75]. Only the Nox family produces ROS as their main enzymatic function [76].

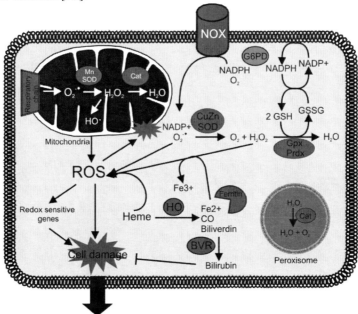

Normal cellular energy metabolism generates mitochondrial ROS that are scavenged by superoxide (Mn-SOD) and catalase (Cat). Nox contributes to cytoplasmic oxidative stress by superoxide (O_2^-) production. Cytoplasmic CuZn-SOD converts superoxide radicals into hydrogen peroxide (H_2O_2) and oxygen (O_2). The generated H_2O_2 is detoxified by Cat and various peroxidases (glutathione peroxidase; Gpx, peroxiredoxin, Prdx). Peroxidases use reduced glutathione (GSH) that concomitantly is oxidized to glutathione disulfide (GSSH). GSSH is reduced to GSH by glutathione reductase in a NADPH-dependent manner. The NADPH reducing power is generated by the pentose phosphate pathway enzyme glucose-6-phosphate dehydrogenase (G6PD) from $NADP^+$. If H_2O_2 is not rapidly detoxified, it can participate in the Fenton reaction, and give rise to the highly cytotoxic hydroxyl (HO•) radical. Free iron (Fe^{2+}) generated by heme degradation by heme oxygenase (HO) can catalyze HO• formation. However, co-induced ferritin efficiently scavenges this metal. HO-activity also generates biliverdin that rapidly is converted by bilirubin reductase (BVR) to bilirubin, the most potent antioxidant in the body. Imbalance of the redox homeostasis towards oxidative stress promotes pathological wound healing and excessive scar formation.
Note that the chemical reactions are not stoichiometrically balanced. Oxidant factors are indicated in red, and antioxidant systems in green. G6PD is indicated in orange due to its association with both oxidative and antioxidant factors.

Figure 2. Different oxidant and antioxidant systems.

Furthermore, free redox active metals, e.g. copper and iron, and their corresponding metal complexes, such as heme, provide catalytic function to (anti)oxidant enzymes [77]. Transition metal homeostasis is regulated on both cellular and systemic levels [78, 79], and metal homeostasis is a central feature of several human diseases including neurodegeneration and genetic disorders like Type-1 hemochromatosis and Wilson's disease characterized by iron and copper overload, respectively, due to defective metal transporters [78-81]. Redox cycling between Cu^+/Cu^{2+} and Fe^{2+}/Fe^{3+} is an integral part of the mitochondrial electron transport chain and ATP generation [82], but unregulated interaction of these metals with molecular oxygen also facilitates excessive ROS generation, predominantly via Fenton chemistry [83].

In the following part, we discuss the role of mitochondrial and Nox-generated ROS in redox balancing and fibrosis. The importance of heme and free iron in ROS formation will be discussed later in this review.

Mitochondrial ROS

Mitochondria are best known for the generation of energy in the form of ATP or heat, but can also produce ROS, regulate calcium homeostasis, synthesize heme, and modulate apoptosis. Evidence is accumulating that mitochondria also function as signaling centre for the control of cytoprotective mechanisms and adaptive responses to various forms of stress [84]. Genes affecting mitochondria are pivotal for human health. Mutations in the proteins within these organelles are recognized to be involved in a growing number of diseases, including diabetes, Parkinson's disease, and cancer [85]. Indeed, mutations in mitochondrial or nuclear DNA encoding for these proteins impair mitochondrial function and have already been found to result in devastating diseases. Also during wound healing several processes are controlled by mitochondria, such as loss of energy, deranged ionic homeostasis, and apoptosis [86].

The oxidative phosphorylation system consists of five multi-protein complexes (I–V) and is essential for mitochondrial function. Electrons from glucose products can pass this respiratory chain and react with oxygen and protons to form water. This results in energy that allows building up a proton gradient that is used by ATP-synthase to produce ATP. A small continuous amount of ROS is always formed as a result of electron carriers reacting directly with oxygen, especially at complex I and at the interface of ubiquinone and complex III [87]. Mitochondrial ROS may contribute to oxidative damage to mitochondrial proteins, membranes, and DNA, and likely exacerbates leakage and oxidative damage to the cell in general [85]. During ageing a slow accumulation of these ROS-mediated mutations ultimately damage cellular integrity and function [85].

Moreover, during circumstances of stress, such as hyperglycemia or the presence of mutated proteins, the mitochondrial electron transport chain (ETC) gets overwhelmed and cannot handle the electron flow sufficiently [88, 89]. For instance, when a protein in complex I is mutated, this may result in blockage of respiration, leading to backed up electrons and hyper-reactive electron carriers, resulting in a small sudden burst of superoxide. This is currently thought to act as a signal for help, the so-called retrograde response [90]. These ROS activate redox-sensitive transcription factors that will signal for a stress response and e.g. for the increased production of mitochondrial proteins [90]. The cell is given some time to repair the damage, however, when this damage cannot be repaired, the amount of ROS will increase, leading to more oxidative damage that ultimately signals for apoptosis [88, 89].

NADPH Oxidases (Nox)

The Nox family consists of 7 members, Nox1-5 and Duox1-2, having a transmembrane, catalytic Nox or Duox domain, respectively. Furthermore, Nox isoforms contain a stabilizing domain (p22phox) and several regulatory subunits [76]. They display differential expression, regulation, subcellular localization and produce different ROS products [91 and references therein]. Nox1, 2 and 5 are the key sources of $O_2^{\bullet-}$, whereas Nox4 mainly produces H_2O_2 from molecular oxygen using NADPH as electron donor [92]. This Nox-dependent ROS generation is activated by a wide range of chemical, physical, environmental, and biological factors [93]. The functions of the different Nox isoforms depend on their cellular localization and mode of activation [94] and have been thoroughly reviewed [94-96]. Nox function has predominantly been studied in phagocytes, as impaired Nox2 function in phagocytes results in chronic granulomatous disease (CGD) characterized by hyperinflammation [97]. Interestingly, neutrophils from CGD patients have a markedly reduced capacity to the respiratory burst, making these patients highly susceptible to bacterial infections [98]. Besides this, the primary biological functioning of the mammalian Nox enzymes is still not completely clear [95]. Nox-induced oxidative stress may contribute to different conditions including chronic inflammation, ischemia-reperfusion injury, septic shock, renal diseases, and cardiovascular complications [see 93 and references therein].

Other studies indicate that Nox participates in different phases of wound healing and tissue regeneration [reviewed by 99]. Nox2-mediated respiratory bursts by neutrophils clean up the wound site, and factors released to stimulate coagulation and hemostasis possibly create a local environment facilitating Nox activation. For example, thrombin stimulates Nox-dependent ROS production in endothelial cells, vascular smooth muscle cells, adventitial fibroblasts and platelets [100-102]. Nox-generated H_2O_2 induces VEGF expression in a mouse excisional wound model leading to facilitated dermal wound closure and tissue remodeling [103], supporting the claim that wound healing is subject to redox control. Active production of H_2O_2 by Duox at the wound margin before cellular recruitment has been demonstrated [37], whereas Duox knockdown reduces H_2O_2 production at the wound site and reduced leukocyte recruitment [37]. These elegantly generated data suggest that ROS generated by Nox may play an important signaling role during the early phase of wound healing for recruitment of inflammatory cells [37, 104].

Nox deficiency has been linked to a state of hyperinflammation. For example, Nox2 KO mice demonstrate an enhanced gene expression of inflammatory mediators and increased neutrophil recruitment to lung and heart after systemic acute inflammation induced by lipopolysaccharide (LPS) exposure [105, 106]. Furthermore, intracheal zymosan or LPS challenging of p47phox KO mice results in exaggerated and progressive lung inflammation, augmented NF-κB activation, and elevated downstream pro-inflammatory cytokine levels compared to wild type mice [107]. A normal lung inflammatory response was restored upon delivery of functional Nox by bone marrow-derived cells [107]. Importantly, monocytes from Nox KO mice produce fewer oxidants accompanied with an enhanced inflammatory response after an inflammatory trigger compared to wild type mice [108]. This is in agreement with the observed hyperinflammation in CGD patients with impaired Nox2 activity [97]. Importantly, studies on macrophages from Nox deficient mice demonstrate inability to activate Nfr2 [107], a redox-sensitive master regulator of several stress-induced genes including HO-1 [109].

Up-regulation of Nox4 is observed after *in vitro* wounding of a vascular endothelial monolayer, whereas Nox4 down-regulation has a negative effect on wound closure *in vitro*

[110, 111]. Vascular Nox function is stimulated by pro-inflammatory mediators including LPS, tumor necrosis factor-α (TNFα), interleukin (IL)-1, interferon (INF)γ, and AngII [112, 113]. Moreover, pro-inflammatory cytokines and AngII upregulate expression of different Nox isoforms in various cell types including vascular smooth muscle cells [114, 115] and human and rat kidney cells [115, 116]. Also, wounds generated in monolayers of human airway epithelial cells close faster after LPS exposure, and this effect is absent in the presence of ROS scavengers or Nox inhibition [117] further supporting the involvement of ROS and Nox in all phases of wound healing. Also during the proliferative phase of wound healing Nox enzymes may play a role, as Nox-derived ROS have been implicated in stimulating keratinocyte proliferation [118], and vascular repair and remodeling [99]. Furthermore, it regulates collagen producing cells, like fibroblasts, kidney mesangial cells, hepatic and pancreatic stellate cells [99], As collagen I and III production and deposition is a key event in fibrosis Nox-mediated stimulation of collagen producing cells may be detrimental to wound healing and contribute to fibrogenesis and excessive scar formation. In fact, down-regulation of Nox expression or activity inhibition may prevent fibrosis in different organ systems including liver, kidney and heart under stress conditions [99]. In liver, activated HSCs are the major suppliers of ECM components and *in vitro* studies have demonstrated Nox involvement in stimulating HSC activation and proliferation [52, 119, 120]. Knockdown of p47phox, a regulatory Nox2 subunit, or knockout (KO) of Nox2 results in attenuated collagen expression and reduced hepatic fibrosis compared to wild type controls in different mouse liver fibrosis models [52, 121]. Also in kidney Nox is important in the wound healing response, as Nox is involved in mediating kidney mesangial cell proliferation, differentiation and collagen deposition *in vitro*. For instance, inhibition of Nox blocks expression of TGFβ-1 [122], whereas stimulation of Nox2 expression increases collagen I deposition [123].

Scavenging of Nox-generated H_2O_2 by superoxide dismutase (SOD) overexpression, mimetics, or Nox inhibition reduces collagen deposition [123, 124]. Also, chemical Nox inhibition suppresses fibrosis *in vivo* in a rat renal fibrotic model [125].

Nox has also been linked to fibrogenesis after cardiac infarction [126]. Similarly to the kidney, inhibition of Nox reduces cardiac collagen deposition in a model of aldosterone-induced cardiac remodeling [127]. Also, Nox2 KO models demonstrate a reduction of cardiac fibrosis in different cardiac injury models [128-130]. Importantly, also Nox4 has been shown to be essential for trans-differentiation of cardiac fibroblasts into myofibroblasts in response to TGFβ-1 [131, 132]. Moreover, Nox4 is a source of TGFβ-1-induced ROS production in cardiac and pulmonary fibroblasts [131, 132] and Nox4 is up-regulated in lung tissue of patients with idiopathic pulmonary fibrosis [133, 134] and in mice subjected to non-infectious lung injury [132]. In mouse pulmonary mesenchymal cells Nox4-derived H_2O_2 is necessary for TGFβ-1-induced myofibroblast differentiation, ECM production, and contractility [132], whereas targeting of Nox4 inhibits fibrogenesis in two mouse lung injury models [132]. Additionally, Nox4-dependent H_2O_2 generation by lung fibroblasts may induce apoptosis [135], epithelial-mesenchymal transition [136] or ECM cross-linking in the presence of extracellular peroxidases [137] thereby increasing fibrotic insults.

Thus, the underlying mechanisms of Nox action in (abnormal) wound healing still needs to be elucidated. However, the above mentioned studies suggest that Nox-generated ROS is involved in regulating the inflammatory response after induction of acute inflammation and may therefore play a central role in proper execution of the different wound healing phases including inflammatory resolution.

IIb. Antioxidant Systems

Oxidative stress occurs due to an imbalance of oxidant production and antioxidant defense. Antioxidant enzymes and molecules control ROS levels by keeping H_2O_2 and Nox-generated $O_2^{\cdot-}$ at low concentrations. NADPH generated by glucose 6-phosphate dehydrogenase (G6PD) is central in regulating this balance. Even though many potential intracellular antioxidants are known, the antioxidant defense system is basically comprised of reduced glutathione (GSH), catalase and SOD, which all depend on NADPH for functional activity. In short, SOD converts $O_2^{\cdot-}$ to H_2O_2 that gets reduced to water by either catalase or by glutathione peroxidase (GPx) and the GSH system. GSH is the most abundant cellular antioxidant, and prevents thiol groups from oxidation either in a direct manner or indirectly through the actions of GPx [138]. Simultaneously with H_2O_2 oxidation GSH is reduced to glutathione disulfide (GSSG) and is being converted back to GSH by glutathione reductase (GR) using NAPDH as reducing power (Figure 2).

Antioxidant compounds like vitamins C and E, bilirubin, and metal binding proteins play important roles in the defense against ROS. Numerous studies have demonstrated a protective role of vitamin C, a water-soluble compound, against cytoplasmic oxidative damage [139, 140], and vitamin E, a fat-soluble antioxidant, acts protective against lipid membrane peroxidation [139, 140]. Bilirubin, generated from heme degradation by HO enzymes, has been demonstrated to be a powerful antioxidant [141], whereas metal-binding proteins, e.g. the iron scavenger ferritin [142], maintain metal homeostasis by regulating cellular metal uptake, trafficking, and sequestration, and thereby keep redox active transition metals within strict physiological concentration levels [143].

Next, we review the role of enzymatic antioxidant systems in wound healing and fibrosis, and later we discuss the role of ferritin and bilirubin in antioxidant defense.

Glucose-6-Phosphate Dehydrogenase (G6PD)

Intracellular redox balance is determined by antioxidant and oxidant concentrations. The principal intracellular reductant in all cells, NADPH, is a critical modulator of the redox balance and is generated from $NADP^+$ by G6PD, the rate-limiting enzyme of the pentose phosphate pathway [144]. G6PD is the principal source of NADPH which is required by many enzymes involved in the antioxidant and oxidant systems including catalase and Nox. Also, NAPDH is essential for the conversion of GSSG to GSH by GR, which, in turn, is an obligate co-substrate for GPxs. This places G6PD in the centre of regulating (anti)oxidant enzyme activity.

G6PD is considered a constitutively expressed housekeeping gene in many tissues, however, in fat tissue, liver and lung G6PD expression is regulated by external stimuli like hormones, growth factors, nutrients, and oxidative stress [144-148]. Many studies have shown that abrogation of G6PD activity dramatically increases cellular sensitivity to oxidative stress *in vitro* [149, 150].

Recently, a G6DP deficient mouse has been generated using chemical mutagenesis displaying a phenotype resembling diabetic kidney disease including increased oxidative stress, albuminuria, and NF-κB activation [151]. Chemical inhibition of G6PD activity in rats also results in a nephrotoxic phenotype, decreased levels of NAPDH and GSH accompanied by reduced activities of GPx, GR, and G6PD [152]. The reduction of antioxidant enzyme activity is believed to be the major cause of ROS-induced kidney damage [152].

Notably, G6DP deficiency in humans is the most commonly occurring enzyme defect and is a X-linked hereditary genetic defect caused by mutations in the G6PD gene [153]. G6PD deficiency is especially affecting erythrocytes as these cells rely on G6PD as sole supplier of NAPDH, and any oxidative stress will result in hemolytic anemia [154]. Ironically, G6PD deficiency protects via the oxidative environment in the erythrocytes against *Plasmodium falciparum* malaria [153]. A few reports link G6PD deficiency to hypertension [155] and diabetes [155-159]. Increased G6PD expression has been reported in pancreatic islets of diabetic rats [158].

High levels of glucose decrease G6PD activity in endothelial cells, kidney, liver, and erythrocytes, leading to oxidative damage, cellular dysfunction, and ultimately organ damage [160-162]. Also, an altered energy metabolism has been demonstrated as response to injury and subsequent wound healing [163, 164]. Moreover, G6PD activity in cutaneous wounds of young rats is reduced during the first days of wound healing compared to unwounded and healed skin [164]. Notably, aged or immunosuppressed rats have lower basal G6PD activity but a higher G6PD activity during early wound healing compared to young animals [164]. The authors suggest that aged and immunosuppressed animals may have a changed NAPDH production what may delay the wound healing process, as impaired wound healing is common complication of aging, diabetes, and immunosuppressive therapy [165]. Unfortunately, no correlation between wound closure and enzyme activity was done in this study to support this hypothesis.

Interestingly, a guinea pig hypertrophic scar model demonstrate increased G6PD activity in hypertrophic scars compared to normal skin or normal scars [166], and several fold higher G6PD activity has been detected in human hypertrophic scars compared to normal skin [167]. Also, increased G6PD levels contribute to generation of $O_2^{-\bullet}$ via Nox during heart failure [168] and ROS accumulation and pro-inflammatory responses in adipocytes [169]. On the contrary, G6PD reduces ROS by activating antioxidant responses in cardiomyocytes, renal cortical cells, and ovary cells [150, 162, 170].

Thus, because NADPH is a cofactor for both oxidant and antioxidant enzymes, G6PD appears to have dual functions in the regulation of the cellular redox balance in a cell- or environmental-dependent manner.

Superoxide Dismutases (SODs)

SOD catalyzes the conversion of $O_2^{-\bullet}$ radicals into H_2O_2 using NAPDH as cofactor [171]. Three isoforms exist: cytosolic Cu/Zn-dependent SOD1, mitochondrial Mn-dependent SOD2, and extracellular SOD3 [172]. SOD2 is the most important form of the SODs during embryogenesis, as SOD2 deficient mice display a neonatal lethal phenotype [173, 174].

SOD1 and SOD2 are up-regulated in healing wounds during the early inflammatory phase [64]. However, contradictive to the expression pattern SOD activity is reduced during wound healing [64], probably because of high ROS levels [64, 175, 176]. Interestingly, this effect gets more pronounced with age [177].

Addition of recombinant SOD to ischemic wounds increases wound breaking strength and reduced wound edema [178]. Moreover, application of SOD1-loaded scaffolds improves wound healing [179]. Importantly, mice with pharmacologically induced diabetes show reduced wound $O_2^{-\bullet}$ levels and normalized wound healing after cutaneous SOD2 gene therapy [180]. Furthermore, ischemic skin wound healing is normalized upon SOD2 gene therapy or use of a SOD2 mimetic [181]. Moreover, SOD injections have been successfully used as anti-fibrotic therapy in treatment of cutaneous radiation-induced fibrosis in humans [182] and in a porcine wound model [183].

Other studies have suggested a central role for SOD in myocardial fibrosis, as SOD inhibition and the resulting increase in $O_2^{\bullet-}$ levels increases the levels of collagen and fibronectin in cardiac fibroblasts, and this effect is reversed by SOD mimetics [184]. Moreover, AngII has been demonstrated to affect the expression and activity levels of the different SOD isoforms in a highly cell-specific manner [185-190] and more specifically, AngII decreases SOD activity in rat cardiac fibroblasts [184, 191]. Thus, these data suggest that SOD counteracts AngII-mediated myocardial fibrosis [50 and references therein].

Thus, it is clear that detoxification of $O_2^{\bullet-}$ by SODs during wound healing is important to ensure proper wound healing and minimize the risk of fibrotic events.

Catalase

H_2O_2 generated by SOD detoxification activity can be further scavenged by catalase and GPx enzymes. Excessive amounts of H_2O_2 are harmful to cells and rapid scavenging hereof is thus important [192]. Catalase, a tetrameric heme protein, is one of the major intracellular antioxidant enzymes that degrades H_2O_2 to oxygen and water.

Studies addressing the role of catalase in wound healing and fibrosis are still limited. Notably, in contrast to GPx and SOD, catalase gene expression is not up-regulated in the wound area after excisional wounding [193]. However, in human fibrotic lungs decreased catalase activity and expression has been reported [194]. Furthermore, acatalasemic mice subjected to bleomycin-induced lung fibrosis demonstrate a temporal increase in fibrotic loading [194] and they are more susceptible to oxidative tissue damage in renal fibrosis [195, 196] and peritoneal fibrosis [197]. Acatalasemic mice demonstrate significantly more tubulointerstitial fibrosis with collagen I and III accumulation after nephrectomy compared to wild type mice until week 18 where after compensatory up-regulation of GPx or SOD occurs [195]. Similarly, unilateral ureteral obstruction in acatalamic mice significantly increased cell infiltration and interstitial fibrosis in the obstructed kidney compared to wild type control mice [196]. In addition, induction of peritoneal fibrosis results in more fibrosis accompanied with increased deposition of collagen I and lipid peroxidation products in acatalamic mice compared to wild type controls [197]. Together, this suggests that sufficient amounts of catalase are necessary for coping with injury-induced ROS generation.

Importantly, treatment with a catalase mimetic or adenoviral over-expression of catalase inhibits H_2O_2-mediated up-regulation of extracellular matrix metalloproteinase inducer, EMMPRIN, in cardiomyocytes [198], a feature also reported for bronchiolar epithelial cells in fibrotic lung tissue [199, 200]. Also, adenoviral over-expression of catalase in excisional wounds of mice is accompanied with reduced angiogenesis and subsequent impaired wound closure [40]. Notably, H_2O_2 has been shown to significantly induce VEGF expression in keratinocytes [103] thereby contributing to a proper wound healing response. The amount catalase and subsequently H_2O_2 levels may have different consequences in different cellular environments as catalase administration and subsequent H_2O_2 scavenging reduced matrix metalloproteinase (MMP) activity and cell proliferation in metastatic cancer cells [201].

Collectively, these observations underscores an important role of catalase in anti-fibrotic protection, probably through regulation of MMP expression and activity.

Glutathione Peroxidase (GPx)

Mammalian cells express 5 isoforms of the GPx selenoprotein [202] that have been described as important cellular antioxidant enzymes [203]. The most prominent isoform is GPx1 that reduces H_2O_2 and a range of organic peroxides [204, 205]. GPx4 has a tissue-dependent subcellular localization [206] and is thought to play a crucial role in counteracting lipid peroxidation and biomembrane damage [202]. In fact, GPx4 appears to be the only life-essential GSH-dependent enzyme [207]. Besides GPx, the glutathione antioxidant system includes GSH and GR [208, 209].

GPx1 expression and activity is up-regulated by ROS [210] and GPx1 but not GPx4 expression is induced after excisional wounding [193, 211]. However, contradicting observations exist, as down-regulation of GPx and SOD after cutaneous injury has been reported [212]. This discrepancy may be explained by the different wound models used and an enzymatic activity saturation due to extreme ROS levels at the wound site [176, 213]. Notably, GPx1 and SOD display similar expression patterns [211] thereby securing an effective detoxification of H_2O_2 generated by SODs and avoiding the generation of HO• radicals.

Studies using GPx1 KO mice have linked GPx to the regulation of acute oxidative stress [214], as GPx1 KO mice are highly susceptible to injury induced by paraquat and H_2O_2 [210], cerebral ischemia-reperfusion, and cold-induced head trauma [214]. Furthermore, GPx1 KO fibroblasts demonstrate increased sensitivity to oxidant-induced apoptosis [214], while activated peritoneal GPx1 KO macrophages display oxidative injury due to increased nitric oxide (NO) production [215]. On the contrary, chemically-induced diabetic GPx1 KO mice have equivalent levels of oxidative renal injury and similar degrees of renal damage and fibrosis to diabetic wild type mice [216], suggesting that GPx1 is not a crucial regulator of oxidative stress injury in the diabetic kidney. Also, no compensatory up-regulation of other GPx isoforms was detected in non-diabetic GPx1-deficient kidneys [216].

Thus, it is clear that the GPx enzymes are important in the antioxidant defense against acute oxidative stress. However, the role of these enzymes in fibrosis and wound healing needs further investigations.

Peroxiredoxins (Prdx)

The peroxiredoxin family consists of 6 members (Prdx1-6) that all catalyze the reduction of H_2O_2 and a wide spectrum of organic peroxides and peroxynitrite. Prdx1-5 use thioredoxin and/or GSH as substrate [217-219], whereas Prdx6, a cytosolic enzyme also known as 1 Cys-peroxiredoxin or nonselenium glutathione peroxidase, uses GSH or ascorbate as reducing agent [220, 221].

Studies have implied an important function for Prdx6 in the cellular stress response. Different cell types are protected from ROS-induced toxicity when over-expressing Prdx6 [222, 223] whereas Prdx6 knockdown results in enhanced sensitivity towards oxidative stress [224-226]. Also, Prdx6 KO mice display increased sensitivity towards paraquat, an inducer of oxidative stress [227] and a higher sensitivity to myocardial ischemia-reperfusion injury [228]

Prdx6 expression is induced after wounding, with keratinocytes having the highest levels [211, 229]. In keratinocytes this expression is induced by keratinocyte growth factor [230], which is also up-regulated after wounding [231]. Keratinocytes isolated from transgenic mice with epidermal Prdx6 over-expression demonstrate enhanced resistance against insults causing oxidative stress [232]. Moreover, these keratinocytes are less sensitive towards UV radiation-induced apoptosis [232].

Also, a strong up-regulation of Prdx6 expression after cutaneous wounding in a mouse injury model has been demonstrated predominantly in the hyper-proliferative epidermis of wound edges [229]. Interestingly, high levels of Prdx6 have been found in psoriatic skin [230]. Moreover, aged mice over-expressing Prdx6 in the epidermis demonstrate accelerated dermal wound closure compared to age-matched wild type mice suggesting that high levels of Prdx6 counteract build-up of ROS normally responsible for age-related defects in wound healing [232]. Importantly, Prdx6 KO mice do not have impaired re-epithelization suggesting a compensating expression of other antioxidant systems during wound healing [226]. However, no differences in gene transcription levels of Prdx, GPx, catalase or SOD is observed between Prdx6 KO and wild type mice [226]. However, Prdx6 KO mice show severe hemorrhage in the granulation tissue correlating with the degree of oxidative stress in the tissue due to enhanced ROS sensitivity of endothelial cells combined with increased ROS production by Prdx6-deficient macrophages [226].

Together, Prdx6 is important in dermal antioxidant defense and acts cytoprotective in especially keratinocytes. One could imagine that regulated activation of Prdx6 could contribute to improved wound healing or skin protection after e.g. sun burns.

IIc. The Heme-Heme Oxygenase (HO) System

Heme is crucial as the functional group of various hemoproteins, such as hemoglobin, cytochromes, peroxidases, and catalases [233]. In addition, heme can act as signaling molecule [Reviewed by 234]. However, large amounts of free heme may be injurious to cells, since heme catalyzes the formation of ROS via the Fenton reaction [235]. After injury, large amounts of free heme is released from hemoproteins and may aggravate tissue damage [236-239]. High local accumulation of heme in blood clots may overwhelm the cellular ROS detoxification systems and prolongs oxidative stress and cellular injury [238, 240-242]. Moreover, increased heme levels have been associated with fibrogenesis [243, 244]. In addition, several studies have indicated that free heme besides acting as an oxidant when present in high concentrations also possesses pro-inflammatory properties [245-248]. Additionally, studies have indicated a beneficial role for heme in wound healing, as moderate concentrations of heme stimulates vasoconstriction, coagulation and cell differentiation [249]. At lower concentrations free heme contributes to inflammatory resolution by down-regulating inflammatory mediators probably via induction of HO-activity [250-252]. Thus, heme has been suggested to be a molecular switch due to its opposite, concentration-dependent effects [253].

HO enzymes comprise the inducible HO-1 and the predominantly constitutively expressed HO-2 isoforms [254, 255] and are the rate-limiting enzymes in the degradation of heme into carbon monoxide (CO), iron, and biliverdin. Biliverdin is rapidly converted to bilirubin by biliverdin reductase (BVR) [256, 257]. Besides the classical ROS detoxifying enzymes discussed earlier, the HO system also exhibits potent antioxidant functions [258]. The HO system contributes to the cellular antioxidant defense by both the generation of protective effector molecules and by the degradation of free redox active heme. In low concentrations, free heme confers essential cellular functions and cytoprotection via HO-1 induction, whereas high concentrations of free heme cause cytotoxic cellular insults [259]. Thus, a beneficial effect of HO activity on the cellular redox balance can be directly ascribed to its active heme detoxification. However, iron released from degraded heme is itself also a redox active molecule and can participate in Fenton chemistry just like heme, leading to ROS formation and subsequent biomolecular damage [143]. Thus, iron chelation to keep the free iron levels low is important, and HO-1-induction is indeed paralleled by co-induction of the iron scavenger ferritin [253].

Numerous studies have linked the HO system to the regulation of various (patho)physiological processes, including cellular adaptation of oxidative stress, inflammatory resolution, and wound healing responses [recently reviewed in 245] and HO activity confers cytoprotection, reduces oxidative stress and inflammation in numerous cell and animal models [253, 259-265]. Moreover, HO-1 over-expression counteracts the cytotoxic effects caused by high concentrations of free heme [234, 247, 263, 266], whereas HO-1 activity inhibition intensifies heme-mediated cellular damage [263, 267-270]. Importantly, numerous studies have demonstrated a positive effect of HO-1 expression on controlling inflammation and counteracting fibrogenesis [271]. For example, transgenic HO-1 mice demonstrate better protection against oxidative stress and fibrotic tissue formation post-infarction [272]. Research using HO-1 and HO-2 KO mice underscores the central role for the HO system and redox status in wound healing, as these mice show delayed wound closure due to a poor response towards oxidative and inflammatory stress [244, 273-280], and administration of biliverdin has shown to ameliorate wound healing [277, 278]. Pharmacological inhibition of HO-activity confirms the findings in HO-KO animals on the wound healing process [281]. In cutaneous wound healing, the duality of heme is important, as local free heme accumulation may promote ROS formation and oxidative injury [238-240]. To cope with this stress fibroblasts rapidly can induce HO-1 expression as a feedback response, whereas keratinocytes express high levels of HO-2 [282]. Moreover, keratinocyte-specific over-expression of HO-1 in transgenic mice improve neovascularization and accelerate wound healing after injury. This effect is also evident with adenoviral HO-1 delivery [281] suggesting that increasing levels of HO-1 counteract dermal fibrosis. Indeed, pre-induction of HO-1 in a mouse excisional wound model accelerates wound closure by increasing cellular proliferation and collagen synthesis as reflected by an increased hydroxyproline content and reducing transcription of inflammatory mediators [283]. Thus, low levels of heme are postulated to promote wound healing via induction of HO-1, whereas high heme levels prolong oxidative stress what favors a pro-fibrotic wound environment.

Preclinical and epidemiological evidence indicate that the cytoprotective and oxidative effects of the HO system are mediated via the actions of the generated effector molecules CO, bilirubin/biliverdin, and by co-induced ferritin [For a recent review, see 284]. The expression of HO-1 is induced by various cell stresses [284 and references therein] including ROS generation by heme [285], UV light [282], H_2O_2 [286], and heavy metals [285]. Also, oxidative stress-mediated induction of HIF-1 stimulates HO-1 activity in many tissues [287].

CO is a versatile gaseous molecule that acts as an endogenous neural transmitter as well as a regulator of vascular tone [288-292] via cGMP formation by guanylyl cyclase (GC) activity [293, 294]. During the last decade the many regulatory functions of CO have received great attention due to its promising therapeutic properties, and exogenous CO application, either as gas inhalation [295, 296] or CO-releasing molecules (CO-RMs)[297] has been studied intensively in diverse disease settings. For instance, CO therapy has demonstrated cytoprotective effects in different experimental models of inflammation, cardiovascular diseases, and organ transplantation and graft survival [Recently reviewed by 298, 299] via anti-inflammatory [300, 301], vasodilatory [302], anti-coagulant [303], anti-apoptotic [304], and anti-fibrotic [300] mechanisms.

Notably, even though no direct antioxidant properties of CO have been reported, CO has the capacity to react with Fe^{2+} in heme groups of hemoproteins and can thereby modulate the activity of various enzymes, including GC [For a review, see 305]. Moreover, CO prevents the onset of severe malaria by binding cell-free hemoglobin (Hb) that has been released from ruptured erythrocytes that were infected with *Plasmodium falciparum* during malaria disease progression. This leads to the formation of carboxyhemoglobin (COHb) that is less susceptible towards oxidation which subsequently slows down free heme release [306]. This prevents the deleterious effects of high concentrations of free heme in pathologies like severe malaria [307] and sepsis [308].

Intriguingly, it is known that HO-derived CO can reversibly inhibit mitochondrial respiration by binding to the prosthetic heme-group of cytochrome c oxidase, by competing with oxygen [309]. The finding that the body could "poison" one of its own enzymes (cytochrome c oxidase) was initially thought to be an imperfection of nature [90]. However, this blockage in respiration causes the generation of $O_2^{\bullet}$ suggesting the induction of a protective CO-induced *retrograde response* [310]. The pro-survival PI3-K/AKT pathway, which signals for the replication of mitochondrial DNA, is indeed activated by CO [311, 312]. *In vivo* experiments in mouse hearts illustrate that CO activates mitochondrial biogenesis [313-315]. Cardiac mitochondrial protein content for all five ETC complexes was increased following exposure to CO for 24 hours. This new finding suggests a regulatory role for HO-1 in mitochondrial biogenesis and protection against mitochondrial ROS.

In vertebrates most bilirubin originates from erythrocyte turnover and heme catabolism in spleen and liver, but in other tissues a significant smaller quantity is found during normal intracellular turnover of heme. Both biliverdin and bilirubin are strong endogenous antioxidants [316-319] and bilirubin has been implicated in preventing oxidative changes in different diseases including atherosclerosis, neurodegeneration, diabetes mellitus, cancer, and inflammatory and autoimmune diseases [Recently reviewed in 320]. Moreover, recent clinical studies have demonstrated that bilirubin may have protective antioxidant effects *in vivo*, as Gilberts patients with slightly elevated serum bilirubin levels are protected against cardiovascular complications [321]. Also, experimentally-induced mild hyperbilirubinemia has recently been demonstrated to improve both the redox status and the vascular function in diabetes mellitus type-1 patients [322]. Moreover, serum bilirubin levels are associated with reduced development of diabetes-associated complications [323-326]. Besides exerting cytoprotection during organ transplantation by reducing ischemia-reperfusion injury and improving graft survival [327, 328], probably via immunomodulatory and anti-inflammatory effects [260], biliverdin and bilirubin demonstrates antioxidant properties [316, 329]. For instance, bilirubin protects cells against high H_2O_2 concentrations [316, 317, 330, 331]. The antioxidant function of bilirubin is expected to be effective against ROS in lipophilic environments due to the lipophilic nature of bilirubin [320], which may be important in protecting biomembranes [318, 332-334]. Exogenous bilirubin reduces lipid peroxidation in heart and kidney and prevents ROS-mediated apoptosis in thymus cells [335]. Furthermore, bilirubin counteracts free radical-induced peroxidation of low density lipoprotein (LDL) [336]. Nanomolar concentrations of bilirubin suppress Nox activity *in vitro* thereby reducing

ROS levels and subsequent tissue damage [337-339]. Thus, the involvement of biliverdin and bilirubin in antioxidant defense is evident [340]. Additionally, the BVR enzyme has received increasing attention as potential cytoprotective and antioxidant enzyme [316, 317], but more research is warranted [recently reviewed by 341]. Interestingly, HO-1 can translocate from the endoplasmic reticulum to mitochondria [342], suggesting that by producing bilirubin from heme it can also modulate the intramitochondrial redox status.

Ferrous iron (Fe^{2+}) is released during heme degradation by HO enzymes. As mentioned earlier, excess levels of iron can be cytotoxic due to its participation in the Fenton reaction leading to the generation of HO• and subsequently oxidative stress-induced damage to biomolecules [343-345]. Ferritin is an ubiquitous iron-binding protein that can accommodate up to 4500 iron atoms per molecule [343, 346].

The sequestration of free iron by ferritin provides detoxification of a redox active molecule as well as iron storage [343, 345]. Ferritin expression is regulated by iron levels via iron regulatory protein (IRP), but also oxidative stress induces ferritin expression via an antioxidant responsive element (ARE) in the promoter of the ferritin gene [347]. Notably, one of the transcription factors mediating ARE driven transcription of ferritin is Nrf2 [348], a master regulator the anti-oxidant response and mediator of HO-1 induction [reviewed by 109]. Thus, ferritin expression is often induced in parallel with HO-1 expression, and using ferritin over-expression or down-regulation several lines of evidence have demonstrated that ARE-driven ferritin expression is likely responsible for protection against oxidative stress [347].

Thus, from these observations it is clear that the HO system besides its cytoprotective functions contributes significantly to the cellular antioxidant defense by degrading redox active heme and thereby generates ROS scavenging effector molecules further contributing to counteracting oxidative stress and preventing fibrosis.

III. ROS and Disease

ROS are crucial for cellular functions and essential protective mechanisms. The most obvious example is the involvement of ROS in the antibacterial action in the immune defense, but also in signal transduction, ROS have proven important. However, ROS and oxidative stress have also been linked to various disease states including cancer, insulin resistance, diabetes mellitus, cardiovascular diseases, atherosclerosis, and aging [349].

Different theories exist to explain the underlying mechanisms of ROS-mediated damage and its effects in disease progression. A well-balanced redox homeostasis is important, as oxidative stress either by increased levels of ROS and/or by depleted antioxidant systems may modulate protein function due to oxidative modifications and are suspected to be associated with chronic complications of diabetes, aging and aging-related diseases. As illustrated in this chapter, maintenance of homeostasis and tight control of ROS levels by means of different antioxidant systems is essential for proper wound healing and prevention of scarring. Here we discuss the role of ROS in diabetes mellitus and aging as examples of how ROS act as central players in pathology, leading to exacerbation of pathological wound healing.

Diabetes Mellitus

Diabetes mellitus is characterized by excessive levels of extracellular glucose and fatty acids that exert damaging effects leading to several complications including blindness, chronic kidney disease, and cardiovascular problems [350]. Moreover, impaired healing of acute wounds is a well-known complication related to diabetes. Fifteen percent of diabetic patients will develop chronic, non-healing foot ulcers and 84% of them will have to undergo lower-limb amputation [351]. This impaired wound healing is often accompanied by hypoxia [352]. Prolonged hypoxia can exaggerate and/or prolong the inflammatory phase, thereby increasing the levels of ROS and extending the time of exposure [353, 354]. Experimental diabetes models have demonstrated increased cardiovascular and renal ROS levels due to hyperglycemia [355, 356], and diabetes patients present increased plasma levels of ROS biomarkers, and reduced levels of bilirubin, SOD, and antioxidant vitamins [357-360].

Furthermore, decreased antioxidant serum levels in diabetes mellitus patients [361-364], and decreased blood catalase activity has been associated with an increased risk of developing diabetes [365]. Hyperglycemia also contributes to a defective or overwhelmed antioxidant response [366], Hyperglycemia is associated with impaired wound healing in diabetic mice [367], whereas over-expression of cytoprotective genes has been shown to restore delayed wound healing in diabetic mice [180]. Oxidative stress has been demonstrated to play a central role in insulin resistance, impaired insulin secretion, and the development of diabetes-associated complications [364]. Additionally, factors associated with diabetes further contribute to increased ROS production, formation of advanced glucation end-products (AGE), activation of polyol pathway, elevated levels of free fatty acids and leptin [368, 369].

Furthermore, several of the ROS generating mechanisms discussed earlier in this chapter have been directly linked to diabetic pathology. For instance, the renin-angiotensin system has been linked to ROS generation and is associated with cellular damage [370]. AngII contributes to oxidative stress, inflammation, and apoptosis in pancreatic β-cells [370], which leads to ROS-induced insulin resistance, altered insulin signaling and subsequently reduced glucose clearance [reviewed in 370]. Also, AngII is a known stimulator of Nox, and activation of Nox has indeed been proven particularly important in diabetes [371, 372], as increased Nox-mediated ROS production in parallel with Nox up-regulation has been demonstrated in experimental diabetes models [373, 374]. For comprehensive reviews of Nox, AngII and diabetes, we refer to [350, 370].

Excess glucose increases oxidative stress by a wide range of biochemical pathways [375], whereas excess amounts of fatty acids lead to oxidative stress, insulin resistance and lipid accumulation in non-fat tissues including liver and heart [376]. Moreover, this increase in oxidative stress caused by increased levels of glucose and fatty acids contributes to an inflammatory response mediated by metabolic stress-mediated NF-κB activation and expression of NF-κB target genes, including several pro-inflammatory cytokines. This inflammatory response furthermore contributes to aforementioned insulin resistance [377].

Aging

Mammalian aging is characterized by a reduced capacity to adequately restore and maintain tissue homeostasis after injury [378]. The process of aging is predominantly caused by accumulated damage caused by the actions of free radicals including lipid peroxidation, DNA damage, and oxidative protein modifications, and is known as the free radical theory of aging [379]. Also, aging is accompanied by natural dysregulation of immune functioning which may be amplified when it occurs in the presence of chronic stress [380].

It is generally recognized that aging causes a temporal delay in wound healing, whereas the quality of wound healing is unaffected based on wound healing studies in aging animals [381, 382]. Importantly, similar results have been observed in aged human adults and this age-dependent effect was still evident after correction for confounding factors like medication use [383]. As discussed in the introduction of this chapter, wound healing time is a crucial determinant of the wound healing quality and the risk of excessive scar tissue formation. This delay in wound healing is caused by an altered inflammatory response including a delayed resolution of inflammatory cell infiltration into the wound area, chemokine secretion, and reduced phagocytic capacity of macrophages [384], what may contribute to a poorer response against invading pathogens after injury. Indeed, an age-related delay in wound repair has been associated with increased risk of infection and thereby accompanying complications [385]. Furthermore, increased production of the pro-inflammatory cytokine IL-6 has been associated with aging [386] resulting in a chronic low-grade inflammation that has been linked to a number of age-related illnesses including cardiovascular disease, arthritis, diabetes, osteoporosis, periodontal diseases, and cancers [387, 388]. In the context of wound healing chronic oxidative stress would contribute to an exaggerated inflammatory response upon injury and an impaired wound healing response due to prolonged injury.

Aged mice demonstrate delayed re-epithelization, collagen synthesis and angiogenesis compared to young mice [389] and different animal models have demonstrated increased accumulation of oxidative modified proteins due to reduced antioxidant enzyme activity [390]. Moreover, aged rats displayed reduced activities of SOD, catalase and GPx compared to young rats [177] whereas no differences in SOD, GSH, or catalase levels were detected in humans ranging from 35-69 years of age [391].

Concluding Remarks and Future Perspectives

Wound healing is a fine-tuned biological process and multiple factors can impair wound healing by affecting one or more phases of the process. ROS play an important but dual role in wound healing. They are essential for an efficient defense against pathogens and in low concentrations important as cellular signaling molecules. However, excessive ROS production or impaired/overwhelmed ROS detoxification causes oxidative stress that disturbs the wound healing process and exacerbate scar formation. Thus, tight regulation of the redox balance in the wound area is essential for a normal wound healing process. The use of cytoprotective enzymes in the prevention and treatment of these diseases by strengthening the antioxidant defense and reducing ROS-induced damage is now being extensively studied and may ultimately result in novel clinical strategies to prevent scar formation. Although many antioxidants are available as dietary supplements or as prescription, the clinical use of antioxidant therapy in wound healing and as anti-fibrotic therapy is still limited.

Acknowledgments

This work was supported by grants from the Dutch Burn Foundation (#09.110) and TASENE (NWO/WOTRO; W 02.29.101).

References

[1] Clark, R.A.F., The molecular and cellular biology of wound repair. 2nd ed. 1996, New York: Plenum Press.
[2] Behm, B., et al., Cytokines, chemokines and growth factors in wound healing. *J. Eur. Acad. Dermatol. Venereol.,* 2012. 26(7): p. 812-20.
[3] Hubner, G. and S. Werner, Serum growth factors and proinflammatory cytokines are potent inducers of activin expression in cultured fibroblasts and keratinocytes. *Exp. Cell Res.,* 1996. 228(1): p. 106-13.
[4] Gabbiani, G., et al., Collagen and myofibroblasts of granulation tissue. A chemical, ultrastructural and immunologic study. *Virchows Arch. B Cell Pathol.,* 1976. 21(2): p. 133-45.
[5] Martin, P., Wound healing--aiming for perfect skin regeneration. *Science,* 1997. 276(5309): p. 75-81.
[6] Gurtner, G.C., et al., Wound repair and regeneration. *Nature,* 2008. 453(7193): p. 314-21.
[7] Guarino, M., A. Tosoni, and M. Nebuloni, Direct contribution of epithelium to organ fibrosis: epithelial-mesenchymal transition. *Hum. Pathol.,* 2009. 40(10): p. 1365-76.
[8] Franklin, T.J., Therapeutic approaches to organ fibrosis. *Int. J. Biochem. Cell Biol.,* 1997. 29(1): p. 79-89.
[9] Penn, J.W., A.O. Grobbelaar, and K.J. Rolfe, The role of the TGF-beta family in wound healing, burns and scarring: a review. *Int. J. Burns Trauma,* 2012. 2(1): p. 18-28.
[10] Bataller, R. and D.A. Brenner, Liver fibrosis. *J. Clin. Invest.,* 2005. 115(2): p. 209-18.
[11] Thannickal, V.J., et al., Myofibroblast differentiation by transforming growth factor-beta1 is dependent on cell adhesion and integrin signaling via focal adhesion kinase. *J. Biol. Chem.,* 2003. 278(14): p. 12384-9.
[12] Flanders, K.C., Smad3 as a mediator of the fibrotic response. *Int. J. Exp. Pathol.,* 2004. 85(2): p. 47-64.
[13] Kaneto, H., J. Morrissey, and S. Klahr, Increased expression of TGF-beta 1 mRNA in the obstructed kidney of rats with unilateral ureteral ligation. *Kidney Int.,* 1993. 44(2): p. 313-21.
[14] Kopp, J.B., et al., Transgenic mice with increased plasma levels of TGF-beta 1 develop progressive renal disease. *Lab. Invest.,* 1996. 74(6): p. 991-1003.
[15] Koli, K., et al., Bone morphogenetic protein-4 inhibitor gremlin is overexpressed in idiopathic pulmonary fibrosis. *Am. J. Pathol.,* 2006. 169(1): p. 61-71.
[16] Rygiel, K.A., et al., Epithelial-mesenchymal transition contributes to portal tract fibrogenesis during human chronic liver disease. *Lab. Invest.,* 2008. 88(2): p. 112-23.
[17] Droge, W., Free radicals in the physiological control of cell function. *Physiol. Rev.,* 2002. 82(1): p. 47-95.

[18] Forman, H.J., et al., The chemistry of cell signaling by reactive oxygen and nitrogen species and 4-hydroxynonenal. *Arch. Biochem. Biophys.,* 2008. 477(2): p. 183-95.
[19] Kamata, H. and H. Hirata, Redox regulation of cellular signalling. *Cell Signal,* 1999. 11(1): p. 1-14.
[20] Trachootham, D., et al., Redox regulation of cell survival. *Antioxid Redox. Signal.,* 2008. 10(8): p. 1343-74.
[21] Haddad, J.J., Antioxidant and prooxidant mechanisms in the regulation of redox(y)-sensitive transcription factors. *Cell Signal,* 2002. 14(11): p. 879-97.
[22] Pastore, A. and F. Piemonte, S-Glutathionylation signaling in cell biology: progress and prospects. *Eur. J. Pharm. Sci.,* 2012. 46(5): p. 279-92.
[23] Jones, D.P., Radical-free biology of oxidative stress. *Am. J. Physiol. Cell Physiol.,* 2008. 295(4): p. C849-68.
[24] Fritz, G., et al., APE/Ref-1 and the mammalian response to genotoxic stress. *Toxicology,* 2003. 193(1-2): p. 67-78.
[25] Rahman, I., J. Marwick, and P. Kirkham, Redox modulation of chromatin remodeling: impact on histone acetylation and deacetylation, NF-kappaB and pro-inflammatory gene expression. *Biochem. Pharmacol.,* 2004. 68(6): p. 1255-67.
[26] England, K. and T.G. Cotter, Direct oxidative modifications of signalling proteins in mammalian cells and their effects on apoptosis. *Redox. Rep.,* 2005. 10(5): p. 237-45.
[27] Bourdon, E. and D. Blache, The importance of proteins in defense against oxidation. *Antioxid. Redox. Signal,* 2001. 3(2): p. 293-311.
[28] Pantano, C., et al., Redox-sensitive kinases of the nuclear factor-kappaB signaling pathway. *Antioxid. Redox. Signal,* 2006. 8(9-10): p. 1791-806.
[29] Cross, J.V. and D.J. Templeton, Regulation of signal transduction through protein cysteine oxidation. *Antioxid. Redox. Signal,* 2006. 8(9-10): p. 1819-27.
[30] Gilmore, T.D., Introduction to NF-kappaB: players, pathways, perspectives. *Oncogene,* 2006. 25(51): p. 6680-4.
[31] Shlomai, J., Redox control of protein-DNA interactions: from molecular mechanisms to significance in signal transduction, gene expression, and DNA replication. *Antioxid. Redox. Signal,* 2010. 13(9): p. 1429-76.
[32] Dinkova-Kostova, A.T., et al., Direct evidence that sulfhydryl groups of Keap1 are the sensors regulating induction of phase 2 enzymes that protect against carcinogens and oxidants. *Proc. Natl. Acad. Sci. U S A,* 2002. 99(18): p. 11908-13.
[33] Valko, M., et al., Free radicals and antioxidants in normal physiological functions and human disease. Int J Biochem Cell Biol, 2007. 39(1): p. 44-84.
[34] Valko, M., et al., Free radicals, metals and antioxidants in oxidative stress-induced cancer. *Chem. Biol. Interact.,* 2006. 160(1): p. 1-40.
[35] Wlaschek, M. and K. Scharffetter-Kochanek, Oxidative stress in chronic venous leg ulcers. *Wound Repair Regen.,* 2005. 13(5): p. 452-61.
[36] Clark, R.A.F., Wound repair: overview and general considerations., in The molecular and cellular biology of wound repair, R.A.F. Clark, Editor. 1996, Plenum Press: New York, NY.
[37] Niethammer, P., et al., A tissue-scale gradient of hydrogen peroxide mediates rapid wound detection in zebrafish. *Nature,* 2009. 459(7249): p. 996-9.

[38] D'Autreaux, B. and M.B. Toledano, ROS as signalling molecules: mechanisms that generate specificity in ROS homeostasis. *Nat. Rev. Mol. Cell Biol.,* 2007. 8(10): p. 813-24.
[39] Mittler, R., et al., ROS signaling: the new wave? *Trends Plant Sci.,* 2011. 16(6): p. 300-9.
[40] Roy, S., et al., Dermal wound healing is subject to redox control. *Mol. Ther.,* 2006. 13(1): p. 211-20.
[41] Lenaz, G., Mitochondria and reactive oxygen species. Which role in physiology and pathology? *Adv. Exp. Med. Biol.,* 2012. 942: p. 93-136.
[42] Rodriguez, P.G., et al., The role of oxygen in wound healing: a review of the literature. *Dermatol. Surg.,* 2008. 34(9): p. 1159-69.
[43] Zhang, Y., et al., Redox control of the survival of healthy and diseased cells. *Antioxid. Redox. Signal,* 2011. 15(11): p. 2867-908.
[44] Garcia-Bailo, B., et al., Vitamins D, C, and E in the prevention of type 2 diabetes mellitus: modulation of inflammation and oxidative stress. *Biologics,* 2011. 5: p. 7-19.
[45] Wilgus, T.A., et al., Hydrogen peroxide disrupts scarless fetal wound repair. *Wound Repair Regen.,* 2005. 13(5): p. 513-9.
[46] Frantz, F.W., et al., Biology of fetal repair: the presence of bacteria in fetal wounds induces an adult-like healing response. *J. Pediatr. Surg.,* 1993. 28(3): p. 428-33; discussion 433-4.
[47] Touyz, R.M., Reactive oxygen species, vascular oxidative stress, and redox signaling in hypertension: what is the clinical significance? *Hypertension,* 2004. 44(3): p. 248-52.
[48] Redon, J., et al., Antioxidant activities and oxidative stress byproducts in human hypertension. *Hypertension,* 2003. 41(5): p. 1096-101.
[49] Lassegue, B. and K.K. Griendling, Reactive oxygen species in hypertension; An update. *Am. J. Hypertens,* 2004. 17(9): p. 852-60.
[50] Lijnen, P.J., J.F. van Pelt, and R.H. Fagard, Stimulation of reactive oxygen species and collagen synthesis by angiotensin II in cardiac fibroblasts. *Cardiovasc. Ther.,* 2012. 30(1): p. e1-8.
[51] Sun, Y., et al., Angiotensin-converting enzyme and myocardial fibrosis in the rat receiving angiotensin II or aldosterone. *J. Lab. Clin. Med.,* 1993. 122(4): p. 395-403.
[52] Bataller, R., et al., NADPH oxidase signal transduces angiotensin II in hepatic stellate cells and is critical in hepatic fibrosis. *J. Clin. Invest.,* 2003. 112(9): p. 1383-94.
[53] Sancho-Bru, P., et al., Genomic and functional characterization of stellate cells isolated from human cirrhotic livers. *J. Hepatol.,* 2005. 43(2): p. 272-82.
[54] Oakley, F., et al., Angiotensin II activates I kappaB kinase phosphorylation of RelA at Ser 536 to promote myofibroblast survival and liver fibrosis. *Gastroenterology,* 2009. 136(7): p. 2334-2344 e1.
[55] Deitch, E.A., et al., Hypertrophic burn scars: analysis of variables. *J. Trauma,* 1983. 23(10): p. 895-8.
[56] Singer, A.J. and R.A. Clark, Cutaneous wound healing. *N. Engl. J. Med.,* 1999. 341(10): p. 738-46.
[57] Aarabi, S., M.T. Longaker, and G.C. Gurtner, Hypertrophic scar formation following burns and trauma: new approaches to treatment. *PLoS Med.,* 2007. 4(9): p. e234.

[58] Svegliati-Baroni, G., et al., Involvement of reactive oxygen species and nitric oxide radicals in activation and proliferation of rat hepatic stellate cells. *Liver,* 2001. 21(1): p. 1-12.

[59] Piotrowski, W.J. and J. Marczak, Cellular sources of oxidants in the lung. *Int. J. Occup. Med. Environ. Health,* 2000. 13(4): p. 369-85.

[60] Serrano-Mollar, A., et al., In vivo antioxidant treatment protects against bleomycin-induced lung damage in rats. *Br. J. Pharmacol.,* 2003. 138(6): p. 1037-48.

[61] Manoury, B., et al., The absence of reactive oxygen species production protects mice against bleomycin-induced pulmonary fibrosis. *Respir. Res.,* 2005. 6: p. 11.

[62] Kawada, N., et al., Increased oxidative stress in mouse kidneys with unilateral ureteral obstruction. *Kidney Int.,* 1999. 56(3): p. 1004-13.

[63] Kim, J., et al., Reactive oxygen species/oxidative stress contributes to progression of kidney fibrosis following transient ischemic injury in mice. *Am. J. Physiol. Renal. Physiol.,* 2009. 297(2): p. F461-70.

[64] Steiling, H., et al., Different types of ROS-scavenging enzymes are expressed during cutaneous wound repair. *Exp. Cell Res.,* 1999. 247(2): p. 484-94.

[65] Bondi, C.D., et al., NAD(P)H oxidase mediates TGF-beta1-induced activation of kidney myofibroblasts. *J. Am. Soc. Nephrol.,* 2010. 21(1): p. 93-102.

[66] Gorin, Y., et al., Nox4 NAD(P)H oxidase mediates hypertrophy and fibronectin expression in the diabetic kidney. *J. Biol. Chem.,* 2005. 280(47): p. 39616-26.

[67] Lassegue, B. and R.E. Clempus, Vascular NAD(P)H oxidases: specific features, expression, and regulation. *Am. J. Physiol. Regul. Integr. Comp. Physiol.,* 2003. 285(2): p. R277-97.

[68] Haurani, M.J. and P.J. Pagano, Adventitial fibroblast reactive oxygen species as autacrine and paracrine mediators of remodeling: bellwether for vascular disease? *Cardiovasc. Res.,* 2007. 75(4): p. 679-89.

[69] Sachse, A. and G. Wolf, Angiotensin II-induced reactive oxygen species and the kidney. *J. Am. Soc. Nephrol.,* 2007. 18(9): p. 2439-46.

[70] Mailloux, R.J. and M.E. Harper, Uncoupling proteins and the control of mitochondrial reactive oxygen species production. *Free Radic. Biol. Med.,* 2011. 51(6): p. 1106-15.

[71] Agarwal, A., A. Banerjee, and U.C. Banerjee, Xanthine oxidoreductase: a journey from purine metabolism to cardiovascular excitation-contraction coupling. *Crit. Rev. Biotechnol.,* 2011. 31(3): p. 264-80.

[72] Zhang, R., et al., Myeloperoxidase functions as a major enzymatic catalyst for initiation of lipid peroxidation at sites of inflammation. *J. Biol. Chem.,* 2002. 277(48): p. 46116-22.

[73] Fleming, I., et al., Endothelium-derived hyperpolarizing factor synthase (Cytochrome P450 2C9) is a functionally significant source of reactive oxygen species in coronary arteries. *Circ. Res.,* 2001. 88(1): p. 44-51.

[74] Tabima, D.M., S. Frizzell, and M.T. Gladwin, Reactive oxygen and nitrogen species in pulmonary hypertension. *Free Radic. Biol. Med.,* 2012. 52(9): p. 1970-86.

[75] Andrew, P.J. and B. Mayer, Enzymatic function of nitric oxide synthases. *Cardiovasc. Res.,* 1999. 43(3): p. 521-31.

[76] Altenhofer, S., et al., The NOX toolbox: validating the role of NADPH oxidases in physiology and disease. *Cell Mol. Life Sci.,* 2012. 69(14): p. 2327-43.

[77] Harris, E.D., Regulation of antioxidant enzymes. *FASEB J,* 1992. 6(9): p. 2675-83.

[78] Duncan, C. and A.R. White, Copper complexes as therapeutic agents. *Metallomics*, 2012. 4(2): p. 127-38.

[79] Pantopoulos, K., et al., Mechanisms of mammalian iron homeostasis. *Biochemistry*, 2012. 51(29): p. 5705-24.

[80] Bleackley, M.R. and R.T. Macgillivray, Transition metal homeostasis: from yeast to human disease. *Biometals*, 2011. 24(5): p. 785-809.

[81] Andrews, N.C., Metal transporters and disease. *Curr. Opin. Chem. Biol.*, 2002. 6(2): p. 181-6.

[82] Yoshikawa, S., K. Muramoto, and K. Shinzawa-Itoh, The O(2) reduction and proton pumping gate mechanism of bovine heart cytochrome c oxidase. *Biochim. Biophys. Acta*, 2011. 1807(10): p. 1279-86.

[83] Jomova, K. and M. Valko, Advances in metal-induced oxidative stress and human disease. *Toxicology*, 2011. 283(2-3): p. 65-87.

[84] Butow, R.A. and N.G. Avadhani, Mitochondrial signaling: the retrograde response. *Mol. Cell*, 2004. 14(1): p. 1-15.

[85] Lane, N., Power, Sex, Suicide: Mitochondria and the Meaning of Life 2005, New York: Oxford University Press.

[86] Jassem, W., et al., The role of mitochondria in ischemia/reperfusion injury. *Transplantation*, 2002. 73(4): p. 493-9.

[87] Drose, S. and U. Brandt, Molecular mechanisms of superoxide production by the mitochondrial respiratory chain. *Adv. Exp. Med. Biol.*, 2012. 748: p. 145-69.

[88] Scharstuhl, A., et al., Involvement of VDAC, Bax and ceramides in the efflux of AIF from mitochondria during curcumin-induced apoptosis. *PLoS.One*, 2009. 4(8): p. e6688.

[89] Wagener, F.A., et al., The role of reactive oxygen species in apoptosis of the diabetic kidney. *Apoptosis*, 2009. 14(12): p. 1451-8.

[90] Lane, N., Cell biology: power games. *Nature*, 2006. 443(7114): p. 901-3.

[91] Brown, D.I. and K.K. Griendling, Nox proteins in signal transduction. *Free Radic. Biol. Med.*, 2009. 47(9): p. 1239-53.

[92] Takac, I., et al., The E-loop is involved in hydrogen peroxide formation by the NADPH oxidase Nox4. *J. Biol. Chem.*, 2011. 286(15): p. 13304-13.

[93] Jiang, F., Y. Zhang, and G.J. Dusting, NADPH oxidase-mediated redox signaling: roles in cellular stress response, stress tolerance, and tissue repair. *Pharmacol. Rev.*, 2011. 63(1): p. 218-42.

[94] Lambeth, J.D., T. Kawahara, and B. Diebold, Regulation of Nox and Duox enzymatic activity and expression. *Free Radic. Biol. Med.*, 2007. 43(3): p. 319-31.

[95] Bedard, K. and K.H. Krause, The NOX family of ROS-generating NADPH oxidases: physiology and pathophysiology. *Physiol. Rev.*, 2007. 87(1): p. 245-313.

[96] Grandvaux, N., A. Soucy-Faulkner, and K. Fink, Innate host defense: Nox and Duox on phox's tail. *Biochimie*, 2007. 89(9): p. 1113-22.

[97] Royer-Pokora, B., et al., Cloning the gene for an inherited human disorder--chronic granulomatous disease--on the basis of its chromosomal location. *Nature*, 1986. 322(6074): p. 32-8.

[98] Holmes, B., A.R. Page, and R.A. Good, Studies of the metabolic activity of leukocytes from patients with a genetic abnormality of phagocytic function. *J. Clin. Invest.*, 1967. 46(9): p. 1422-32.

[99] Chan, E.C., et al., Regulation of cell proliferation by NADPH oxidase-mediated signaling: potential roles in tissue repair, regenerative medicine and tissue engineering. *Pharmacol. Ther.*, 2009. 122(2): p. 97-108.

[100] Holland, J.A., et al., Thrombin stimulated reactive oxygen species production in cultured human endothelial cells. *Endothelium*, 1998. 6(2): p. 113-21.

[101] Patterson, C., et al., Stimulation of a vascular smooth muscle cell NAD(P)H oxidase by thrombin. Evidence that p47(phox) may participate in forming this oxidase in vitro and in vivo. *J. Biol. Chem.*, 1999. 274(28): p. 19814-22.

[102] Begonja, A.J., et al., Platelet NAD(P)H-oxidase-generated ROS production regulates alphaIIbbeta3-integrin activation independent of the NO/cGMP pathway. *Blood*, 2005. 106(8): p. 2757-60.

[103] Sen, C.K., et al., Oxidant-induced vascular endothelial growth factor expression in human keratinocytes and cutaneous wound healing. *J. Biol. Chem.*, 2002. 277(36): p. 33284-90.

[104] Wong, H.L. and K. Shimamoto, Sending ROS on a bullet train. *Sci. Signal.*, 2009. 2(90): p. pe60.

[105] Zhang, W.J., H. Wei, and B. Frei, Genetic deficiency of NADPH oxidase does not diminish, but rather enhances, LPS-induced acute inflammatory responses in vivo. *Free Radic. Biol. Med.*, 2009. 46(6): p. 791-8.

[106] Koay, M.A., et al., Impaired pulmonary NF-kappaB activation in response to lipopolysaccharide in NADPH oxidase-deficient mice. *Infect. Immun.*, 2001. 69(10): p. 5991-6.

[107] Segal, B.H., et al., NADPH oxidase limits innate immune responses in the lungs in mice. *PLoS One*, 2010. 5(3): p. e9631.

[108] Yang, S., et al., Exuberant inflammation in nicotinamide adenine dinucleotide phosphate-oxidase-deficient mice after allogeneic marrow transplantation. *J. Immunol.*, 2002. 168(11): p. 5840-7.

[109] Magesh, S., Y. Chen, and L. Hu, Small molecule modulators of Keap1-Nrf2-ARE pathway as potential preventive and therapeutic agents. *Med. Res. Rev.*, 2012. 32(4): p. 687-726.

[110] Datla, S.R., et al., Important role of Nox4 type NADPH oxidase in angiogenic responses in human microvascular endothelial cells in vitro. *Arterioscler. Thromb. Vasc. Biol.*, 2007. 27(11): p. 2319-24.

[111] Peshavariya, H., et al., NADPH oxidase isoform selective regulation of endothelial cell proliferation and survival. *Naunyn. Schmiedebergs Arch. Pharmacol.*, 2009. 380(2): p. 193-204.

[112] Griendling, K.K. and M. Ushio-Fukai, Reactive oxygen species as mediators of angiotensin II signaling. *Regul. Pept.*, 2000. 91(1-3): p. 21-7.

[113] Wu, F., et al., Ascorbate inhibits NADPH oxidase subunit p47phox expression in microvascular endothelial cells. *Free Radic. Biol. Med.*, 2007. 42(1): p. 124-31.

[114] Manea, A., et al., AP-1-dependent transcriptional regulation of NADPH oxidase in human aortic smooth muscle cells: role of p22phox subunit. *Arterioscler. Thromb. Vasc. Biol.*, 2008. 28(5): p. 878-85.

[115] Moe, K.T., et al., Differential upregulation of Nox homologues of NADPH oxidase by tumor necrosis factor-alpha in human aortic smooth muscle and embryonic kidney cells. *J. Cell Mol. Med.*, 2006. 10(1): p. 231-9.

[116] Pleskova, M., et al., Nitric oxide down-regulates the expression of the catalytic NADPH oxidase subunit Nox1 in rat renal mesangial cells. *FASEB J.*, 2006. 20(1): p. 139-41.

[117] Koff, J.L., et al., Pseudomonas lipopolysaccharide accelerates wound repair via activation of a novel epithelial cell signaling cascade. *J. Immunol.*, 2006. 177(12): p. 8693-700.

[118] Nakai, K., et al., Angiotensin II enhances EGF receptor expression levels via ROS formation in HaCaT cells. *J. Dermatol. Sci.*, 2008. 51(3): p. 181-9.

[119] Adachi, T., et al., NAD(P)H oxidase plays a crucial role in PDGF-induced proliferation of hepatic stellate cells. *Hepatology*, 2005. 41(6): p. 1272-81.

[120] Sugimoto, R., et al., High glucose stimulates hepatic stellate cells to proliferate and to produce collagen through free radical production and activation of mitogen-activated protein kinase. *Liver Int.*, 2005. 25(5): p. 1018-26.

[121] Novitskiy, G., et al., Influences of reactive oxygen species and nitric oxide on hepatic fibrogenesis. *Liver Int.*, 2006. 26(10): p. 1248-57.

[122] Grewal, J.S., et al., Serotonin 5-HT2A receptor induces TGF-beta1 expression in mesangial cells via ERK: proliferative and fibrotic signals. *Am. J. Physiol.*, 1999. 276(6 Pt 2): p. F922-30.

[123] Yang, Z.Z. and A.P. Zou, Homocysteine enhances TIMP-1 expression and cell proliferation associated with NADH oxidase in rat mesangial cells. *Kidney Int.*, 2003. 63(3): p. 1012-20.

[124] Craven, P.A., et al., Overexpression of manganese superoxide dismutase suppresses increases in collagen accumulation induced by culture of mesangial cells in high-media glucose. *Metabolism*, 2001. 50(9): p. 1043-8.

[125] Zhao, W., et al., Kidney fibrosis in hypertensive rats: role of oxidative stress. *Am. J. Nephrol.*, 2008. 28(4): p. 548-54.

[126] Sirker, A., et al., Involvement of NADPH oxidases in cardiac remodelling and heart failure. *Am. J. Nephrol.*, 2007. 27(6): p. 649-60.

[127] Park, Y.M., et al., NAD(P)H oxidase inhibitor prevents blood pressure elevation and cardiovascular hypertrophy in aldosterone-infused rats. *Biochem. Biophys. Res. Commun.*, 2004. 313(3): p. 812-7.

[128] Grieve, D.J., et al., Involvement of the nicotinamide adenosine dinucleotide phosphate oxidase isoform Nox2 in cardiac contractile dysfunction occurring in response to pressure overload. *J. Am. Coll. Cardiol.*, 2006. 47(4): p. 817-26.

[129] Touyz, R.M., et al., Angiotensin II-dependent chronic hypertension and cardiac hypertrophy are unaffected by gp91phox-containing NADPH oxidase. *Hypertension*, 2005. 45(4): p. 530-7.

[130] Looi, Y.H., et al., Involvement of Nox2 NADPH oxidase in adverse cardiac remodeling after myocardial infarction. *Hypertension*, 2008. 51(2): p. 319-25.

[131] Cucoranu, I., et al., NAD(P)H oxidase 4 mediates transforming growth factor-beta1-induced differentiation of cardiac fibroblasts into myofibroblasts. *Circ. Res.*, 2005. 97(9): p. 900-7.

[132] Hecker, L., et al., NADPH oxidase-4 mediates myofibroblast activation and fibrogenic responses to lung injury. *Nat. Med.*, 2009. 15(9): p. 1077-81.

[133] Amara, N., et al., NOX4/NADPH oxidase expression is increased in pulmonary fibroblasts from patients with idiopathic pulmonary fibrosis and mediates TGFbeta1-induced fibroblast differentiation into myofibroblasts. *Thorax*, 2010. 65(8): p. 733-8.

[134] Carnesecchi, S., et al., A key role for NOX4 in epithelial cell death during development of lung fibrosis. *Antioxid. Redox. Signal.*, 2011. 15(3): p. 607-19.

[135] Waghray, M., et al., Hydrogen peroxide is a diffusible paracrine signal for the induction of epithelial cell death by activated myofibroblasts. *FASEB J.*, 2005. 19(7): p. 854-6.

[136] Rhyu, D.Y., et al., Role of reactive oxygen species in TGF-beta1-induced mitogen-activated protein kinase activation and epithelial-mesenchymal transition in renal tubular epithelial cells. *J. Am. Soc. Nephrol.*, 2005. 16(3): p. 667-75.

[137] Larios, J.M., et al., Oxidative protein cross-linking reactions involving L-tyrosine in transforming growth factor-beta1-stimulated fibroblasts. *J. Biol. Chem.*, 2001. 276(20): p. 17437-41.

[138] Townsend, D.M., K.D. Tew, and H. Tapiero, The importance of glutathione in human disease. *Biomed. Pharmacother.*, 2003. 57(3-4): p. 145-55.

[139] Jialal, I. and C.J. Fuller, Effect of vitamin E, vitamin C and beta-carotene on LDL oxidation and atherosclerosis. *Can. J. Cardiol.*, 1995. 11 Suppl G: p. 97G-103G.

[140] Heller, F.R., O. Descamps, and J.C. Hondekijn, LDL oxidation: therapeutic perspectives. *Atherosclerosis*, 1998. 137 Suppl: p. S25-31.

[141] Siow, R.C., H. Sato, and G.E. Mann, Heme oxygenase-carbon monoxide signalling pathway in atherosclerosis: anti-atherogenic actions of bilirubin and carbon monoxide? *Cardiovasc. Res.*, 1999. 41(2): p. 385-94.

[142] Wang, J. and K. Pantopoulos, Regulation of cellular iron metabolism. *Biochem. J.*, 2011. 434(3): p. 365-81.

[143] Jomova, K. and M. Valko, Importance of iron chelation in free radical-induced oxidative stress and human disease. *Curr. Pharm. Des.*, 2011. 17(31): p. 3460-73.

[144] Kletzien, R.F., P.K. Harris, and L.A. Foellmi, Glucose-6-phosphate dehydrogenase: a "housekeeping" enzyme subject to tissue-specific regulation by hormones, nutrients, and oxidant stress. *FASEB J.*, 1994. 8(2): p. 174-81.

[145] Iritani, N., et al., Regulation of hepatic lipogenic enzyme gene expression by diet quantity in rats fed a fat-free, high carbohydrate diet. *J. Nutr.*, 1992. 122(1): p. 28-36.

[146] Stapleton, S.R., et al., Effects of acetaldehyde on glucose-6-phosphate dehydrogenase activity and mRNA levels in primary rat hepatocytes in culture. *Biochimie*, 1993. 75(11): p. 971-6.

[147] Fico, A., et al., Glucose-6-phosphate dehydrogenase plays a crucial role in protection from redox-stress-induced apoptosis. *Cell Death Differ.*, 2004. 11(8): p. 823-31.

[148] Katsurada, A., et al., Effects of nutrients and insulin on transcriptional and post-transcriptional regulation of glucose-6-phosphate dehydrogenase synthesis in rat liver. *Biochim. Biophys. Acta*, 1989. 1006(1): p. 104-10.

[149] Pandolfi, P.P., et al., Targeted disruption of the housekeeping gene encoding glucose 6-phosphate dehydrogenase (G6PD): G6PD is dispensable for pentose synthesis but essential for defense against oxidative stress. *EMBO J.*, 1995. 14(21): p. 5209-15.

[150] Rosenstraus, M. and L.A. Chasin, Isolation of mammalian cell mutants deficient in glucose-6-phosphate dehydrogenase activity: linkage to hypoxanthine phosphoribosyl transferase. *Proc. Natl. Acad. Sci. U S A*, 1975. 72(2): p. 493-7.

[151] Xu, Y., et al., Glucose-6-phosphate dehydrogenase-deficient mice have increased renal oxidative stress and increased albuminuria. *FASEB J.*, 2010. 24(2): p. 609-16.

[152] Suzuki, Y. and J. Sudo, Changes in glutathione peroxidase system and pyridine nucleotide phosphate levels in kidneys of cephaloridine-administered rats. *Jpn. J. Pharmacol.,* 1989. 51(2): p. 181-9.

[153] Cappellini, M.D. and G. Fiorelli, Glucose-6-phosphate dehydrogenase deficiency. *Lancet,* 2008. 371(9606): p. 64-74.

[154] Elyassi, A.R. and M.H.H. Rowshan, Perioperative Management of the Glucose-6-Phosphate Dehydrogenase Deficient Patient: A Review of Literature. *Anesth. Prog.,* 2009. 56: p. 86-91.

[155] Gaskin, R.S., D. Estwick, and R. Peddi, G6PD deficiency: its role in the high prevalence of hypertension and diabetes mellitus. *Ethn. Dis.,* 2001. 11(4): p. 749-54.

[156] Nkhoma, E.T., et al., The global prevalence of glucose-6-phosphate dehydrogenase deficiency: a systematic review and meta-analysis. *Blood Cells Mol. Dis.,* 2009. 42(3): p. 267-78.

[157] Cappai, G., et al., Increased prevalence of proliferative retinopathy in patients with type 1 diabetes who are deficient in glucose-6-phosphate dehydrogenase. *Diabetologia,* 2011. 54(6): p. 1539-42.

[158] Lee, J.W., et al., G6PD up-regulation promotes pancreatic beta-cell dysfunction. *Endocrinology,* 2011. 152(3): p. 793-803.

[159] Heymann, A.D., Y. Cohen, and G. Chodick, Glucose-6-phosphate dehydrogenase deficiency and type 2 diabetes. *Diabetes Care,* 2012. 35(8): p. e58.

[160] Zhang, Z., et al., High glucose inhibits glucose-6-phosphate dehydrogenase via cAMP in aortic endothelial cells. *J. Biol. Chem.,* 2000. 275(51): p. 40042-7.

[161] Diaz-Flores, M., et al., Glucose-6-phosphate dehydrogenase activity and NADPH/NADP+ ratio in liver and pancreas are dependent on the severity of hyperglycemia in rat. *Life Sci.,* 2006. 78(22): p. 2601-7.

[162] Xu, Y., B.W. Osborne, and R.C. Stanton, Diabetes causes inhibition of glucose-6-phosphate dehydrogenase via activation of PKA, which contributes to oxidative stress in rat kidney cortex. *Am. J. Physiol. Renal. Physiol.,* 2005. 289(5): p. F1040-7.

[163] Arturson, G. and M. Hjelm, Concentration of adenine nucleotides and glycolytic intermediates in erythrocytes, liver and muscle tissue in rats after thermal injury. *Scand. J. Plast. Reconstr. Surg.,* 1984. 18(1): p. 21-31.

[164] Gupta, A., N. Manhas, and R. Raghubir, Energy metabolism during cutaneous wound healing in immunocompromised and aged rats. *Mol. Cell Biochem.,* 2004. 259(1-2): p. 9-14.

[165] Guo, S. and L.A. Dipietro, Factors affecting wound healing. *J. Dent. Res.,* 2010. 89(3): p. 219-29.

[166] Aksoy, M.H., et al., A new experimental hypertrophic scar model in guinea pigs. *Aesthetic. Plast. Surg.,* 2002. 26(5): p. 388-96.

[167] Hoopes, J.E., C.T. Su, and M.J. Im, Enzyme activities in hypertrophic scars and keloids. *Plast. Reconstr. Surg.,* 1971. 47(2): p. 132-7.

[168] Gupte, R.S., et al., Upregulation of glucose-6-phosphate dehydrogenase and NAD(P)H oxidase activity increases oxidative stress in failing human heart. *J. Card Fail,* 2007. 13(6): p. 497-506.

[169] Park, J., et al., Increase in glucose-6-phosphate dehydrogenase in adipocytes stimulates oxidative stress and inflammatory signals. *Diabetes,* 2006. 55(11): p. 2939-49.

[170] Jain, M., et al., Glucose-6-phosphate dehydrogenase modulates cytosolic redox status and contractile phenotype in adult cardiomyocytes. *Circ. Res.,* 2003. 93(2): p. e9-16.

[171] Spolarics, Z., Endotoxemia, pentose cycle, and the oxidant/antioxidant balance in the hepatic sinusoid. *J. Leukoc. Biol.,* 1998. 63(5): p. 534-41.

[172] Zelko, I.N., T.J. Mariani, and R.J. Folz, Superoxide dismutase multigene family: a comparison of the CuZn-SOD (SOD1), Mn-SOD (SOD2), and EC-SOD (SOD3) gene structures, evolution, and expression. *Free Radic. Biol. Med.,* 2002. 33(3): p. 337-49.

[173] Huang, T.T., et al., Genetic modification of prenatal lethality and dilated cardiomyopathy in Mn superoxide dismutase mutant mice. *Free Radic. Biol. Med.,* 2001. 31(9): p. 1101-10.

[174] Li, Y., et al., Dilated cardiomyopathy and neonatal lethality in mutant mice lacking manganese superoxide dismutase. *Nat. Genet.,* 1995. 11(4): p. 376-81.

[175] Vessey, D.A., K.H. Lee, and K.L. Blacker, Characterization of the oxidative stress initiated in cultured human keratinocytes by treatment with peroxides. *J. Invest. Dermatol.,* 1992. 99(6): p. 859-63.

[176] Pigeolet, E., et al., Glutathione peroxidase, superoxide dismutase, and catalase inactivation by peroxides and oxygen derived free radicals. *Mech. Ageing. Dev.,* 1990. 51(3): p. 283-97.

[177] Rasik, A.M. and A. Shukla, Antioxidant status in delayed healing type of wounds. *Int. J. Exp. Pathol.,* 2000. 81(4): p. 257-63.

[178] Senel, O., et al., Oxygen free radicals impair wound healing in ischemic rat skin. *Ann. Plast. Surg.,* 1997. 39(5): p. 516-23.

[179] Chiumiento, A., et al., Anti-inflammatory properties of superoxide dismutase modified with carboxymetil-cellulose polymer and hydrogel. *J. Mater. Sci. Mater. Med.,* 2006. 17(5): p. 427-35.

[180] Luo, J.D., et al., Gene therapy of endothelial nitric oxide synthase and manganese superoxide dismutase restores delayed wound healing in type 1 diabetic mice. *Circulation,* 2004. 110(16): p. 2484-93.

[181] Ceradini, D.J., et al., Decreasing intracellular superoxide corrects defective ischemia-induced new vessel formation in diabetic mice. *J. Biol. Chem.,* 2008. 283(16): p. 10930-8.

[182] Delanian, S., et al., Successful treatment of radiation-induced fibrosis using liposomal Cu/Zn superoxide dismutase: clinical trial. *Radiother Oncol.,* 1994. 32(1): p. 12-20.

[183] Lefaix, J.L., et al., Successful treatment of radiation-induced fibrosis using Cu/Zn-SOD and Mn-SOD: an experimental study. *Int. J. Radiat. Oncol. Biol. Phys.,* 1996. 35(2): p. 305-12.

[184] Lijnen, P., et al., Inhibition of superoxide dismutase induces collagen production in cardiac fibroblasts. *Am. J. Hypertens,* 2008. 21(10): p. 1129-36.

[185] Chabrashvili, T., et al., Effects of ANG II type 1 and 2 receptors on oxidative stress, renal NADPH oxidase, and SOD expression. *Am. J. Physiol. Regul. Integr. Comp. Physiol.,* 2003. 285(1): p. R117-24.

[186] Welch, W.J., et al., Role of extracellular superoxide dismutase in the mouse angiotensin slow pressor response. *Hypertension,* 2006. 48(5): p. 934-41.

[187] Zhao, W., et al., ANG II-induced cardiac molecular and cellular events: role of aldosterone. *Am. J. Physiol. Heart Circ. Physiol.,* 2006. 291(1): p. H336-43.

[188] Fukai, T., et al., Modulation of extracellular superoxide dismutase expression by angiotensin II and hypertension. *Circ. Res.,* 1999. 85(1): p. 23-8.

[189] Stralin, P. and S.L. Marklund, Vasoactive factors and growth factors alter vascular smooth muscle cell EC-SOD expression. *Am. J. Physiol. Heart Circ. Physiol.,* 2001. 281(4): p. H1621-9.

[190] Didion, S.P., D.A. Kinzenbaw, and F.M. Faraci, Critical role for CuZn-superoxide dismutase in preventing angiotensin II-induced endothelial dysfunction. *Hypertension,* 2005. 46(5): p. 1147-53.

[191] Lijnen, P.J., J.F. van Pelt, and R.H. Fagard, Downregulation of manganese superoxide dismutase by angiotensin II in cardiac fibroblasts of rats: Association with oxidative stress in myocardium. *Am. J. Hypertens,* 2010. 23(10): p. 1128-35.

[192] Zamocky, M., et al., The peroxidase-cyclooxygenase superfamily: Reconstructed evolution of critical enzymes of the innate immune system. *Proteins,* 2008. 72(2): p. 589-605.

[193] Steiling, H., et al., Different types of ROS-scavenging enzymes are expressed during cutaneous wound repair. *Exp .Cell Res.,* 1999. 247(2): p. 484-494.

[194] Odajima, N., et al., The role of catalase in pulmonary fibrosis. *Respir. Res.,* 2010. 11: p. 183.

[195] Kobayashi, M., et al., Catalase deficiency renders remnant kidneys more susceptible to oxidant tissue injury and renal fibrosis in mice. *Kidney Int.,* 2005. 68(3): p. 1018-31.

[196] Sunami, R., et al., Acatalasemia sensitizes renal tubular epithelial cells to apoptosis and exacerbates renal fibrosis after unilateral ureteral obstruction. *Am. J. Physiol. Renal. Physiol.,* 2004. 286(6): p. F1030-8.

[197] Fukuoka, N., et al., Increased susceptibility to oxidant-mediated tissue injury and peritoneal fibrosis in acatalasemic mice. *Am. J. Nephrol.,* 2008. 28(4): p. 661-8.

[198] Siwik, D.A., et al., EMMPRIN mediates beta-adrenergic receptor-stimulated matrix metalloproteinase activity in cardiac myocytes. *J. Mol. Cell Cardiol.,* 2008. 44(1): p. 210-7.

[199] Odajima, N., et al., Extracellular matrix metalloproteinase inducer in interstitial pneumonias. *Hum. Pathol.,* 2006. 37(8): p. 1058-65.

[200] Odajima, N., et al., Loss of caveolin-1 in bronchiolization in lung fibrosis. *J. Histochem. Cytochem.,* 2007. 55(9): p. 899-909.

[201] Nishikawa, M., et al., Inhibition of experimental hepatic metastasis by targeted delivery of catalase in mice. *Clin. Exp. Metastasis,* 2004. 21(3): p. 213-21.

[202] Brigelius-Flohe, R., Glutathione peroxidases and redox-regulated transcription factors. *Biol. Chem.,* 2006. 387(10-11): p. 1329-35.

[203] Reeves, M.A. and P.R. Hoffmann, The human selenoproteome: recent insights into functions and regulation. *Cell Mol. Life Sci.,* 2009. 66(15): p. 2457-78.

[204] Sunde, R.A., et al., Selenium regulation of selenium-dependent glutathione peroxidases in animals and transfected CHO cells. *Biomed. Environ. Sci.,* 1997. 10(2-3): p. 346-55.

[205] Arthur, J.R., The glutathione peroxidases. *Cell Mol. Life Sci.,* 2000. 57(13-14): p. 1825-35.

[206] Conrad, M., et al., Physiological role of phospholipid hydroperoxide glutathione peroxidase in mammals. *Biol. Chem.,* 2007. 388(10): p. 1019-25.

[207] Yant, L.J., et al., The selenoprotein GPX4 is essential for mouse development and protects from radiation and oxidative damage insults. *Free Radic. Biol. Med.*, 2003. 34(4): p. 496-502.
[208] Dringen, R., Glutathione metabolism and oxidative stress in neurodegeneration. *Eur. J. Biochem.*, 2000. 267(16): p. 4903.
[209] Dringen, R., Metabolism and functions of glutathione in brain. *Prog. Neurobiol.*, 2000. 62(6): p. 649-71.
[210] de Haan, J.B., et al., Mice with a homozygous null mutation for the most abundant glutathione peroxidase, Gpx1, show increased susceptibility to the oxidative stress-inducing agents paraquat and hydrogen peroxide. *J. Biol. Chem.*, 1998. 273(35): p. 22528-36.
[211] auf dem Keller, U., et al., Reactive oxygen species and their detoxification in healing skin wounds. *J. Investig. Dermatol. Symp. Proc.*, 2006. 11(1): p. 106-11.
[212] Shukla, A., A.M. Rasik, and G.K. Patnaik, Depletion of reduced glutathione, ascorbic acid, vitamin E and antioxidant defence enzymes in a healing cutaneous wound. *Free Radic. Res.*, 1997. 26(2): p. 93-101.
[213] Vessey, D.A. and K.H. Lee, Inactivation of enzymes of the glutathione antioxidant system by treatment of cultured human keratinocytes with peroxides. *J. Invest. Dermatol.*, 1993. 100(6): p. 829-33.
[214] De Haan, J.B., et al., An imbalance in antioxidant defense affects cellular function: the pathophysiological consequences of a reduction in antioxidant defense in the glutathione peroxidase-1 (Gpx1) knockout mouse. *Redox. Rep.*, 2003. 8(2): p. 69-79.
[215] Fu, Y., et al., Lipopolysaccharide and interferon-gamma-induced nitric oxide production and protein oxidation in mouse peritoneal macrophages are affected by glutathione peroxidase-1 gene knockout. *Free Radic. Biol. Med.*, 2001. 31(4): p. 450-9.
[216] de Haan, J.B., et al., Kidney expression of glutathione peroxidase-1 is not protective against streptozotocin-induced diabetic nephropathy. *Am. J. Physiol. Renal. Physiol.*, 2005. 289(3): p. F544-51.
[217] Rhee, S.G., et al., Peroxiredoxin, a novel family of peroxidases. *IUBMB Life*, 2001. 52(1-2): p. 35-41.
[218] Fujii, J. and Y. Ikeda, Advances in our understanding of peroxiredoxin, a multifunctional, mammalian redox protein. *Redox. Rep.*, 2002. 7(3): p. 123-30.
[219] Wood, Z.A., et al., Structure, mechanism and regulation of peroxiredoxins. *Trends Biochem. Sci.*, 2003. 28(1): p. 32-40.
[220] Monteiro, G., et al., Reduction of 1-Cys peroxiredoxins by ascorbate changes the thiol-specific antioxidant paradigm, revealing another function of vitamin C. *Proc. Natl. Acad. Sci. U S A*, 2007. 104(12): p. 4886-91.
[221] Manevich, Y., S.I. Feinstein, and A.B. Fisher, Activation of the antioxidant enzyme 1-CYS peroxiredoxin requires glutathionylation mediated by heterodimerization with pi GST. *Proc. Natl. Acad. Sci. U S A*, 2004. 101(11): p. 3780-5.
[222] Manevich, Y., et al., 1-Cys peroxiredoxin overexpression protects cells against phospholipid peroxidation-mediated membrane damage. *Proc. Natl. Acad. Sci. U S A*, 2002. 99(18): p. 11599-604.
[223] Wang, Y., et al., Adenovirus-mediated transfer of the 1-cys peroxiredoxin gene to mouse lung protects against hyperoxic injury. *Am. J. Physiol. Lung Cell Mol. Physiol.*, 2004. 286(6): p. L1188-93.

[224] Pak, J.H., et al., An antisense oligonucleotide to 1-cys peroxiredoxin causes lipid peroxidation and apoptosis in lung epithelial cells. *J. Biol. Chem.,* 2002. 277(51): p. 49927-34.
[225] Mo, Y., et al., 1-Cys peroxiredoxin knock-out mice express mRNA but not protein for a highly related intronless gene. *FEBS Lett.,* 2003. 555(2): p. 192-8.
[226] Wang, X., et al., Mice with targeted mutation of peroxiredoxin 6 develop normally but are susceptible to oxidative stress. *J. Biol. Chem.,* 2003. 278(27): p. 25179-90.
[227] Wang, Y., et al., Lung injury and mortality with hyperoxia are increased in peroxiredoxin 6 gene-targeted mice. *Free Radic. Biol. Med.,* 2004. 37(11): p. 1736-43.
[228] Nagy, N., et al., Targeted disruption of peroxiredoxin 6 gene renders the heart vulnerable to ischemia-reperfusion injury. *Am. J. Physiol. Heart Circ. Physiol.,* 2006. 291(6): p. H2636-40.
[229] Munz, B., et al., A novel type of glutathione peroxidase: expression and regulation during wound repair. *Biochem. J.,* 1997. 326 (Pt 2): p. 579-85.
[230] Frank, S., B. Munz, and S. Werner, The human homologue of a bovine non-selenium glutathione peroxidase is a novel keratinocyte growth factor-regulated gene. *Oncogene,* 1997. 14(8): p. 915-21.
[231] Werner, S., et al., Large induction of keratinocyte growth factor expression in the dermis during wound healing. *Proc. Natl. Acad. Sci. U S A,* 1992. 89(15): p. 6896-900.
[232] Kumin, A., et al., Peroxiredoxin 6 is a potent cytoprotective enzyme in the epidermis. *Am. J. Pathol.,* 2006. 169(4): p. 1194-205.
[233] Tsiftsoglou, A.S., A.I. Tsamadou, and L.C. Papadopoulou, Heme as key regulator of major mammalian cellular functions: molecular, cellular, and pharmacological aspects. *Pharmacol. Ther.,* 2006. 111(2): p. 327-45.
[234] Wagener, F.A., et al., Different faces of the heme-heme oxygenase system in inflammation. *Pharmacol. Rev.,* 2003. 55(3): p. 551-571.
[235] Halliwell, B. and J.M. Gutteridge, Oxygen toxicity, oxygen radicals, transition metals and disease. *Biochem. J.,* 1984. 219(1): p. 1-14.
[236] Nath, K.A., et al., Heme protein-mediated renal injury: a protective role for 21-aminosteroids in vitro and in vivo. *Kidney Int.,* 1995. 47(2): p. 592-602.
[237] Ryter, S.W. and R.M. Tyrrell, The heme synthesis and degradation pathways: role in oxidant sensitivity. Heme oxygenase has both pro- and antioxidant properties. *Free Radic. Biol. Med.,* 2000. 28(2): p. 289-309.
[238] Jeney, V., et al., Pro-oxidant and cytotoxic effects of circulating heme. *Blood,* 2002. 100(3): p. 879-887.
[239] Balla, J., et al., Ferriporphyrins and endothelium: a 2-edged sword-promotion of oxidation and induction of cytoprotectants. *Blood,* 2000. 95(11): p. 3442-50.
[240] Balla, G., et al., Hemin: a possible physiological mediator of low density lipoprotein oxidation and endothelial injury. *Arterioscler. Thromb.,* 1991. 11(6): p. 1700-1711.
[241] Balla, J., et al., Endothelial-cell heme uptake from heme proteins: induction of sensitization and desensitization to oxidant damage. *Proc. Natl. Acad. Sci. U.S.A,* 1993. 90(20): p. 9285-9289.
[242] Eipel, C., et al., Inhibition of heme oxygenase-1 protects against tissue injury in carbon tetrachloride exposed livers. *J. Surg. Res.,* 2007. 139(1): p. 113-20.

[243] Tolosano, E., et al., Enhanced splenomegaly and severe liver inflammation in haptoglobin/hemopexin double-null mice after acute hemolysis. *Blood,* 2002. 100(12): p. 4201-4208.

[244] Kovtunovych, G., et al., Dysfunction of the heme recycling system in heme oxygenase 1-deficient mice: effects on macrophage viability and tissue iron distribution. *Blood,* 2010. 116(26): p. 6054-6062.

[245] Lundvig, D.M., S. Immenschuh, and F.A. Wagener, Heme oxygenase, inflammation, and fibrosis: the good, the bad, and the ugly? *Front Pharmacol.,* 2012. 3: p. 81.

[246] Wagener, F.A., et al., Heme-induced cell adhesion in the pathogenesis of sickle-cell disease and inflammation. *Trends Pharmacol. Sci.,* 2001. 22(2): p. 52-54.

[247] Wagener, F.A., et al., Differential effects of heme oxygenase isoforms on heme mediation of endothelial intracellular adhesion molecule 1 expression. *J. Pharmacol. Exp. Ther.,* 1999. 291(1): p. 416-423.

[248] Wagener, F.A., et al., Heme induces the expression of adhesion molecules ICAM-1, VCAM-1, and E selectin in vascular endothelial cells. *Proc. Soc. Exp. Biol. Med.,* 1997. 216(3): p. 456-463.

[249] Nakajima, O., et al., Heme deficiency in erythroid lineage causes differentiation arrest and cytoplasmic iron overload. *EMBO J.,* 1999. 18(22): p. 6282-6289.

[250] Ma, J.L., et al., Hemin modulates cytokine expressions in macrophage-derived foam cells via heme oxygenase-1 induction. *J. Pharmacol. Sci.,* 2007. 103(3): p. 261-6.

[251] Cambos, M., et al., The IL-12p70/IL-10 interplay is differentially regulated by free heme and hemozoin in murine bone-marrow-derived macrophages. *Int. J. Parasitol.,* 2010. 40(9): p. 1003-12.

[252] Cambos, M. and T. Scorza, Robust erythrophagocytosis leads to macrophage apoptosis via a hemin-mediated redox imbalance: role in hemolytic disorders. *J. Leukoc. Biol.,* 2011. 89(1): p. 159-71.

[253] Wagener, F.A., et al., The heme-heme oxygenase system: a molecular switch in wound healing. *Blood,* 2003. 102(2): p. 521-8.

[254] Abraham, N.G. and A. Kappas, Pharmacological and clinical aspects of heme oxygenase. *Pharmacol. Rev.,* 2008. 60(1): p. 79-127.

[255] Kinobe, R.T., R.A. Dercho, and K. Nakatsu, Inhibitors of the heme oxygenase - carbon monoxide system: on the doorstep of the clinic? *Can. J. Physiol. Pharmacol.,* 2008. 86(9): p. 577-99.

[256] Maines, M.D., Heme oxygenase: function, multiplicity, regulatory mechanisms, and clinical applications. *FASEB J.,* 1988. 2(10): p. 2557-2568.

[257] Tenhunen, R., H.S. Marver, and R. Schmid, The enzymatic conversion of heme to bilirubin by microsomal heme oxygenase. *Proc. Natl. Acad. Sci. U.S.A,* 1968. 61(2): p. 748-755.

[258] Haines, D.D., et al., Role of haeme oxygenase-1 in resolution of oxidative stress-related pathologies: focus on cardiovascular, lung, neurological and kidney disorders. *Acta Physiol.,* (Oxf), 2012. 204(4): p. 487-501.

[259] Wagener, F.A., et al., The heme-heme oxygenase system in wound healing; implications for scar formation. *Curr. Drug Targets.,* 2010. 11(12): p. 1571-1585.

[260] Willis, D., et al., Heme oxygenase: a novel target for the modulation of the inflammatory response. *Nat. Med.,* 1996. 2(1): p. 87-90.

[261] Soares, M.P. and F.H. Bach, Heme oxygenase-1 in organ transplantation. *Front. Biosci.*, 2007. 12: p. 4932-4945.

[262] Brouard, S., et al., Carbon monoxide generated by heme oxygenase 1 suppresses endothelial cell apoptosis. *J. Exp. Med.*, 2000. 192(7): p. 1015-26.

[263] Rucker, M., et al., Reduction of inflammatory response in composite flap transfer by local stress conditioning-induced heat-shock protein 32. *Surgery*, 2001. 129(3): p. 292-301.

[264] Ryter, S.W. and A.M. Choi, Heme oxygenase-1/carbon monoxide: from metabolism to molecular therapy. *Am. J. Respir. Cell Mol. Biol.*, 2009. 41(3): p. 251-60.

[265] Gozzelino, R., V. Jeney, and M.P. Soares, Mechanisms of cell protection by heme oxygenase-1. *Annu. Rev. Pharmacol. Toxicol.*, 2010. 50: p. 323-54.

[266] Wagener, F.A., et al., Heme is a potent inducer of inflammation in mice and is counteracted by heme oxygenase. *Blood*, 2001. 98(6): p. 1802-1811.

[267] Hayashi, S., et al., Induction of heme oxygenase-1 suppresses venular leukocyte adhesion elicited by oxidative stress: role of bilirubin generated by the enzyme. *Circ. Res.*, 1999. 85(8): p. 663-71.

[268] Vachharajani, T.J., et al., Heme oxygenase modulates selectin expression in different regional vascular beds. *Am. J. Physiol. Heart Circ. Physiol.*, 2000. 278(5): p. H1613-7.

[269] Takahashi, T., et al., Heme oxygenase-1: a fundamental guardian against oxidative tissue injuries in acute inflammation. *Mini Rev. Med. Chem.*, 2007. 7(7): p. 745-53.

[270] Takahashi, T., et al., Heme Oxygenase-1 is an Essential Cytoprotective Component in Oxidative Tissue Injury Induced by Hemorrhagic Shock. *J. Clin. Biochem. Nutr.*, 2009. 44(1): p. 28-40.

[271] Bauer, M., et al., The heme oxygenase-carbon monoxide system: regulation and role in stress response and organ failure. *Intensive Care Med.*, 2008. 34(4): p. 640-8.

[272] Wang, G., et al., Cardioprotective and antiapoptotic effects of heme oxygenase-1 in the failing heart. *Circulation*, 2010. 121(17): p. 1912-1925.

[273] Braun, S., et al., Nrf2 transcription factor, a novel target of keratinocyte growth factor action which regulates gene expression and inflammation in the healing skin wound. *Mol. Cell Biol.*, 2002. 22(15): p. 5492-505.

[274] Seta, F., et al., Heme oxygenase-2 is a critical determinant for execution of an acute inflammatory and reparative response. *Am. J. Pathol.*, 2006. 169(5): p. 1612-1623.

[275] Deshane, J., et al., Stromal cell-derived factor 1 promotes angiogenesis via a heme oxygenase 1-dependent mechanism. *J. Exp. Med.*, 2007. 204(3): p. 605-618.

[276] Bellner, L., et al., Heme oxygenase-2 deletion causes endothelial cell activation marked by oxidative stress, inflammation, and angiogenesis. *J. Pharmacol. Exp. Ther.*, 2009. 331(3): p. 925-932.

[277] Bellner, L., et al., Exacerbated corneal inflammation and neovascularization in the HO-2 null mice is ameliorated by biliverdin. *Exp. Eye Res.*, 2008. 87(3): p. 268-278.

[278] Bellner, L., et al., Biliverdin Rescues the HO-2 Null Mouse Phenotype of Unresolved Chronic Inflammation Following Corneal Epithelial Injury. *Invest. Ophthalmol. Vis. Sci.*, 2011. 52(6): p. 3246-53.

[279] Patil, K., et al., Heme oxygenase-1 induction attenuates corneal inflammation and accelerates wound healing after epithelial injury. *Invest. Ophthalmol. Vis. Sci.*, 2008. 49(8): p. 3379-3386.

[280] Halilovic, A., et al., Knockdown of heme oxygenase-2 impairs corneal epithelial cell wound healing. *J. Cell Physiol.*, 2011. 226(7): p. 1732-1740.
[281] Grochot-Przeczek, A., et al., Heme oxygenase-1 accelerates cutaneous wound healing in mice. *PLoS.One*, 2009. 4(6): p. e5803.
[282] Applegate, L.A., et al., Two genes contribute to different extents to the heme oxygenase enzyme activity measured in cultured human skin fibroblasts and keratinocytes: implications for protection against oxidant stress. *Photochem. Photobiol.*, 1995. 61(3): p. 285-91.
[283] Ahanger, A.A., et al., Pro-healing potential of hemin: an inducer of heme oxygenase-1. *Eur. J. Pharmacol.*, 2010. 645(1-3): p. 165-170.
[284] Grochot-Przeczek, A., J. Dulak, and A. Jozkowicz, Haem oxygenase-1: non-canonical roles in physiology and pathology. *Clin. Sci. (Lond)*, 2012. 122(3): p. 93-103.
[285] Alam, J., S. Shibahara, and A. Smith, Transcriptional activation of the heme oxygenase gene by heme and cadmium in mouse hepatoma cells. *J. Biol. Chem.*, 1989. 264(11): p. 6371-5.
[286] Cisowski, J., et al., Role of heme oxygenase-1 in hydrogen peroxide-induced VEGF synthesis: effect of HO-1 knockout. Biochem. *Biophys. Res. Commun.*, 2005. 326(3): p. 670-6.
[287] Tosaki, A. and D.K. Das, The role of heme oxygenase signaling in various disorders. *Mol. Cell Biochem.*, 2002. 232(1-2): p. 149-57.
[288] Rattan, S. and S. Chakder, Inhibitory effect of CO on internal anal sphincter: heme oxygenase inhibitor inhibits NANC relaxation. *Am. J. Physiol.*, 1993. 265(4 Pt 1): p. G799-804.
[289] Watkins, C.C., et al., Carbon monoxide mediates vasoactive intestinal polypeptide-associated nonadrenergic/noncholinergic neurotransmission. *Proc. Natl. Acad. Sci. USA*, 2004. 101(8): p. 2631-5.
[290] Suematsu, M., et al., Carbon monoxide: an endogenous modulator of sinusoidal tone in the perfused rat liver. *J. Clin. Invest.*, 1995. 96(5): p. 2431-7.
[291] Sylvester, J.T. and C. McGowan, The effects of agents that bind to cytochrome P-450 on hypoxic pulmonary vasoconstriction. *Circ. Res.*, 1978. 43(3): p. 429-37.
[292] Wang, R., Z. Wang, and L. Wu, Carbon monoxide-induced vasorelaxation and the underlying mechanisms. *Br. J. Pharmacol.*, 1997. 121(5): p. 927-34.
[293] Verma, A., et al., Carbon monoxide: a putative neural messenger. *Science*, 1993. 259(5093): p. 381-4.
[294] Kim, H.P., S.W. Ryter, and A.M. Choi, CO as a cellular signaling molecule. *Annu. Rev. Pharmacol. Toxicol.*, 2006. 46: p. 411-49.
[295] Mayr, F.B., et al., Effects of carbon monoxide inhalation during experimental endotoxemia in humans. *Am. J. Respir. Crit. Care Med.*, 2005. 171(4): p. 354-60.
[296] Moore, B.A., et al., Brief inhalation of low-dose carbon monoxide protects rodents and swine from postoperative ileus. *Crit. Care Med.*, 2005. 33(6): p. 1317-26.
[297] Motterlini, R., et al., Carbon monoxide-releasing molecules: characterization of biochemical and vascular activities. *Circ. Res.*, 2002. 90(2): p. E17-24.
[298] Motterlini, R. and L.E. Otterbein, The therapeutic potential of carbon monoxide. *Nat. Rev. Drug Discov.*, 2010. 9(9): p. 728-43.

[299] Ozaki, K.S., S. Kimura, and N. Murase, Use of carbon monoxide in minimizing ischemia/reperfusion injury in transplantation. *Transplant. Rev. (Orlando),* 2012. 26(2): p. 125-39.

[300] Neto, J.S., et al., Low-dose carbon monoxide inhalation prevents development of chronic allograft nephropathy. *Am. J. Physiol. Renal. Physiol.,* 2006. 290(2): p. F324-34.

[301] Chora, A.A., et al., Heme oxygenase-1 and carbon monoxide suppress autoimmune neuroinflammation. *J. Clin. Invest.,* 2007. 117(2): p. 438-47.

[302] Sammut, I.A., et al., Carbon monoxide is a major contributor to the regulation of vascular tone in aortas expressing high levels of haeme oxygenase-1. *Br. J. Pharmacol.,* 1998. 125(7): p. 1437-44.

[303] Chlopicki, S., et al., Carbon monoxide released by CORM-3 inhibits human platelets by a mechanism independent of soluble guanylate cyclase. *Cardiovasc. Res.,* 2006. 71(2): p. 393-401.

[304] Wang, X., et al., Carbon monoxide protects against hyperoxia-induced endothelial cell apoptosis by inhibiting reactive oxygen species formation. *J. Biol. Chem.,* 2007. 282(3): p. 1718-26.

[305] Bilban, M., et al., Heme oxygenase and carbon monoxide initiate homeostatic signaling. *J. Mol. Med. (Berl),* 2008. 86(3): p. 267-79.

[306] Pamplona, A., et al., Heme oxygenase-1 and carbon monoxide suppress the pathogenesis of experimental cerebral malaria. *Nat. Med.,* 2007. 13(6): p. 703-10.

[307] Ferreira, A., et al., A central role for free heme in the pathogenesis of severe malaria: the missing link? *J. Mol. Med. (Berl),* 2008. 86(10): p. 1097-111.

[308] Larsen, R., et al., A central role for free heme in the pathogenesis of severe sepsis. *Sci. Transl. Med.,* 2010. 2(51): p. 51ra71.

[309] D'Amico, G., et al., Inhibition of cellular respiration by endogenously produced carbon monoxide. *J. Cell Sci.,* 2006. 119(Pt 11): p. 2291-8.

[310] Zuckerbraun, B.S., et al., Carbon monoxide signals via inhibition of cytochrome c oxidase and generation of mitochondrial reactive oxygen species. *Faseb. J.,* 2007. 21(4): p. 1099-106.

[311] Zhang, J. and C.A. Piantadosi, Mitochondrial oxidative stress after carbon monoxide hypoxia in the rat brain. *J. Clin. Invest.,* 1992. 90(4): p. 1193-9.

[312] Cantley, L.C., The phosphoinositide 3-kinase pathway. *Science,* 2002. 296(5573): p. 1655-7.

[313] Piantadosi, C.A., et al., Heme Oxygenase-1 Regulates Cardiac Mitochondrial Biogenesis via Nrf2-Mediated Transcriptional Control of Nuclear Respiratory Factor-1. *Circ. Res.,* 2008. 103(11): p. 1232-40.

[314] Suliman, H.B., et al., The CO/HO system reverses inhibition of mitochondrial biogenesis and prevents murine doxorubicin cardiomyopathy. *J. Clin. Invest.,* 2007. 117(12): p. 3730-41.

[315] Suliman, H.B., et al., A new activating role for CO in cardiac mitochondrial biogenesis. *J. Cell Sci.,* 2007. 120(Pt 2): p. 299-308.

[316] Baranano, D.E., et al., Biliverdin reductase: a major physiologic cytoprotectant. *Proc. Natl. Acad. Sci. USA,* 2002. 99(25): p. 16093-8.

[317] Sedlak, T.W. and S.H. Snyder, Bilirubin benefits: cellular protection by a biliverdin reductase antioxidant cycle. *Pediatrics,* 2004. 113(6): p. 1776-82.

[318] Stocker, R., et al., Bilirubin is an antioxidant of possible physiological importance. *Science,* 1987. 235(4792): p. 1043-6.
[319] Jansen, T., et al., Conversion of biliverdin to bilirubin by biliverdin reductase contributes to endothelial cell protection by heme oxygenase-1-evidence for direct and indirect antioxidant actions of bilirubin. *J. Mol. Cell Cardiol.,* 2010. 49(2): p. 186-95.
[320] Kim, S.Y. and S.C. Park, Physiological antioxidative network of the bilirubin system in aging and age-related diseases. *Front. Pharmacol.,* 2012. 3: p. 45.
[321] Schwertner, H.A. and L. Vitek, Gilbert syndrome, UGT1A1*28 allele, and cardiovascular disease risk: possible protective effects and therapeutic applications of bilirubin. *Atherosclerosis,* 2008. 198(1): p. 1-11.
[322] Dekker, D., et al., The bilirubin-increasing drug atazanavir improves endothelial function in patients with type 2 diabetes mellitus. *Arterioscler. Thromb. Vasc. Biol.,* 2011. 31(2): p. 458-63.
[323] Fukui, M., et al., Relationship between serum bilirubin and albuminuria in patients with type 2 diabetes. *Kidney Int.,* 2008. 74(9): p. 1197-201.
[324] Fukui, M., et al., Low serum bilirubin concentration in haemodialysis patients with Type 2 diabetes. *Diabet. Med.,* 2011. 28(1): p. 96-9.
[325] Han, S.S., et al., High serum bilirubin is associated with the reduced risk of diabetes mellitus and diabetic nephropathy. *Tohoku. J. Exp. Med.,* 2010. 221(2): p. 133-40.
[326] Cheriyath, P., et al., High Total Bilirubin as a Protective Factor for Diabetes Mellitus: An Analysis of NHANES Data From 1999 - 2006. *J. Clin. Med. Res.,* 2010. 2(5): p. 201-6.
[327] Clark, J.E., et al., Heme oxygenase-1-derived bilirubin ameliorates postischemic myocardial dysfunction. *Am. J. Physiol. Heart Circ. Physiol.,* 2000. 278(2): p. H643-51.
[328] Fondevila, C., et al., Biliverdin therapy protects rat livers from ischemia and reperfusion injury. *Hepatology,* 2004. 40(6): p. 1333-1341.
[329] Sedlak, T.W., et al., Bilirubin and glutathione have complementary antioxidant and cytoprotective roles. *Proc. Natl. Acad. Sci. USA,* 2009. 106(13): p. 5171-6.
[330] Dore, S. and S.H. Snyder, Neuroprotective action of bilirubin against oxidative stress in primary hippocampal cultures. *Ann. NY Acad. Sci.,* 1999. 890: p. 167-72.
[331] Dore, S., et al., Bilirubin, formed by activation of heme oxygenase-2, protects neurons against oxidative stress injury. *Proc. Natl. Acad. Sci. USA,* 1999. 96(5): p. 2445-50.
[332] Stocker, R. and B.N. Ames, Potential role of conjugated bilirubin and copper in the metabolism of lipid peroxides in bile. *Proc. Natl. Acad. Sci. USA,* 1987. 84(22): p. 8130-4.
[333] Stocker, R., et al., Antioxidant activities of bile pigments: biliverdin and bilirubin. *Methods Enzymol.,* 1990. 186: p. 301-9.
[334] Dudnik, L.B. and N.G. Khrapova, Characterization of bilirubin inhibitory properties in free radical oxidation reactions. *Membr. Cell Biol.,* 1998. 12(2): p. 233-40.
[335] Dudnik, L.B., et al., Effect of bilirubin on lipid peroxidation, sphingomyelinase activity, and apoptosis induced by sphingosine and UV irradiation. *Biochemistry (Mosc),* 2001. 66(9): p. 1019-27.
[336] Wu, T.W., et al., Antioxidation of human low density lipoprotein by unconjugated and conjugated bilirubins. *Biochem. Pharmacol.,* 1996. 51(6): p. 859-62.

[337] Lanone, S., et al., Bilirubin decreases nos2 expression via inhibition of NAD(P)H oxidase: implications for protection against endotoxic shock in rats. *FASEB J.,* 2005. 19(13): p. 1890-2.

[338] Jiang, F., et al., NO modulates NADPH oxidase function via heme oxygenase-1 in human endothelial cells. *Hypertension,* 2006. 48(5): p. 950-7.

[339] Matsumoto, H., et al., Carbon monoxide and bilirubin from heme oxygenase-1 suppresses reactive oxygen species generation and plasminogen activator inhibitor-1 induction. *Mol. Cell Biochem.,* 2006. 291(1-2): p. 21-8.

[340] McDonagh, A.F., The biliverdin-bilirubin antioxidant cycle of cellular protection: Missing a wheel? *Free Radic. Biol. Med.,* 2010. 49(5): p. 814-20.

[341] Jansen, T. and A. Daiber, Direct Antioxidant Properties of Bilirubin and Biliverdin. Is there a Role for Biliverdin Reductase? *Front. Pharmacol.,* 2012. 3: p. 30.

[342] Bindu, S., et al., Translocation of heme oxygenase-1 to mitochondria is a novel cytoprotective mechanism against non-steroidal anti-inflammatory drug-induced mitochondrial oxidative stress, apoptosis, and gastric mucosal injury. *J. Biol. Chem.,* 2011. 286(45): p. 39387-402.

[343] Harrison, P.M. and P. Arosio, The ferritins: molecular properties, iron storage function and cellular regulation. *Biochim. Biophys. Acta,* 1996. 1275(3): p. 161-203.

[344] McCord, J.M., Effects of positive iron status at a cellular level. *Nutr. Rev.,* 1996. 54(3): p. 85-8.

[345] Torti, F.M. and S.V. Torti, Regulation of ferritin genes and protein. *Blood,* 2002. 99(10): p. 3505-16.

[346] Theil, E.C., Ferritin: structure, gene regulation, and cellular function in animals, plants, and microorganisms. *Annu. Rev. Biochem.,* 1987. 56: p. 289-315.

[347] Orino, K. and K. Watanabe, Molecular, physiological and clinical aspects of the iron storage protein ferritin. *Vet. J.,* 2008. 178(2): p. 191-201.

[348] Chen, X.L. and C. Kunsch, Induction of cytoprotective genes through Nrf2/antioxidant response element pathway: a new therapeutic approach for the treatment of inflammatory diseases. *Curr. Pharm. Des.,* 2004. 10(8): p. 879-91.

[349] Alfadda, A.A. and R.M. Sallam, Reactive oxygen species in health and disease. *J. Biomed. Biotechnol.,* 2012. 2012: p. 936486.

[350] Sedeek, M., et al., Oxidative stress, Nox isoforms and complications of diabetes--potential targets for novel therapies. *J. Cardiovasc. Transl. Res.,* 2012. 5(4): p. 509-18.

[351] Brem, H. and M. Tomic-Canic, Cellular and molecular basis of wound healing in diabetes. *J. Clin. Invest.,* 2007. 117(5): p. 1219-22.

[352] Tandara, A.A. and T.A. Mustoe, Oxygen in wound healing--more than a nutrient. *World J. Surg.,* 2004. 28(3): p. 294-300.

[353] Eltzschig, H.K., Targeting Hypoxia-induced Inflammation. *Anesthesiology,* 2011. 114(2): p. 239-42.

[354] Woo, K., E.A. Ayello, and R.G. Sibbald, The edge effect: current therapeutic options to advance the wound edge. *Adv. Skin Wound Care,* 2007. 20(2): p. 99-117; quiz 118-9.

[355] Huang, A., et al., Exacerbation of endothelial dysfunction during the progression of diabetes: role of oxidative stress. *Am. J. Physiol. Regul. Integr. Comp. Physiol.,* 2012. 302(6): p. R674-81.

[356] Tikellis, C., et al., Interaction of diabetes and ACE2 in the pathogenesis of cardiovascular disease in experimental diabetes. *Clin. Sci. (Lond)*, 2012. 123(8): p. 519-29.

[357] Chang, C.M., et al., Acute and chronic fluctuations in blood glucose levels can increase oxidative stress in type 2 diabetes mellitus. Acta Diabetol, 2012.

[358] Tang, W.H., K.A. Martin, and J. Hwa, Aldose reductase, oxidative stress, and diabetic mellitus. *Front Pharmacol.*, 2012. 3: p. 87.

[359] Whaley-Connell, A. and J.R. Sowers, Oxidative stress in the cardiorenal metabolic syndrome. *Curr. Hypertens Rep.*, 2012. 14(4): p. 360-5.

[360] Styskal, J., et al., Oxidative stress and diabetes: what can we learn about insulin resistance from antioxidant mutant mouse models? *Free Radic. Biol. Med.*, 2012. 52(1): p. 46-58.

[361] Marra, G., et al., Early increase of oxidative stress and reduced antioxidant defenses in patients with uncomplicated type 1 diabetes: a case for gender difference. *Diabetes Care*, 2002. 25(2): p. 370-5.

[362] Vessby, J., et al., Oxidative stress and antioxidant status in type 1 diabetes mellitus. *J. Intern. Med.*, 2002. 251(1): p. 69-76.

[363] Opara, E.C., et al., Depletion of total antioxidant capacity in type 2 diabetes. *Metabolism*, 1999. 48(11): p. 1414-7.

[364] Rahimi, R., et al., A review on the role of antioxidants in the management of diabetes and its complications. *Biomed. Pharmacother.*, 2005. 59(7): p. 365-73.

[365] Goth, L. and T. Nagy, Acatalasemia and diabetes mellitus. *Arch. Biochem. Biophys.*, 2012. 525(2): p. 195-200.

[366] Vincent, A.M., et al., Oxidative stress in the pathogenesis of diabetic neuropathy. *Endocr. Rev.*, 2004. 25(4): p. 612-28.

[367] Huijberts, M.S., N.C. Schaper, and C.G. Schalkwijk, Advanced glycation end products and diabetic foot disease. *Diabetes Metab. Res. Rev.*, 2008. 24 Suppl 1: p. S19-24.

[368] Coughlan, M.T., et al., Advanced glycation urinary protein-bound biomarkers and severity of diabetic nephropathy in man. *Am. J. Nephrol.*, 2011. 34(4): p. 347-55.

[369] Jay, D., H. Hitomi, and K.K. Griendling, Oxidative stress and diabetic cardiovascular complications. *Free Radic. Biol. Med.*, 2006. 40(2): p. 183-92.

[370] Luther, J.M. and N.J. Brown, The renin-angiotensin-aldosterone system and glucose homeostasis. *Trends Pharmacol. Sci.*, 2011. 32(12): p. 734-9.

[371] Shen, G.X., Oxidative stress and diabetic cardiovascular disorders: roles of mitochondria and NADPH oxidase. *Can. J. Physiol. Pharmacol.*, 2010. 88(3): p. 241-8.

[372] Thum, T., et al., Endothelial nitric oxide synthase uncoupling impairs endothelial progenitor cell mobilization and function in diabetes. *Diabetes*, 2007. 56(3): p. 666-74.

[373] Forbes, J.M., M.T. Coughlan, and M.E. Cooper, Oxidative stress as a major culprit in kidney disease in diabetes. *Diabetes*, 2008. 57(6): p. 1446-54.

[374] Sedeek, M., et al., Critical role of Nox4-based NADPH oxidase in glucose-induced oxidative stress in the kidney: implications in type 2 diabetic nephropathy. *Am. J. Physiol. Renal. Physiol.*, 2010. 299(6): p. F1348-58.

[375] Robertson, R.P., Chronic oxidative stress as a central mechanism for glucose toxicity in pancreatic islet beta cells in diabetes. *J. Biol. Chem.*, 2004. 279(41): p. 42351-4.

[376] Brookheart, R.T., et al., The non-coding RNA gadd7 is a regulator of lipid-induced oxidative and endoplasmic reticulum stress. *J. Biol. Chem.*, 2009. 284(12): p. 7446-54.

[377] Donath, M.Y. and S.E. Shoelson, Type 2 diabetes as an inflammatory disease. *Nat. Rev. Immunol., 2011.* 11(2): p. 98-107.

[378] Jeyapalan, J.C. and J.M. Sedivy, Cellular senescence and organismal aging. *Mech. Ageing. Dev.,* 2008. 129(7-8): p. 467-74.

[379] Harman, D., Aging: a theory based on free radical and radiation chemistry. *J. Gerontol.,* 1956. 11(3): p. 298-300.

[380] Gouin, J.P., L. Hantsoo, and J.K. Kiecolt-Glaser, Immune dysregulation and chronic stress among older adults: a review. *Neuroimmunomodulation,* 2008. 15(4-6): p. 251-9.

[381] Gosain, A. and L.A. DiPietro, Aging and wound healing. *World J. Surg.,* 2004. 28(3): p. 321-6.

[382] Keylock, K.T., et al., Exercise accelerates cutaneous wound healing and decreases wound inflammation in aged mice. *Am. J. Physiol. Regul. Integr. Comp. Physiol.,* 2008. 294(1): p. R179-84.

[383] Engeland, C.G., et al., Mucosal wound healing: the roles of age and sex. *Arch. Surg.,* 2006. 141(12): p. 1193-7; discussion 1198.

[384] Swift, M.E., et al., Age-related alterations in the inflammatory response to dermal injury. *J. Invest. Dermatol.,* 2001. 117(5): p. 1027-35.

[385] Ghadially, R., et al., The aged epidermal permeability barrier. Structural, functional, and lipid biochemical abnormalities in humans and a senescent murine model. *J. Clin. Invest.,* 1995. 95(5): p. 2281-90.

[386] Ershler, W.B., Interleukin-6: a cytokine for gerontologists. *J. Am. Geriatr. Soc.,* 1993. 41(2): p. 176-81.

[387] Maggio, M., et al., Interleukin-6 in aging and chronic disease: a magnificent pathway. *J. Gerontol. A Biol. Sci. Med. Sci.,* 2006. 61(6): p. 575-84.

[388] Ershler, W.B. and E.T. Keller, Age-associated increased interleukin-6 gene expression, late-life diseases, and frailty. *Annu. Rev. Med.,* 2000. 51: p. 245-70.

[389] Swift, M.E., H.K. Kleinman, and L.A. DiPietro, Impaired wound repair and delayed angiogenesis in aged mice. *Lab. Invest.,* 1999. 79(12): p. 1479-87.

[390] Stadtman, E.R., Role of oxidant species in aging. *Curr. Med. Chem.,* 2004. 11(9): p. 1105-12.

[391] Barnett, Y.A. and C.M. King, An investigation of antioxidant status, DNA repair capacity and mutation as a function of age in humans. *Mutat. Res.,* 1995. 338(1-6): p. 115-28.

In: Scars and Scarring
Editor: Yongsoo Lee

ISBN: 978-1-62808-005-6
© 2013 Nova Science Publishers, Inc.

Chapter 5

Moving Beyond Inflammation in Cutaneous Scar Formation

*Victor W. Wong and Geoffrey C. Gurtner**
Hagey Laboratory for Pediatric Regenerative Medicine
Department of Surgery, Stanford University, Stanford, CA, US

Abstract

Scar formation following injury causes substantial morbidity and mortality. Despite decades of research, there remains a lack of effective clinical therapies to block scar formation and promote skin regeneration. Inflammatory mediators play an important role in driving fibrosis but non-specific interventions such as corticosteroids have limited efficacy and significant side effects. Traditional concepts in scar formation are based largely on observations using in vitro systems, surrogate animal models, and histologic assays that capture only static biologic events. In spite of these limitations, recent basic science and clinical studies suggest that non-cellular components of the wound including extracellular matrix and transmitted mechanical forces are also important in pathologic scarring. Future challenges in scar research include integrating advances in molecular imaging, in vivo cell-specific targeting, and bioinformatics to better understand the dynamic nature of scar formation and to develop rational mechanism-based therapeutics.

Expert Commentary

Introduction: Traditional Paradigms in Scar Formation

Wound healing has traditionally been described as a progressive sequence of inflammatory cell recruitment, wound cell proliferation, and extracellular matrix production and remodeling [1]. These overlapping stages are activated immediately following injury and result in varying degrees of scar formation to restore skin integrity. Wound fibrosis is a normal part of human wound healing and scar phenotype can vary tremendously from a thin, fine line to the tumor-like appearance of keloids [2]. The primary factor driving wound fibroproliferation is thought to be prolonged inflammation which continuously activates collagen production by fibroblasts [3, 4]. This inability to turn off pro-fibrotic signaling results in a dysfunctional repair state characterized by an imbalance between matrix deposition and proteolysis [3, 5].

Modern strategies to treat and prevent excess scar formation have focused on blocking this inflammatory cascade by modulating cytokine secretion and/or cellular function [6]. For example, corticosteroid treatments inhibit cytokine signaling, laser/radiation treatments diminish cellular activity, and compression therapy is thought to induce cellular apoptosis [7]. Basic science studies have implicated several cytokines in scar formation including the family of transforming growth factors (TGF)-β, platelet-derived growth factor (PDGF), interleukins, and connective tissue growth factor (CTGF) [2, 3, 6, 8]. Although antagonists of these cytokines have demonstrated benefits in animal models, clinical studies have failed to show any significant benefits in humans (e.g. recent failure of recombinant TGF-β3 in Phase III clinical trials). These studies highlight the inadequate understanding of scar pathogenesis and suggest that blockade of inflammation alone is adequate to prevent pathologic scarring.

Evolving Concepts in Wound Fibrosis

The myriad pathways activated following injury can be understood in the context of "seed" and "soil" [1]. The "seeds" are the local and systemic cells in the healing wound and "soil" describes the non-cellular wound environment including matrix components, cytokines, mechanical forces, pH, and oxygen tension. Numerous studies have demonstrated the importance of these forces in regulating cell activity including survival, proliferation, morphology, and migration. Similarly, the term "dynamic reciprocity" has been coined to characterize the bidirectional relationship between cells and their immediate environment [9]. Matrix components are actively modulating cell biology and conversely, cells such as fibroblasts are constantly modifying the extracellular matrix [10].

The majority of extracellular matrix content consists of collagen, specifically types I and III. Accordingly, wound healing and scar formation are discussed mainly in the context of these two collagen subtypes. However, the entire collagen superfamily includes 27 unique members that may play distinct roles in cutaneous disease [11]. Other components of the extracellular matrix that have been implicated in pathologic scarring include glycosaminoglycans and elastin fibers [12, 13]. Abnormalities in matrix glycoproteins including tenascin and fibronectin may drive collagen production in fibroblasts. Moreover, "matricellular" proteins such as periostin and thrombospondins may have a (non-structural) regulatory role in fibroblast-matrix interactions [14, 15]. The importance of these myriad matrix components in scar formation and remodeling remains to be determined.

Basic science and clinical studies have increasingly recognized the importance of mechanical forces in scar formation [16-19]. We have recently described a mechanism through which mechanical forces activate fibroblast secretion of the chemokine monocyte chemoattractant protein-1 to sustain a pro-fibrotic inflammatory state [20, 21]. This pathway is critically dependent on fibroblast mechanosensing via focal adhesion kinase, a focal adhesion component involved in cell-matrix communication. Conversely, attenuation of mechanical force has been shown to reduce incisional scar formation in both a large animal model and early clinical trials in surgical patients [16]. These studies strongly suggest that biophysical approaches to modulate fibrosis may prove effective to minimize cutaneous scarring.

In addition to fibroblasts (the end effector of collagen production), other wound cells are also likely involved in abnormal fibroproliferation. For example, keratinocytes have been demonstrated to regulate fibroblast activity and dysfunctional epithelial-mesenchymal interactions may activate pathologic scar formation [22, 23]. There is also accumulating evidence that both epithelial and endothelial cells transdifferentiate into fibroblasts following injury via processes known as epithelial-mesenchymal and endothelial-mesenchymal transition, respectively [24, 25]. Skin stem cells have been described in human scar tissue and are thought to play a role in scarring via epidermal stem cell-related mechanisms [26, 27]. Inflammatory cells such as macrophages regulate matrix remodeling and are increasingly implicated in wound fibrosis [28, 29]. Moreover, differential activation of helper T cells may modulate scar formation, potentially through the recruitment of circulating fibroblast precursors [20, 30, 31]. Collectively, these studies illustrate the diversity of the wound environment and demonstrate why scar pathogenesis cannot be understood solely in the context of fibroblasts and collagen production.

Future Challenges

Although fibroblasts have been extensively studied in vitro, their behavior in vivo remains unclear. One major obstacle to investigating fibroblasts in living tissues is the lack of fibroblast-specific markers [32]. Several biomarkers have been described, but none are entirely specific for detecting fibroblasts. For example, alpha-smooth muscle actin is thought to define the "activated" myofibroblast, but this marker is also expressed on smooth muscle cells, endothelial cells, and pericytes. Various surface membrane (e.g. integrins), intracellular (e.g. vimentin, fibroblast-specific protein-1) and collagen biosynthesis (e.g. heat shock protein-47, procollagen) targets have been proposed to identify fibroblasts, but these markers lack specificity and reliability [32]. It has also been suggested that fibroblasts exhibit remarkable heterogeneity and multiple cell types may be capable of transdifferentiating into collagen-producing fibroblasts [33], further underscoring the need for specific biomarkers to track fibroblast activity in vivo.

Modern molecular technologies have permitted researchers to target discrete components of the wound environment. For example, transgenic knockout mice have been developed that lack specific genes in fibroblasts alone [34, 35]. Our laboratory has utilized the Cre/loxP recombinase system to generate fibroblast-specific knockout mice that lack a critical intracellular mechanosensor during scar formation [21]. Another group has demonstrated that fibroblast-specific hypoxia-inducible factor-1 alpha regulates tumor vascularization [36], suggesting that scar vascularity may be directly modified by fibroblasts. Novel fluorescent markers have also been designed to follow fibroblast activity in vivo. For example, liver fibroblasts that were monitored using dual collagen and alpha-smooth muscle reporters demonstrated significant heterogeneity during active fibrogenesis [37]. Using similar tracking technology, researchers found that circulating fibroblast precursors did not contribute to skin fibrosis or wound healing in mice [38, 39], raising questions about the relevance of these cells to human scarring. These molecular tools are an important early step in understanding how fibroblasts behave during wound healing and fibrosis.

The study of disease processes has traditionally relied on static histologic techniques that are prone to artifact. This lack of real-time, in vivo imaging has limited our ability to understand dynamic processes such as scar formation and fibrosis on a tissue/organ level. However, recent developments in high resolution imaging offer promising new approaches to investigate wound fibrosis on increasingly fine spatiotemporal scales. Microscopic systems based on intra-tissue fluorescence and second harmonic detection have allowed researchers to track stem cells in living animals over extended time periods [40]. For example, multiphoton imaging techniques have permitted real-time visualization of dermal cells and hair follicle stem cells [41, 42]. Intravital fluorescence microscopy has been used to study the role of mesenchymal stem cells in skin revascularization [43] and confocal microscopy-based techniques have also been utilized to track real-time interleukin production and therapeutic molecule delivery in skin [44-46].

In addition to imaging of cells and biomolecules, novel systems have been designed to study matrix remodeling. Fibrillar collagen exhibits anisotropic properties that are amenable to submicron examination using second harmonic generation microscopy [47]. These techniques have been applied to study collagen ultrastructure during liver fibrogenesis and tumor formation [48, 49]. The matrix composition of human hypertrophic scar can also be effectively assessed using these imaging modalities [50], demonstrating the potential to follow scar formation non-invasively. Recently, innovative molecular ultrasound techniques have been used to track matrix metalloproteinase-mediated remodeling during ischemic-reperfusion injury [51], suggesting that similar methods can be applied to study scar remodeling. Taken together, these studies suggest that non-invasive, high resolution imaging modalities are poised to transform how we understand cell and matrix activity during scar pathogenesis.

Conclusion

An abundance of studies on organ fibrosis over the last decade has produced a growing list of molecular targets implicated in abnormal scar formation [3, 4]. However, recent bioinformatics studies have focused more on establishing common transcriptional networks to identify core and regulatory pathways that may underlie organ fibrosis [52, 53]. Application of these techniques to study cutaneous scarring may reveal fundamental biologic networks encompassing cellular, cytokine, and matrix-associated pathways that drive wound fibroproliferation. Although traditional concepts in scarring have proven useful to begin understanding what scar formation *is*, many questions remain as to *why* humans scar. However, scientists are better equipped than ever with an expanding armamentarium of research tools to elucidate the molecular pathways driving pathologic scarring. The ongoing challenge for wound fibrosis research is integrating technologic advances across disciplines to develop effective clinical therapies with a rational mechanistic basis.

Conflicts of Interest

Drs. Wong and Gurtner hold equity in Neodyne Biosciences, Inc. (Menlo Park, CA, USA), a company that markets surgical dressings to prevent and treat abnormal scar formation. Dr. Gurtner is also a founder of Neodyne Biosciences, Inc.

References

[1] Gurtner GC, Werner S, Barrandon Y, Longaker MT. Wound repair and regeneration. *Nature,* 2008;453:314-21.
[2] Aarabi S, Longaker MT, Gurtner GC. Hypertrophic scar formation following burns and trauma: new approaches to treatment. *PLoS Med.,* 2007;4:e234.
[3] Wynn TA. Common and unique mechanisms regulate fibrosis in various fibroproliferative diseases. *J. Clin. Invest.,* 2007;117:524-9.
[4] Wynn TA. Cellular and molecular mechanisms of fibrosis. J Pathol. 2008;214:199-210.
[5] Eckes B, Nischt R, Krieg T. Cell-matrix interactions in dermal repair and scarring. Fibrogenesis *Tissue Repair,* 2010;3:4.
[6] Wynn TA. Fibrotic disease and the T(H)1/T(H)2 paradigm. *Nat. Rev. Immunol.,* 2004;4:583-94.
[7] Mustoe TA, Cooter RD, Gold MH, Hobbs FDR, Ramelet A-A, Shakespeare PG, et al. International clinical recommendations on scar management. *Plast. Reconstr. Surg.,* 2002;110:560-71.
[8] Alster TS, Tanzi EL. Hypertrophic scars and keloids: etiology and management. *Am. J. Clin. Derm.,* 2003;4:235-43.
[9] Schultz GS, Davidson JM, Kirsner RS, Bornstein P, Herman IM. Dynamic reciprocity in the wound microenvironment. *Wound Repair Regen.,* 2011;19:134-48.
[10] Hynes RO. The extracellular matrix: not just pretty fibrils. Science. 2009;326:1216-9.
[11] Krieg T, Aumailley M. The extracellular matrix of the dermis: flexible structures with dynamic functions. *Exp. Dermatol.,* 2011;20:689-95.
[12] Knight KR, Horne RS, Lepore DA, Kumta S, Ritz M, Hurley JV, et al. Glycosaminoglycan composition of uninjured skin and of scar tissue in fetal, newborn and adult sheep. *Res. Exp. Med. (Berl),* 1994;194:119-27.
[13] Amadeu TP, Braune AS, Porto LC, Desmouliere A, Costa AM. Fibrillin-1 and elastin are differentially expressed in hypertrophic scars and keloids. *Wound Repair Regen.,* 2004;12:169-74.
[14] Schultz GS, Wysocki A. Interactions between extracellular matrix and growth factors in wound healing. *Wound Repair Regen.,* 2009;17:153-62.
[15] Bornstein P, Sage EH. Matricellular proteins: extracellular modulators of cell function. *Curr. Opin. Cell Biol.,* 2002;14:608-16.
[16] Gurtner GC, Dauskardt RH, Wong VW, Bhatt KA, Wu K, Vial IN, et al. Improving cutaneous scar formation by controlling the mechanical environment: large animal and phase I studies. *Ann. Surg.,* 2011;254:217-25.

[17] Wong VW, Akaishi S, Longaker MT, Gurtner GC. Pushing back: wound mechanotransduction in repair and regeneration. *J. Invest. Dermatol.,* 2011;131:2186-96.
[18] Akaishi S, Akimoto M, Ogawa R, Hyakusoku H. The relationship between keloid growth pattern and stretching tension: visual analysis using the finite element method. *Ann. Plast. Surg.,* 2008;60.
[19] Ogawa R. Mechanobiology of scarring. *Wound Repair Regen.,* 2011;19 Suppl 1:s2-9.
[20] Wong VW, Rustad KC, Glotzbach JP, Sorkin M, Inayathullah M, Major MR, et al. Pullulan hydrogels improve mesenchymal stem cell delivery into high-oxidative-stress wounds. *Macromol. Biosci.,* 2011;11:1458-66.
[21] Wong VW, Rustad KC, Akaishi S, Sorkin M, Glotzbach JP, Januszyk M, et al. Focal adhesion kinase links mechanical force to skin fibrosis via inflammatory signaling. *Nat. Med.,* 2012;18:148-52.
[22] Quaggin SE, Kapus A. Scar wars: mapping the fate of epithelial-mesenchymal-myofibroblast transition. *Kidney Int.,* 2011;80:41-50.
[23] Ghahary A, Ghaffari A. Role of keratinocyte-fibroblast cross-talk in development of hypertrophic scar. *Wound Rep. Regen.,* 2007;15 Suppl 1:S46-53.
[24] Guarino M, Tosoni A, Nebuloni M. Direct contribution of epithelium to organ fibrosis: epithelial-mesenchymal transition. *Hum. Pathol.,* 2009;40:1365-76.
[25] Piera-Velazquez S, Li Z, Jimenez SA. Role of endothelial-mesenchymal transition (EndoMT) in the pathogenesis of fibrotic disorders. *Am. J. Pathol.,* 2011;179:1074-80.
[26] Yang JH, Shim SW, Lee BY, Lee HT. Skin-derived stem cells in human scar tissues: a novel isolation and proliferation technique and their differentiation potential to neurogenic progenitor cells. *Tissue Eng. Part C Methods,* 2010;16:619-29.
[27] Zhang GY, Li X, Chen XL, Li ZJ, Yu Q, Jiang LF, et al. Contribution of epidermal stem cells to hypertrophic scars pathogenesis. *Med. Hypotheses,* 2009;73:332-3.
[28] Wynn TA, Barron L. Macrophages: master regulators of inflammation and fibrosis. *Semin. Liver Dis.,* 2010;30:245-57.
[29] Mahdavian Delavary B, van der Veer WM, van Egmond M, Niessen FB, Beelen RH. Macrophages in skin injury and repair. *Immunobiology,* 2011;216:753-62.
[30] Niedermeier M, Reich B, Rodriguez Gomez M, Denzel A, Schmidbauer K, Gobel N, et al. CD4+ T cells control the differentiation of Gr1+ monocytes into fibrocytes. *Proc. Natl. Acad. Sci. USA,* 2009;106:17892-7.
[31] Quan T, Cowper S, Bucala R. The role of circulating fibrocytes in fibrosis. *Current Rheumatology Reports,* 2006;8:145-50.
[32] Kalluri R, Zeisberg M. Fibroblasts in cancer. *Nat. Rev. Cancer,* 2006;6:392-401.
[33] Postlethwaite AE, Shigemitsu H, Kanangat S. Cellular origins of fibroblasts: possible implications for organ fibrosis in systemic sclerosis. *Curr. Opin. Rheumatol.,* 2004;16:733-8.
[34] Zheng B, Zhang Z, Black CM, de Crombrugghe B, Denton CP. Ligand-dependent genetic recombination in fibroblasts : a potentially powerful technique for investigating gene function in fibrosis. *Am. J. Pathol.,* 2002;160:1609-17.
[35] Florin L, Alter H, Grone HJ, Szabowski A, Schutz G, Angel P. Cre recombinase-mediated gene targeting of mesenchymal cells. *Genesis,* 2004;38:139-44.
[36] Kim JW, Evans C, Weidemann A, Takeda N, Lee YS, Stockmann C, et al. Loss of fibroblast HIF-1alpha accelerates tumorigenesis. *Cancer Res.,* 2012;72:3187-95.

[37] Magness ST, Bataller R, Yang L, Brenner DA. A dual reporter gene transgenic mouse demonstrates heterogeneity in hepatic fibrogenic cell populations. *Hepatology,* 2004;40:1151-9.

[38] Boban I, Barisic-Dujmovic T, Clark SH. Parabiosis and transplantation models show no evidence of circulating dermal fibroblast progenitors in bleomycin-induced skin fibrosis. *J. Cell Physiol.,* 2008;214:230-7.

[39] Barisic-Dujmovic T, Boban I, Clark SH. Fibroblasts/myofibroblasts that participate in cutaneous wound healing are not derived from circulating progenitor cells. *J. Cell Physiol.,* 2010;222:703-12.

[40] Uchugonova A, Hoffman RM, Weinigel M, Koenig K. Watching stem cells in the skin of living mice noninvasively. *Cell Cycle,* 2011;10:2017-20.

[41] Uchugonova A, Duong J, Zhang N, Konig K, Hoffman RM. The bulge area is the origin of nestin-expressing pluripotent stem cells of the hair follicle. *J. Cell Biochem.,* 2011;112:2046-50.

[42] Flesken-Nikitin A, Williams RM, Zipfel WR, Webb WW, Nikitin AY. Use of multiphoton imaging for studying cell migration in the mouse. *Methods Mol. Biol.,* 2005;294:335-45.

[43] Schlosser S, Dennler C, Schweizer R, Eberli D, Stein JV, Enzmann V, et al. Paracrine effects of mesenchymal stem cells enhance vascular regeneration in ischemic murine skin. *Microvasc. Res.,* 2012;83:267-75.

[44] Matsushima H, Ogawa Y, Miyazaki T, Tanaka H, Nishibu A, Takashima A. Intravital imaging of IL-1beta production in skin. *J. Invest. Dermatol.,* 2010;130:1571-80.

[45] Ra H, Gonzalez-Gonzalez E, Smith BR, Gambhir SS, Kino GS, Solgaard O, et al. Assessing delivery and quantifying efficacy of small interfering ribonucleic acid therapeutics in the skin using a dual-axis confocal microscope. *J. Biomed. Opt.,* 2010;15:036027.

[46] Ra H, Piyawattanametha W, Gonzalez-Gonzalez E, Mandella MJ, Kino GS, Solgaard O, et al. In vivo imaging of human and mouse skin with a handheld dual-axis confocal fluorescence microscope. *J. Invest. Dermatol.,* 2011;131:1061-6.

[47] Chen X, Nadiarynkh O, Plotnikov S, Campagnola PJ. Second harmonic generation microscopy for quantitative analysis of collagen fibrillar structure. *Nat. Protoc.,* 2012;7:654-69.

[48] Gailhouste L, Le Grand Y, Odin C, Guyader D, Turlin B, Ezan F, et al. Fibrillar collagen scoring by second harmonic microscopy: a new tool in the assessment of liver fibrosis. *J. Hepatol.,* 2010;52:398-406.

[49] Sahai E, Wyckoff J, Philippar U, Segall JE, Gertler F, Condeelis J. Simultaneous imaging of GFP, CFP and collagen in tumors in vivo using multiphoton microscopy. *BMC Biotechnol.,* 2005;5:14.

[50] Chen G, Chen J, Zhuo S, Xiong S, Zeng H, Jiang X, et al. Nonlinear spectral imaging of human hypertrophic scar based on two-photon excited fluorescence and second-harmonic generation. *Br. J. Dermatol.,* 2009;161:48-55.

[51] Su H, Du Y, Qian Y, Zong Y, Li J, Zhuang R, et al. Targeted ultrasound contrast imaging of matrix metalloproteinase-2 in ischemia-reperfusion rat model: ex vivo and in vivo studies. *Mol. Imaging Biol.,* 2011;13:293-302.

[52] Wenzke KE, Cantemir-Stone C, Zhang J, Marsh CB, Huang K. Identifying common genes and networks in multi-organ fibrosis. *AMIA Summits Transl. Sci. Proc.,* 2012;2012:106-15.

[53] Mehal WZ, Iredale J, Friedman SL. Scraping fibrosis: expressway to the core of fibrosis. *Nat. Med.,* 2011;17:552-3.

Prevention

Chapter 6

Prevention of Scars

*Rei Ogawa**
Department of Plastic, Reconstructive and Aesthetic Surgery,
Nippon Medical School, Tokyo, Japan

Abstract

Site-specificity of noticeable scar development suggests that mechanical forces may not only promote scar growth, but they may also be a primary trigger of their generation. While strong and prolonged inflammation is another trigger for the generation of scars, it is suggested that mechanical forces play a more significant role in this process.

Surgery: Since keloids and hypertrophic scars arise from the dermis, it is suggested that eliminating mechanical forces on the dermis could reduce the risk of heavy scar formation after surgery. One approach is to apply a specific type of suturing technique.

Postoperative care: It is very important to stabilize the wound to prevent extrinsic mechanical forces being placed on the wound.

This is because when skin resident cells such as fibroblasts and endothelial cells perceive mechanical forces, they can promote the excessive growth of blood vessels, nerve fibers, and collagens and prolongs and increase inflammation, and also increases the possibility of developing immature scars with redness, after which hypertrophic scars with pigmentation can arise.To prevent pigmentation, sunscreen lotion and cream should be used on the scars.

These topical agents can be used over the surgical tapes. It has been suggested that vitamins B2, B6 and C, and tranexamic acid may be able to prevent the overproduction of melanin and accelerate the skin metabolism that results in the egestion of melanin granules.

In addition, Vaseline-based, heparinoid, and urea ointments are useful for accelerating scar maturation.

---

[*] Address correspondence to: Tel: +81-3-5814-6208, Fax: +81-3-5685-3076, E-Mail: r.ogawa@nms.ac.jp.

Preoperative Assessment - Diagnosis of Genetic Predisposition, Systemic and Local Factors of Heavy Scarring

Cutaneous wound healing normally closes skin gaps and re-establishes an effective epidermal barrier. This phenomenon involves complex biochemical events that have been categorized into four general processes, namely, coagulation, inflammation, proliferation, and remodeling.

The result of these processes is the formation of scars. However, various genetic, systemic, and local factors influence the quality and quantity of scars. These factors shape the development of mature scars, atrophic scars and pathological scars (heavy scars) such as hypertrophic scars and keloids.

1. Genetic Factors

At present, physicians cannot control the genetic factors of patients but it is important to determine whether a patient is predisposed to heavy scarring, as this risk will shape the perioperative scar management.

Thus, the patient should be interviewed to determine whether there is a history and/or familial tendency to develop heavy scars. If the patient has heavy scars on the body, special attention and care will be needed in the perioperative period.

The genetic links to heavy scar development may relate to single nucleotide polymorphisms (SNPs). A genome-wide association study [1] has shown that in the Japanese population, four SNP loci (rs873549, rs1511412, rs940187, and rs8032158) in three chromosomal regions (1q41, 3q22.3-23 and 15q21.3) associate significantly with keloids. Another genetic link may relate to racial differences. There is clinical evidence that patients with darker skin are 15 times more likely to develop pathological scars, primarily keloids; moreover, these scars are absent in albinos [2].

2. Systemic Factors

It has been suggested that adolescence and pregnancy are associated with a higher risk of developing heavy scars [3]. A recent study also revealed that hypertension is associated with the development of severe keloids [4].

Another interesting fact is that scars tend to be hypertrophic in the 1–2 years after an extensive burn was received. Thus, heavy scar generation may be related to systemic factors such as hormones, cytokines, chemokines, growth factors, and/or circulating inflammatory cells. Physicians should determine whether the patient has such risks preoperatively. It should also be remembered that patients who are being treated with immunosuppressive agents or corticosteroid tend to have delayed wound healing that can result in abnormal scars such as atrophic scars.

3. Local Factors

There are several primary factors that hamper proper cutaneous wound healing, such as an inadequately moist environment (either too dry or too wet), strong and cyclical mechanical forces on the wound, foreign body reactions and allergy, and infection [5]. If these factors cause strong and continuous/repeated inflammation, then noticeable and/or growing pathological scars can develop. In addition, radiation-treated regions such as those treated for malignancy tend to form atrophic depressed scars.

Inadequately Moist Environment

Rapid wound healing results in inconspicuous mature scars. Cell growth requires an adequately moist environment as it facilitates cell proliferation and migration at a rate that yields optimal tissue regeneration.

Moreover, the wound exudate serves as a transport medium for a variety of bioactive molecules such as enzymes, growth factors, and hormones. The different cells in the wound area communicate with each other *via* these mediators. To ensure the wound environment is adequately moist after surgery, it is necessary to eliminate dead spaces and place adequate drains intraoperatively, and to absorb excess exudate by applying sufficient wound dressings postoperatively.

For this purpose, foams, hydrogels, hydrocolloids, and alginates have all been found to promote favorable outcomes.

The wound exudate also provides the different immune cells with the ideal conditions needed to destroy invading pathogens such as bacteria, foreign bodies and necrotic tissues, thereby reducing the chance of infection. Thus, to promote rapid wound healing for making inconspicuous scars, it is important to ensure an adequate balance between wound moistness and dryness after surgery.

Strong and Cyclical Mechanical Forces

During wound healing after surgery, fibroblasts, myofibroblasts, endothelial cells, and epithelial cells are affected by intrinsic and extrinsic mechanical stimuli [6]. The wound itself contracts due to forces produced by myofibroblasts. It is also affected by many extrinsic forces, including the natural tension within the skin. Moreover, fibroblasts secrete collagen and fibronectin and regulate the volume of the extracellular matrix (ECM) by secreting collagenase, and it has been suggested that this molecular regulatory process is largely controlled by mechanical forces. If the balance between the synthesis and degradation of collagen is not carefully maintained, scars can either become hypertrophic or atrophic. Cells convert mechanical stimuli, such as tension and shear force, into electrical signals that are transmitted by mechanoreceptors (mechanosensors), such as mechanosensitive ion channels, cell adhesion molecules (including integrins), and actin filaments in the cytoskeleton. The recognition of these mechanical stimuli then promotes cell proliferation, angiogenesis, and epithelization.

This means that strong mechanical forces can increase inflammation, thereby inducing heavy scarring. In addition to these cellular responses, the response to mechanical stimuli (including hypoxia) by the tissue itself strongly affects wound healing. Thus, it is important to control the mechanical forces on the wound during surgery and to minimize such forces after surgery.

Foreign Body Reaction and Allergy

Injections or implantation of foreign body materials have the potential to induce immunological reactions and late-onset complications, including heavy scar formation. Once these complications arise, the inflammation can continue for a long time and induce obvious scars around the wound or injected/implanted areas. Such cases require scar revision with the removal of the implanted/injected materials.

Infection

Infection can result from unhygenic intraoperative procedures or inadequate wound dressings. It can also develop later from a hematogenous origin in cases with implanted foreign bodies. Surgical site infections (SSIs) occur at the site of surgery within 30 days of an operation or within 1 year of an operation if a foreign body is implanted as part of the surgery. While most SSIs are superficial infections that only involve the skin, in other cases the infections are more serious and can involve tissues under the skin, organs, or the implanted material. It has been suggested that wound ischemia caused by faulty suture techniques may be one of the mechanisms that generate SSI. Indeed, a good suturing technique improves such ischemia. Since infection delays wound healing, it can promote the development of obvious scars with pigmentation.

Thus, to prevent noticeable scars, it is necessary to use clean procedures and careful suture techniques intraoperatively and to provide proper care postoperatively. The local factors described above are influenced by the body regions and skin structures. For example, the eyelid and back differ markedly in terms of skin thickness, which will shape the perception of various local conditions.

Thus, the surgical methods should be selected on the basis of the site. Notably, the anterior neck and chest, the scapular region, the suprapubic region, and the joints are constantly or frequently subjected to mechanical forces, including skin stretching due to daily body movements. Special attention is needed when performing surgery on these regions. By contrast, noticeable scars occur very rarely on the parietal region, the anterior lower leg, the eyelids, and the palm, even in patients with multiple keloids or hypertrophic scars on other parts of their body [7]. With regard to both the parietal region and the anterior lower leg sites, the bones lie directly under the skin, which means the skin at these sites is rarely subjected to mechanical forces.

Moreover, although the eyelids are moved frequently due to blinking, the tension on this site does not increase during these movements, even when the eyelid is fully closed. With regard to the palm, it has a thick keratin layer that may hamper the transmission to the dermis of the extrinsic forces that produce scars. This site-specificity of noticeable scar development suggests that mechanical forces may not only promote scar growth, they may also be a primary trigger of their generation [6, 7]. While strong and prolonged inflammation is another trigger for the generation of scars, it has been suggested that mechanical forces play a more significant role in this process. Thus, operations on high-risk sites should be conducted carefully.

Intraoperative Technique

Since pathological scars arise from the dermis, it has been speculated that eliminating mechanical forces on the dermis could reduce the risk of heavy scar formation after surgery. Superficial injury that includes the epidermis and papillary layer of the dermis does not cause severe scars.

Therefore, one way to prevent pathological scar development is to use a specific type of suturing technique. In plastic surgery, three-layered sutures consisting of separate subcutaneous/dermal/superficial sutures are conventionally used; these sutures are associated with a clear decrease in the risk of both SSIs and hypertrophic scars.

However, to prevent the development of severe hypertrophic scars and keloids, further modifications of suture techniques are needed because even three-layered sutures place tension on the dermis.

Consequently, we use subcutaneous/fascial tension reduction sutures where the tension is placed on the layer of deep fascia and superficial fascia (Figure 1) [8]. This means that the use of dermal sutures is minimized; indeed, dermal sutures can be avoided altogether if the wound edges can be joined together naturally under very small tension. We prefer 0, 2-0 or 3-0 polydioxanone sutures for subcutaneous/fascial sutures, 4-0 or 5-0 for dermal sutures (if they are necessary), and 6-0 or 7-0 polypropylene or nylon sutures for superficial sutures. The consequence of such suturing is that the wound edges are elevated smoothly with minimal tension on the dermis. This appears to prevent the development of large scars.

Sometimes, after suturing, there are small nodules under the skin that can be sensed when the wound surface is touched.

These are likely to reflect surgical damage to the dermis. We have noticed that keloids and hypertrophic scars tend to recur from these nodules: indeed, it seems that keloid recurrence usually starts from the suture marks rather than from the sutured surfaces. For this reason, we ensure that we do not nick the dermal layer during surgery.

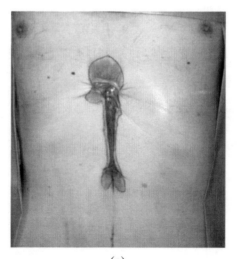

(a)

A keloid on the chest and upper abdomen that is due to be excised.

Figure 1. (Continued).

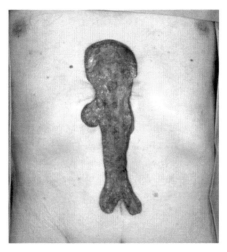

(b)

The contracture was released completely and the wound was opened.

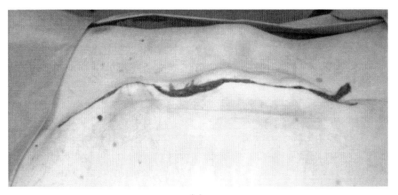

(c)

After deep and superficial fascia suturing, the wound edges attached to each other naturally. This meant that there was only minimal tension on the dermis.

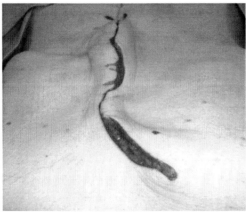

(d)

The wound surface was gently elevated to release tension on the dermis.

Figure 1. (Continued).

Prevention of Scars 115

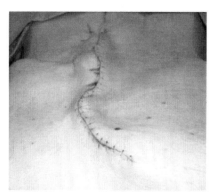

(e)

After the fascial sutures were placed, minimal dermal and superficial sutures were placed to fix the wound edges.

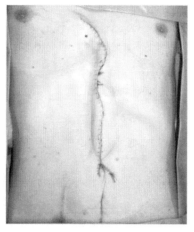

(f)

The keloid was removed and sutured with gentle elevation of the wound surface.

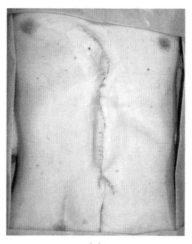

(g)

Non-adhesive gauze was applied with an ointment to keep the wound surface moist.

Figure 1. (Continued).

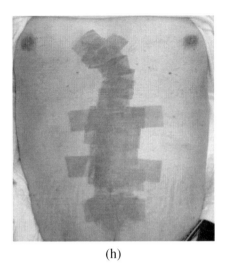

(h)

After removing the sutures, taping fixation was performed for 6 months. Ointment can be applied on top of the tape if the patient feels an itch caused by contact dermatitis. The ointment can penetrate into the tape and reach the skin.

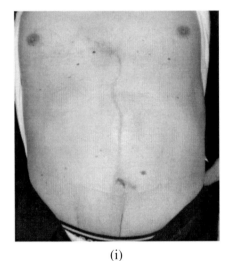

(i)

There was no recurrence of pathological scarring 2 years after the operation.

Figure 1. Suture techniques used to reduce tension on the dermis.

Postoperative Care

1. Within 1-2 Weeks After Surgery

This period is associated with the beginning of the proliferation phase and the end of the inflammation phase of wound healing. To decrease inflammation, it is important to stabilize the wound to prevent extrinsic mechanical forces being placed on the wound.

This is because when skin resident cells such as fibroblasts and endothelial cells perceive mechanical forces, they can promote the excessive growth of blood vessels, nerve fibers, and collagens, thereby prolonging and increasing inflammation. It also increases the possibility that immature scars with redness develop, after which hypertrophic scars with pigmentation can arise.

To stabilize the wound before suture removal, skin closure tape can be combined with a skin adhesive. Bandages, splints, garments are also helpful. To ensure that the wound environment is moist, one can apply moist wound dressing materials or a Vaseline-based ointment.

2. Within 1 Month After Surgery

This period is associated with the beginning of the remodeling phase of wound healing. At this stage, the sutures have been removed and external fixation with surgical tape, silicone gel sheet, polyethylene gel sheet, soft silicone tape, bandages, or foam compression should be considered (Figure 2, 3).

To prevent pigmentation, sunscreen lotion and cream should be used on the scars. These topical agents can be used over the surgical tapes. It has been suggested that vitamins B2, B6 and C, and tranexamic acid may be able to prevent the overproduction of melanin and accelerate the skin metabolism that results in the egestion of melanin granules. In addition, Vaseline-based, heparinoid, and urea ointments and silicone creams or gels are useful for accelerating scar maturation.

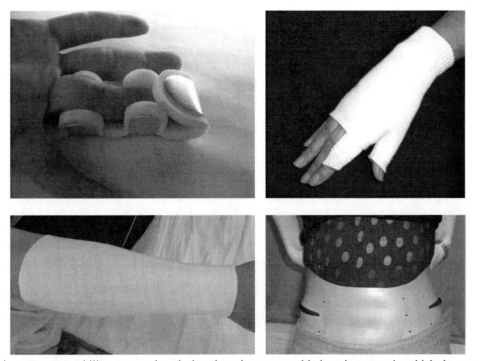

It is important to stabilize a wound such that there is an untroubled environment in which the wound healing process can progress normally.

Figure 2. Methods used to stabilize a sutured wound.

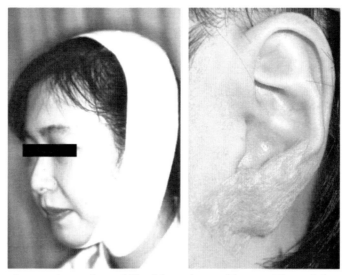

Lower jaw and neck wounds can be stabilized by using a chin cap. The earlobe can be fixed with surgical tape.

Figure 3. Methods of fixing wounds on the face and neck.

3. Within 6 Months After Surgery

This period is associated with the end of the scar maturation stage. Unless there are special reasons such as a genetic predisposition towards keloids or hypertrophic scars, minimum protection from ultraviolet rays is sufficient for scar management. Vitamins B2, B6, and C and tranexamic acid can still decrease melanin levels at this stage.

4. Six Months After Surgery

If scars and/or pigmentation/depigmentation are noticeable at this stage, it means that the natural recovery process will take a long time. If this is the case, aggressive treatments such as scar revision surgery and laser treatment can be started.

Appropriate materials should be selected on a case-by-case basis. Materials that are typically used are described below.

Skin Closure Tape and Surgical Adhesive

Skin closure tape and skin adhesive are helpful for stabilizing sutured wounds. Since neither the tape nor the adhesive can provide sufficient stabilization alone, it is best to use them in combination with sutures. Sticking on the tape in a reticular pattern yields superior stabilization.

The tape in combination with surgical adhesive also effectively stabilizes sutured wounds.

Wound Dressings

Before removing the sutures, wound dressings such as polyurethane films help to protect the wound and keep it moist. A change every 2–3 days is sufficient to keep the wound clean. It is also useful to apply non-adhesive gauze or absorbent dressings for the first 1–3 days to absorb small bleeds that may continue.

Surgical Tapes

Surgical tapes are useful for stabilizing the wound after suture removal. For the high-risk sites mentioned above, taping fixation should be continued for at least 3–6 months. Patients do not need to change the tapes every day, even if they take a bath every day; rather, the tape should only be changed when it becomes unstuck naturally. This will prevent epidermal injury arising from the removal of the tapes. In general, most patients tend to change the tapes every 1–2 weeks. If contact dermatitis occurs, corticosteroid ointment can be applied on the top of the tapes. This agent can penetrate into the tapes and reach the skin.

Gel Sheet

Silicone gel or the cheaper polyethylene gel sheets are available. Gel sheets effectively keep the wound moist; they also reduce the tension on the border between the scar and the normal skin. It has been suggested that gel sheets transfer the tension from the border of the scar to the lateral edge of the sheet. Moreover, gel sheets can protect wounds from extrinsic mechanical forces and are easy to use. However, it is difficult to use gel sheets in weather that induces sweating. In such cases, silicone gel is an alternative choice, although it does not have a mechanical force-reduction effect.

Bandages, Garments, Foams, and Sponges

Bandages, garments, foams and sponges can stabilize and compress the wound, although the mechanisms by which compression improves wound healing have not yet been analyzed precisely. They are effective for wounds on a joint or a movable region.

Moisturizer

To accelerate scar healing, moisturizers such as Vaseline-based, heparinoid and urea ointments are useful. Moreover, silicone gels and creams are widely used, especially in Asian countries, because gel sheets are difficult to use in conditions that induce sweating.

References

[1] Nakashima M, Chung S, Takahashi A, Kamatani N, Kawaguchi T, Tsunoda T, Hosono N, Kubo M, Nakamura Y, Zembutsu H. A genome-wide association study identifies four susceptibility loci for keloid in the Japanese population. *Nat. Genet.,* 2010 Sep;42(9):768-71.

[2] Miller MC, Nanchahal J. Advances in the modulation of cutaneous wound healing and scarring. *BioDrugs,* 2005;19(6):363-81.

[3] Park TH, Chang CH. Keloid recurrence in pregnancy. *Aesthetic Plast Surg.,* 2012 Oct;36(5):1271-2.

[4] Arima J, Ogawa R, Iimura T, Azuma H, Hyakusoku H. Relationship between Hypertension and Aggravation of Keloid. The 55th Annual Meeting of Japan Society of Plastic and Reconstructive Surgery, 2012.4.

[5] Ogawa R. The most current algorithms for the treatment and prevention of hypertrophic scars and keloids. *Plast. Reconstr. Surg.*, 2010 Feb;125(2):557-68.

[6] Ogawa R. Mechanobiology of scarring. *Wound Repair Regen.*, 2011 Sep;19 Suppl 1:s2-9.

[7] Ogawa R, Okai K, Tokumura F, Mori K, Ohmori Y, Huang C, Hyakusoku H, Akaishi S. The relationship between skin stretching/contraction and pathologic scarring: the important role of mechanical forces in keloid generation. *Wound Repair Regen.*, 2012 Mar-Apr;20(2):149-57.

[8] Ogawa R, Akaishi S, Huang C, Dohi T, Aoki M, Omori Y, Koike S, Kobe K, Akimoto M, Hyakusoku H. Clinical applications of basic research that shows reducing skin tension could prevent and treat abnormal scarring: the importance of fascial/subcutaneous tensile reduction sutures and flap surgery for keloid and hypertrophic scar reconstruction. *J. Nippon. Med. Sch.*, 2011;78(2):68-76.

Treatment Options

In: Scars and Scarring
Editor: Yongsoo Lee
ISBN: 978-1-62808-005-6
© 2013 Nova Science Publishers, Inc.

Chapter 7

Radiation Therapy for Scars

Rei Ogawa[*]
Department of Plastic, Reconstructive and Aesthetic Surgery,
Nippon Medical School, Tokyo, Japan

Abstract

Keloids have been treated by using radiation for a century. Freund reported in 1898, three years after X-rays were first detected by Wilhelm Conrad Röntgen, that hypertrophic scars could be restored to normal skin by roentgen treatment. Thereafter, different radiation protocols were developed for keloid treatment. Some of these involved external irradiation using superficial and orthovoltage X-rays (photons) and β-rays (electron-beams). Others were brachytherapies employing β-rays (32P or 90Sr/90Y), and γ-rays (60Co or 192Ir). In addition, radiation therapy has been employed as a monotherapy, or in combination with adjuvant therapy delivered on its own preoperatively, or postoperatively. However, it is generally believed that keloids are best treated by a combination of surgery and postoperative radiation therapy, although it should be noted that this notion has not yet been tested by randomized control trials (RCTs). While it is difficult to determine the effectiveness of irradiation for the treatment of keloids because of variations between studies in patient human race, age and sex, keloid area and size, radiation source and dose, result assessment strategies and follow-up term, the reported postoperative radiation response rates (the rate of recurrences regardless of patient satisfaction) generally fall between 67% and 98%.Thus, it is currently suggested that keloids can be treated effectively by a combination of surgery and radiation therapy.

---

[*] Address correspondence to: Rei Ogawa, M. D., Ph. D., F. A. C. S., Department of Plastic, Reconstructive and Aesthetic Surgery, Nippon Medical School, 1-1-5 Sendagi Bunkyo-ku, Tokyo 113-8603, Japan. Tel: +81-3-5814-6208. Fax: +81-3-5685-3076. E-Mail: r.ogawa@nms.ac.jp.

Introduction

Recent advances in radiation therapy have led to modern radiation therapies that successfully and safely treat keloids. Keloids have been treated with radiation for a century [1]. Freund reported in 1898, 3 years after X-rays were first detected by Wilhelm Conrad Röntgen, that hypertrophic scars could be restored to normal skin by roentgen treatment. Subsequently, in 1901, Harris reported that keloids could be treated preoperatively by roentgen exposure. Freund then, in 1909, described the first combination treatment protocol that involved surgery and postoperative roentgen treatment. Thereafter, different radiation protocols were developed for keloid treatment. Some involved external irradiation with superficial and orthovoltage X-rays (photons) and β-rays (electron-beams). Other protocols were brachytherapies employing β-rays (32P or 90Sr/90Y) and γ-rays (60Co or 192Ir). Intra-tissue or superficial irradiation has been used to treat keloids.

Radiation therapy is employed as a monotherapy (primary radiation therapy) or in combination with adjuvant therapy delivered on its own, preoperatively, or postoperatively [2]. However, it is generally believed that keloids are best treated by a combination of surgery and postoperative radiation therapy, although it should be noted that this notion has not yet been tested by randomized controlled trials (RCTs). The reported postoperative radiation response rates (the rate of no recurrences regardless of patient satisfaction) generally range from 67% to 98% [2]. However, we have also used primary radiation therapy with older patients or patients with severe acne keloids (Figure 1) [3]. The total radiation dose needed is higher than that used for postoperative radiation therapy. Therefore, it is necessary to apply the radiation carefully to prevent secondary radiation carcinogenesis. It is also important to obtain the well-informed consent of the patient. However, the benefit of primary radiation therapy is tremendous. Subjective symptoms such as pain and itch decrease immediately, and the color and thickness of the scars normalize progressively over a year.

In general, physicians tend to avoid radiation therapy for keloids for fear of inducing malignant tumors. Thus, it is important to understand the effectiveness and risk of radiation treatment.

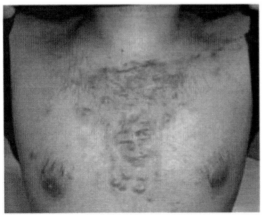 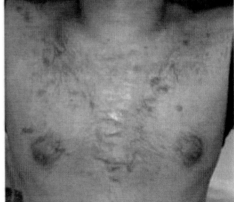

Figure 1. Primary radiation therapy for severe keloids. 24 Gy/5 fractions of radiation therapy were administered for 5 days. The keloids improved dramatically.

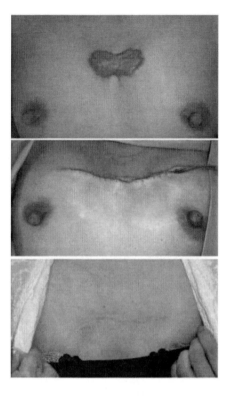

Figure 2. An anterior chest keloid that was treated by surgical excision and 20 Gy/4 fractions/4 days of radiation therapy. There was no recurrence in more than 2 years after surgery.

Optimal Dose for Radiation Therapy for Keloids

From our review of the literature, it appears that for maximal efficacy and safety, postoperative radiation therapy for keloids in adults should involve the application of 10 to 20 Gy delivered as 5 Gy per fraction. When Kal *et al*. [4, 5] calculated the biologically effective doses (BEDs) of various radiation regimens for keloid therapy by using the linear-quadratic concept, they observed that when the BEDs were less than 10 Gy, them recurrence rate decreased as a function of the BED. However, when the BEDs exceeded 30 Gy, the recurrence rate was less than 10%. A BED value of 30 Gy can be obtained with, for instance, a single fraction dose of 13 Gy, two fractions of 8 Gy, three fractions of 6 Gy, or a single dose of 27 Gy administered at a low dose rate. Kal *et al*. [4, 5] also concluded that the radiation treatment should be administered within 2 days after surgery.

The survey by Leer [6] showed that a total dose of 15 Gy is used most frequently throughout the world. Moreover, it has been recommended in the literature that there should be site-dependent dose protocols for the treatment of keloids, as these protocols may vary regarding the total dose of radiation that should be delivered [7]. This concept is based on an analysis of the therapeutic outcomes of radiation that showed that sites with high stretch tension, such as the chest wall and the scapular and suprapubic regions, have significantly higher recurrence rates than sites without high tension. The following radiation doses and procedures have been recommended: 20 Gy in four fractions over 4 days for the anterior chest wall, shoulder-scapular region and suprapubic region (Figure 2), 10 Gy in two fractions over 2 days for the ear lobe (Figure 3), and 15 Gy in three fractions over 3 days for other sites (Figure 4) [7].

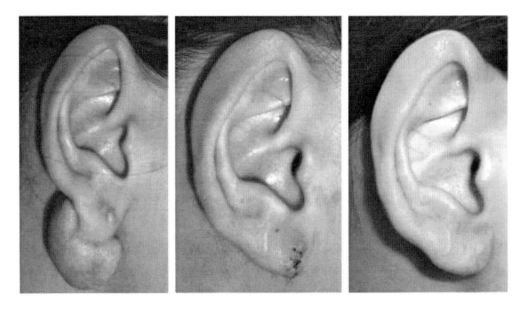

Figure 3. An ear lobe keloid was treated by surgical wedge excision and 10 Gy/2 fractions/2 days of radiation therapy. There were no recurrences in more than 2 years after surgery.

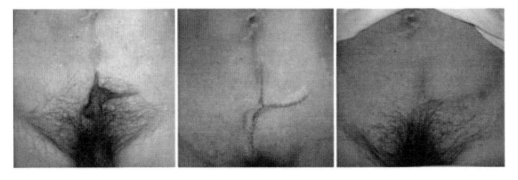

Figure 4. A lower abdominal keloid was treated by surgical wedge excision and 15 Gy/3 fractions/3 days of radiation therapy. There were no recurrence in more than 2 years after surgery.

Complications of Radiation Therapy for Keloids

Since the target of radiation therapy for keloids is the skin, especially the dermis, the reaction of the skin to radiation therapy is of primary interest. Acute skin reactions to radiation therapy occur during the first 7–10 days after treatment and are characterized initially by erythema that then progresses to pigmentation, epilation and desquamation, particularly when higher doses are applied. Subacute and late complications occur several weeks after radiation therapy. Scarring, permanent pigmentation, depigmentation, atrophy, telangiectasis, subcutaneous fibrosis and necrosis can develop and progress for long periods. Other potential complications of radiation therapy for keloids include wound dehiscence in a postoperative radiation setting and, importantly, carcinogenesis. However, while previous reports of radiation therapy of keloids have noted the occurrence of erythema, pigmentation, depigmentation and telangiectasia, ulceration and wound dehiscence have not been mentioned.

Evidence-based Opinions about Carcinogenesis Associated with Radiation Therapy for Keloids

In 2007, the International Commission on Radiological Protection (ICRP) recommended that radiation-sensitive tissues, such as the mammary gland and thyroid, should be protected as much as possible during radiotherapy to prevent the development of radiation-induced breast and thyroid carcinomas [8]. However, the cutaneous malignant changes that could potentially arise from radiation therapy, such as the BCC reported by Horton [9], can be detected early and consequently cured rapidly. This suggests that when surrounding tissues are adequately protected, the risk of radiation-induced carcinogenesis is low. Indeed, Leer *et al.* have stated that "the risk of the induction of secondary tumors had been overestimated in the past" [10]. However, they also commented that it is important that radiation therapy should be performed with an appropriate source, dose and irradiation field, and only after the patient is informed according to the "standard opinion of radiotherapy of non-malignant disorders" and consents to the treatment. There is sufficient evidence that radiotherapy is effective for keloids and that there should be no age limit on this treatment, provided that alternatives are not effective.

However, we should not deny the possibility that radiation therapy for keloids could induce secondary tumors, and patients should not be forced to receive radiation therapy. Moreover, additional caution is still required with regard to the radiation treatment of young patients, and children should only be treated in emergency situations where no other therapeutic solutions seem possible. Supporting this position are the studies by Lundell *et al.* [11, 12], who showed that people irradiated as infants suffer an increased excess relative risk (ERR) of radiation-induced carcinogenesis in the thyroid and mammary gland. This was determined by two cohort studies, one examining thyroid cancer rates in patients who were irradiated as infants and the other measuring breast cancer rates in 9,675 individuals who were irradiated as infants. It was observed that for thyroid cancer, the ERR per gray was 4.92 (95% CI 1.26–10.2) per person-year gray; this effect lasted for at least 40 years after the irradiation. In addition, for breast cancer, the ERR increased significantly over time after exposure, with the ERR at 1 Gy at 50 or more years after exposure being 2.25 (95% CI 0.59–5.62). These observations indicate that X Gy irradiation to Y% area of the thyroid and mammary gland in infancy results in a $1 + 4.92^* X^* 0.01^* Y^*$ and $1 + 2.25^* X^* 0.01^* Y^*$ fold increase in risk of radiation-induced carcinogenesis, respectively. Thus, for example, 20 Gy of irradiation to 5% of the thyroid or mammary gland results in a 5.92- and 3.25-fold increased risk of thyroid and breast carcinogenesis, respectively. Thus, it is essential that the thyroid and mammary gland should be protected when children are to be irradiated, and that radiation therapy for keloids should not be used in infancy when it is likely that these organs will be exposed to radiation.

There is also a report stating that 670 per 10,000 18- to 64-year-old people (6.7%) will have a skin cancer if the whole body is irradiated with 1 Gy [13]. In general, cancer of the skin kills one in 500 patients. Thus, the mortality rate associated with 1 Gy of whole body irradiation would be 6.7% x 1/500 = 0.0134%, namely, one per 7,500 people. Let us apply this to the case of earlobe keloid radiotherapy, where 0.05% of the skin of the whole body is irradiated with 10 Gy. Thus, the incidence of cancer associated with this treatment would be 6.7 x 10 x 0.05 /100 = 0.0335%, namely, one per 3,000 people. The mortality rate of secondary carcinogenesis of earlobe keloid treatment would be 0.0335/500 = 0.000067%, namely, one per 1,500,000 people. As another example, let us say that a chest wall keloid is treated by irradiation of 2.5 cm x 25 cm of skin (1/240 of the whole skin) with 20 Gy. The incidence of cancer would be 0.56%, or one per 180 people, and the mortality rate would be 0.0011%, namely, one per 90,000 people.

Conclusion

At this point, both postoperative adjuvant radiation therapy and primarily radiation therapy seem to be effective for treating keloids. The risk of carcinogenesis due to keloid radiation therapy is very low if it is performed with adequate doses and under conditions that adequately protect the surrounding tissues, including the thyroid and mammary glands (especially in children and infants). Thus, it seems that radiation therapy is acceptable as a keloid treatment modality. However, RCTs of radiation therapy are needed to determine the influence of factors such as patient race, age and sex, keloid area and size, radiation source and dose, result assessment strategies, follow-up duration, response rates, recurrence rate, and patient satisfaction.

References

[1] Ogawa R., Yoshitatsu S., Yoshida K., Miyashita T. Is radiation therapy for keloids acceptable? The risk of radiation-induced carcinogenesis. *Plast Reconstr Surg.* 2009 Oct;124(4):1196-201.

[2] Ogawa R. The most current algorithms for the treatment and prevention of hypertrophic scars and keloids. *Plast Reconstr Surg.* 2010 Feb;125(2):557-68.

[3] Ogawa R. Current Keloid and Hypertrophic Scar Treatment Algorithms and Our Recent Trials. *Journal of Wound Technology* 15: 28-29, 2012.

[4] Kal H. B., Veen R. E. Biologically effective doses of postoperative radiotherapy in the prevention of keloids. Dose-effect relationship. *Strahlenther Onkol.* 2005 Nov;181(11): 717-23.

[5] Kal H. B., Veen R. E., Jürgenliemk-Schulz I. M. Dose-effect relationships for recurrence of keloid and pterygium after surgery and radiotherapy. *Int J Radiat Oncol Biol Phys.* 2009 May 1;74(1):245-51.

[6] Leer J. W., van Houtte P., Davelaar J. Indications and treatment schedules for irradiation of benign diseases: a survey. *Radiother Oncol.* 1998 Sep;48(3):249-57.

[7] Ogawa R., Miyashita T., Hyakusoku H., Akaishi S., Kuribayashi S., Tateno A. Postoperative radiation protocol for keloids and hypertrophic scars: statistical analysis of 370 sites followed for over 18 months. *Ann Plast Surg.* 2007 Dec;59(6):688-91.

[8] ICRP 2007 Recommendations of the International Commission on Radiological Protection ICRP Publication 103; *Ann.* ICRP 37: 2–4, 2007.

[9] Horton, C. E., Crawford, J., Oakey, R. S. Malignant change in keloids. *Plast Reconstr Surg.* 12: 86-89, 1953.

[10] Leer, J. W., van Houtte, P., Seegenschmiedt, H. Radiotherapy of non-malignant disorders: where do we stand? *Radiother Oncol.* 83: 175-177, 2007.

[11] Lundell, M., Hakulinen, T., Holm, L. E.: Thyroid cancer after radiotherapy for skin hemangioma in infancy. *Radiat Res.* 140: 334-339, 1994.

[12] Lundell M., Mattsson A., Hakulinen T., Holm L. E. Breast cancer after radiotherapy for skin hemangioma in infancy. *Radiat Res.* 1996 Feb; 145(2):225-30.

[13] Preston D. L., Ron E. et al. Solid cancer incidence in atomic bomb survivors: 1958-1998. *Radiation Research* 2007; 168:1-64.

In: Scars and Scarring
Editor: Yongsoo Lee

ISBN: 978-1-62808-005-6
© 2013 Nova Science Publishers, Inc.

Chapter 8

Surgical Therapy for Scars

Rei Ogawa[*]
Department of Plastic, Reconstructive and Aesthetic Surgery,
Nippon Medical School, Tokyo, Japan

Abstract

There are two purposes of surgical scar revision, namely, to improve the aesthetic appearance and to restore function. The choice of surgical method depends on whether scar contractures (especially joint contractures) are present. If they are, surgical approaches that release contractures (tension) should be performed. These include z-plasties, w-plasties, skin grafts, and skin flaps. There are two types of scar contractures, namely, linear contractures and broad-band contractures. In the case of linear contractures, healthy skin is available, and thus z-plasty or w-plasty are sufficient for the reconstruction. However, in broad-band contractures, healthy skin is lacking and skin grafting or skin flaps should be transferred from different areas. Another issue when planning surgical scar revision is genetic predisposition or systemic factors. Various genetic, systemic and local factors influence the quality and quantity of scars. Mature scars, atrophic scars and pathological scars (heavy scars) such as hypertrophic scars and keloids result from such factors. Thus, radiation or corticosteroid adjuvant therapies should be added if the patient bears risk factors that promote the development of heavy scars.

Introduction

There are two purposes of surgical scar revision, namely, to improve the aesthetic appearance and to restore function. The choice of surgical method depends on whether scar contractures (especially joint contractures) are present. If they are, surgical approaches that

---

[*] Address correspondence to: Rei Ogawa, M. D., Ph.D., F. A. C. S., Department of Plastic, Reconstructive and Aesthetic Surgery, Nippon Medical School, 1-1-5 Sendagi Bunkyo-ku, Tokyo 113-8603, Japan. Tel: +81-3-5814-6208. Fax: +81-3-5685-3076. E-Mail: r.ogawa@nms.ac.jp.

release contractures (tension) should be performed. These include z-plasties, w-plasties, skin grafts, and skin flaps. There are two types of scar contractures, namely, linear contractures and broad-band contractures. In the case of linear contractures, healthy skin is available, and thus z-plasty or w-plasty are sufficient for the reconstruction. However, in broad-band contractures, healthy skin is lacking and skin grafting or skin flaps should be transferred from different areas.

Another issue when planning surgical scar revision is genetic predisposition or systemic factors. Various genetic, systemic and local factors influence the quality and quantity of scars. Mature scars, atrophic scars and pathological scars (heavy scars) such as hypertrophic scars and keloids result from such factors. Thus, radiation or corticosteroid adjuvant therapies should be added if the patient bears risk factors that promote the development of heavy scars.

Incision Lines

To generate invisible scars, it is important to decide the direction of incision. The Langer line, wrinkle (Kraissl) line, and Borges' relaxed skin tension line (RSTL) are well-known lines that are used to indicate the direction of sutures. However, since the wrinkle line and RSTL have both advantages and disadvantages, the choice regarding the incision line should be made on a case-by-case basis. For example, the wrinkle line and RSTL match on the limbs and trunk but not on the face. Moreover, the situation will differ depending on the size of excised tissues. Thus, the following suture indications are recommended:

1. Forehead: transverse incision according to the wrinkle of the forehead
2. Periorbital and perioral regions: circular incision according to the orbicular muscles
3. Cheek: incisions that are horizontal to the nasolabial line
4. Lower jaw: incisions that are horizontal to the jawline (the line between the ear and the medial mandible region)
5. Neck: transverse lines
6. Shoulder, elbow, wrist, inguinal, knee, ankle, finger, toe joints of limbs: the short axis that is horizontal to the wrinkle of the joints (the joint must not be sutured straight according to the long axis)
7. Regions between joints on limbs: this must be assessed on a case-by-case basis
8. Trunk: transverse lines but vertical lines in the case of the just mid line

Moreover, the contour lines on the border of noticeable structures are important. These include the border of the hairy region and the forehead, and the border of the nose and cheek. These borders can serve as incision lines.

Tension Reduction Sutures

Since heavy scars arise from the dermis, eliminating mechanical forces on the dermis can reduce the risk of pathological scar formation after surgery. In general surgery (e.g., cardiac, abdominal, and gynecological surgery), the epidermis and dermis tend to be sutured together after subcutaneous sutures have been placed. By contrast, three-layered sutures consisting of separate subcutaneous/dermal/superficial sutures are used in plastic surgery: these sutures clearly decrease the risk of hypertrophic scars. Hypertrophic scars occur frequently on particular sites, including the anterior chest wall after cardiac surgery, the abdomen after abdominal surgery, the suprapubic region after gynecological surgery, and the shoulder/thigh after orthopedic surgery. These sites all share the fact that they are frequently subjected to cyclical skin stretching caused by the natural daily movements of the body. Since three-layered sutures reduce tension to some degree, it may be possible to prevent mild hypertrophic scars from developing by using this technique.

However, further modifications of suture techniques are needed to prevent the development of severe pathological scars such as keloids because even three-layered sutures place tension on the dermis. Consequently, we use subcutaneous/fascial tensile reduction sutures, where the tension is placed on the layer of the deep fascia and superficial fascia [1]. This minimizes the use of dermal sutures. Indeed, dermal sutures can be avoided altogether if the wound edges can be joined naturally under very small tension. We prefer 0 or 2-0 PDSII® (Ethicon Japan, Tokyo) or 3-0 PDSII® for the subcutaneous/fascial sutures, 4-0 or 5-0 PDSII® for dermal sutures (if they are necessary), and 6-0 or 7-0 Proline® or Ethilon (Ethicon Japan, Tokyo) for superficial sutures. The consequence of such suturing is that the wound edges are elevated smoothly with minimal tension on the dermis. This appears to prevent the development of large scars.

Sometimes, after suturing, there are small nodules under the skin that can be sensed when the wound surface is touched. These are likely to reflect surgical damage to the dermis. We have noticed that pathological scars tend to recur from these nodules: indeed, keloid recurrence usually starts from the suture marks rather than the sutured surfaces. Therefore, we ensure that we do not nick the dermal layer during surgery.

Z-Plasty

Z-plasty, multiple z-plasties, and planimetric z-plasty are good for releasing linear scar contractures. A few z-plasties should be used for long scars (multiple z-plasties) and planimetric z-plasty should be used for relatively wide scars that cannot be excised and closed primarily. A major benefit of z-plasties is that segmented scars mature faster than long scars (Figure 1). The biggest advantage of z-plasties is that the direct separation force on the incision is 100% of that of the direct separation force in the RSTL direction [2].

Z-plasty has four advantages. First, it releases contractures. Second, shortened skin can be elongated. Third, three-dimensional reconstruction can be performed on an uneven surface. Fourth, structures, including triangular flaps, can be transposed. A disadvantage is that the blood flow in the corner of triangular flaps may be decreased and flaps may develop epithelial necrosis if the flap is designed on the scar or the angle of the corner of triangle flaps is too narrow. Special attention and tips about how not to make narrow angle flaps are needed. Another disadvantage of the z-plasty is that it leaves a geometric scar. Geometric scars may be an aesthetic problem if the z-plasty is used in an inappropriate region.

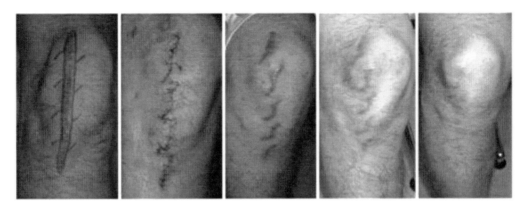

Figure 1. Correction of a segmented linear scar by using multiple z-plasties. The scar had disappeared almost completely 1 year after surgery.

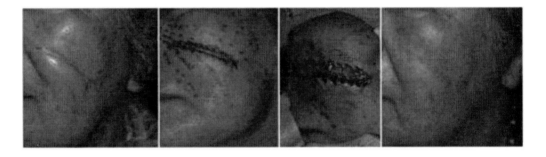

Figure 2. Reconstruction of a trap door deformity by using w-plasty. The depressed scars had disappeared almost completely 6 months after surgery.

W-Plasty

The W-plasty consists of segments less than 5 mm long that are arranged in a zig-zag pattern. W-plasty is especially good for the face (Figure 2). It has both accordion and broken line effects. The accordion effect relates to the fact that linear scars that are reconstructed by w-plasty will expand little by little after surgery and the contracture will be released naturally. The broken line effect is that the regular irregularity of the scar after w-plasty makes the scar less noticeable than a linear scar would be. However, a disadvantage of w-plasty is that healthy skin adjacent to the scar must be excised. Thus, it is not suitable for relatively wide scars.

Skin Grafting

Skin grafting is an established and commonly used method to release scar contractures or replace scar tissues with normal skin (Figure 3). It is important to adjust the thickness of the flap and ensure appropriate donor site selection. A full thickness skin graft should be the first choice for scar contracture release because partial thickness skin grafts tend to result in secondary contractures. The shape of the recipient site is also important: it should not be circular; rather, it should have a zig-zag shape because secondary contractures occur easily on circular recipient sites.

To fix grafted skin, tie-over fixation is the standard method. External wire frame fixation also has some advantages (Figure 4), as follows. First, it secures the graft to the wound bed. Second, it prevents the graft edges from lifting. Third, it is useful for regions that have a free margin (e.g., eyelid grafts) as it overcomes the disadvantages of tarsorrhaphy. Fourth, the digital joints do not need to be fixed by pinning, which is particularly useful when grafting the palmar surfaces of fingers [3]. This method is performed as follows. A wire frame consisting of 1.0 mm-diameter Kirschner wire is first made in the shape of the graft itself. The skin graft is then fixed with sutures and the wire is attached to the edges of the graft with these sutures. Tie-over fixation is performed in the usual way. The skin graft then covers the entire site, even if it involves application to a free edge.

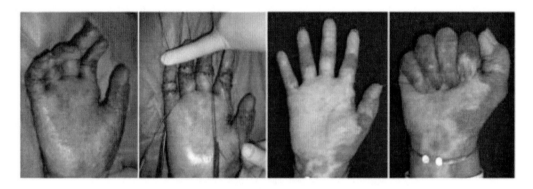

Figure 3. Reconstruction of digital joints with contractures by using full thickness skin grafts. The range of motion had improved markedly 6 months after surgery.

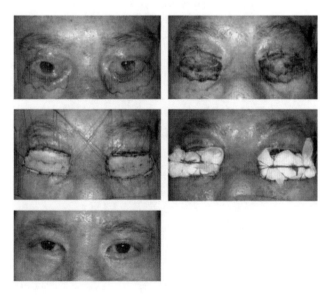

Figure 4. External wire frame fixation for skin grafting. This patient could open and close his eyes even after tie-over fixation had been performed.

Skin Flaps

Various local flaps are useful for releasing scar contractures. They are also important for preventing contractures because skin flaps expand naturally after surgery, unlike skin grafts (Figure 5) [4].

It has been thought that keloids generally should not be reconstructed by skin grafts or flaps because the donor site will be at risk of developing a keloid. However, the recent development of safer postoperative adjuvant radiation therapy has encouraged the use of various flaps to reconstruct keloids [1, 5]. Keloids can be treated surgically in two ways: they can either be radically resected or undergo mass reduction. For both approaches, skin grafting or flap transfer with postoperative radiotherapy may be required if the keloid is difficult to excise completely and suture directly. However, two problems are associated with skin grafting, namely, keloid recurrence at the margins of the skin graft and depigmentation of the center of the skin graft. Computer simulation studies have suggested that the tension on the edge of the keloid will be reduced if there is soft tissue under the keloid (data not shown). Therefore, to reduce the tension on the flap used to reconstruct keloids, skin flaps with fat under the skin may be effective. In particular, since perforator flaps (especially the perforator pedicled propeller flap) are associated with little donor site morbidity, such flaps are suitable for reconstructing huge keloids (Figure 6).

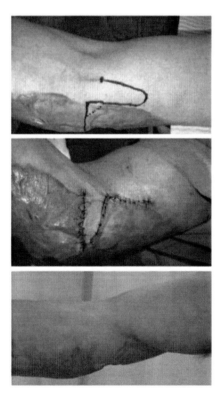

Figure 5. Reconstruction of an elbow joint with contractures by using a transposition flap. The width of the flap widened dramatically after surgery and the contracture had been released completely 6 months after surgery.

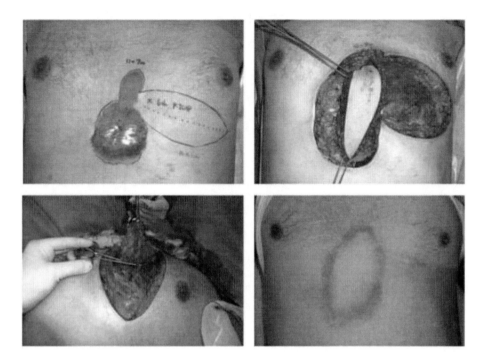

Figure 6. Reconstruction of a keloid by using a perforator pedicled propeller flap. Since the width of the flap can expand after surgery, flap surgery is ideal for releasing tension. However, special attention should be paid to donor site selection.

References

[1] Ogawa R., Akaishi S., Huang C., Dohi T., Aoki M., Omori Y., Koike S., Kobe K., Akimoto M., Hyakusoku H. Clinical applications of basic research that shows reducing skin tension could prevent and treat abnormal scarring: the importance of fascial/subcutaneous tensile reduction sutures and flap surgery for keloid and hypertrophic scar reconstruction. *J Nippon Med Sch.* 2011;78(2):68-76.

[2] Huang C., Ono S., Hyakusoku H, Ogawa R. Small-wave incision method for linear hypertrophic scar reconstruction: a parallel-group randomized controlled study. *Aesthetic Plast Surg.* 2012 Apr;36(2):387-95.

[3] Ogawa R., Hyakusoku H., Ono S. Useful tips for successful skin grafting. *J Nippon Med Sch.* 2007 Dec;74(6):386-92.

[4] Ogawa R., Hyakusoku H. Effectiveness of Super-thin Flaps in Burn Reconstructive Surgery. *Journal of Wound Technology* 15: 67-68, 2012.

[5] Dohi T., Akaishi S., Ono S., Nara S., Iimura T., Hyakusoku H, Ogawa R. Flap Surgery for Severe Keloids: Our Trials of Flap Surgery Performed For the Purpose of Tension Reduction. *Journal of Wound Technology* 15: 92, 2012.

In: Scars and Scarring
Editor: Yongsoo Lee

ISBN: 978-1-62808-005-6
© 2013 Nova Science Publishers, Inc.

Chapter 9

Non/minimally Invasive Treatment Options

Jennifer Ledon[1]*, Jessica Savas[1], Katlein Franca[1], Anna Chacon[1], Yongsoo Lee[2] and Keyvan Nouri[3]

[1]University of Miami Leonard M. Miller School of Medicine,
Department of Dermatology and Cutaneous Surgery
[2]Oracle Dermatology Clinic, Dunsan-dong, Soe-gu, Daejeon, South Korea
[3]Dermatology, Ophthalmology & Otolaryngology
Louis C. Skinner, Jr., M.D. Endowed Chair in Dermatology
Richard Helfman Professor of Dermatologic Surgery
University of Miami Medical Group
Sylvester Comprehensive Cancer Center/University of Miami Hospital and Clinics
Mohs, Dermatologic & Laser Surgery
Surgical Training
Department of Dermatology & Cutaneous Surgery
University of Miami Leonard M. Miller School of Medicine
Sylvester Comprehensive Cancer Center, Mohs/Laser Unit
Miami, FL, USA

Abstract

As dermatologic procedures become more advanced and patients become more and more time constricted due to busy schedules and fast-paced living, the need for non- or minimally invasive treatment modalities is growing. Patients are no longer able to devote days and weeks to the recovery process required of certain more invasive options. Scarring, however, is still a psychologically and physically debilitating problem that requires safe and effective treatment. Several non- or minimally invasive treatment options for all kinds of scars exist, including but not limited to topical therapies, cryosurgery, microdermabrasion, chemical peels, microneedling, intralesional agents and

---

* JLedon1@med.miami.edu.

fillers. When treating patients for scars, moreover, it is important to communicate the expectations of both physician and patient, as these modalities may be better for certain types of scars over others and although non- or minimally invasive, there are certain side effects associated with each. Complete resolution of all scars is also unlikely. In this situation, techniques to help camouflage scars are helpful to have in one's armamentarium. This chapter will address many of the currently available non/minimally invasive treatment options for scars in addition to their indications, relative efficacy, cost and side effect profiles in order for physicians to make more appropriate therapeutic decisions when treating a patient with scars.

Introduction

As dermatologic procedures become more advanced and patients become more and more time constricted due to busy schedules and fast-paced living, the need for non- or minimally invasive treatment modalities is growing. Patients are no longer able to devote days and weeks to the recovery process required of certain more invasive options. Scarring, however, is still a psychologically and physically debilitating problem that requires safe and effective treatment. Several non- or minimally invasive treatment options for all kinds of scars exist, including but not limited to topical therapies, cryosurgery, microdermabrasion, chemical peels, microneedling, intralesional agents and fillers. When treating patients for scars, moreover, it is important to communicate the expectations of both physician and patient, as these modalities may be better for certain types of scars over others and although non- or minimally invasive, there are certain side effects associated with each. Complete resolution of all scars is also unlikely. In this situation, techniques to help camouflage scars are helpful to have in one's armamentarium. This chapter will address many of the currently available non/minimally invasive treatment options for scars in addition to their indications, relative efficacy, cost and side effect profiles in order for physicians to make more appropriate therapeutic decisions when treating a patient with scars.

Topical Therapies

Topical therapies for scars are ideal for both physicians and patients due to their ease-of-use, widespread availability, and relatively low cost. While a myriad of topical therapies have been tried, pressure therapy, silicone sheeting, onion-extract gels, topical vitamin preparations, imiquimod cream and topical corticosteroids are the most common modalities.

Indications

Topical therapies may be potentially used for all kinds of scars, yet they have been found to be more effective in reducing and preventing hypertrophic scars and keloids. Patients who are highly averse to other more invasive options, albeit still minimal, may be better candidates for topical therapy. Atrophic or depressed scars are not typically treated with topical agents.

Pressure Therapy

Despite a lack of evidence supporting its efficacy, pressure dressings are common in the prevention and minimization of hypertrophic scars and keloids. [1] The hypoxic environment created by continuous pressure is thought to decrease collagen formation and increase collagen destruction through the induction of enzymes and cytokines that promote extracellular matrix remodeling. [2] Thus, through several mechanisms, including thinning of the dermis, decreased edema, and reduction of blood flow and oxygen through the compression of small vessels, pressure dressings may help prevent wounds from healing abnormally. [3]

Pressure dressings are most appropriately used in the early, active stages of wound healing and scarring, decreasing in effectiveness with scar maturation. These custom-made elastic garments are worn for approximately one year during which dressings are replaced every six to eight weeks. Despite being one of the more inexpensive options for the management of scarring, patients are not always amenable to this form of therapy due to discomfort and inconvenience. The dressings must be worn at all times and are cumbersome in certain anatomic locations, especially those associated with frequent motion, such as flexural areas. Additionally, they carry the potential to cause skin breakdown and ulceration if the pressure is too great or unevenly distributed. Furthermore, there is no consensus on the optimal pressure to achieve maximal efficacy while maintaining minimal adverse effects. It is currently believed that a pressure of 25mm Hg is necessary; however, recent evidence has shown that pressures much less than this have been associated with improved clinical outcomes. [4]

Silicone Elastomer Sheeting

Silicone elastomer (gel) sheeting has been used as a treatment for scars since the early 1980s. [5] The exact mechanism by which silicone sheeting improves hypertrophic scars and keloids is not completely understood, yet it is hypothesized that the effect is a result of occlusion and hydration. Decreases in capillary activity, hyperemia, and fibroblast-induced collagen deposition aid in extracellular matrix remodeling and improvement in the clinical appearance of scars. [6]

Silicone gel sheeting should be applied for 12-24 hours a day (over 2-3 months) to be effective. Daily changing may be required to prevent irritation. [7]

Although large clinical trials supporting the efficacy of silicone sheeting are lacking, several smaller studies have documented its potential benefit in improving the appearance of scars. Silicone gel sheeting may also be beneficial for scar prophylaxis. Clinically, silicone sheeting appears to be an effective means of treating and possibly preventing abnormal scar maturation while posing minimal risk to the patient. Side effects include rash, skin maceration, and pruritis have been reported, however these are more likely if the sheeting is not changed regularly.

Onion Extract

Onion-extract based products can be found over-the-counter and are inexpensive and easy-to-use. While many studies do not show a significant clinical benefit, a recent randomized, double-blinded study showed a statistically significant difference in mean improvement of lesion induration, pigmentation, tenderness, and overall cosmetic appearance when compared to placebo. [8] *Allium cepa*, the active ingredient derived from quercetin, is thought to possess natural anti-inflammatory, antibacterial, and anti-collagenesis properties that may help scar remodeling. [9] Due to its low cost and low risk for adverse effects, onion-extract based gels can be considered for the topical treatment of scars, either as adjunct or monotherapy.

Onion extract has also been combined with heparin and allantoin commercially for the treatment of scars. This product (Contractubex®) has been clinically and experimentally proven to improve scars by inhibiting fibroblast proliferation and downregulating glycosaminoglycan synthesis. [10] In 2006, this preparation was significantly more effective than topical corticosteroids in regards to improving erythema, pruritus and overall consistency of scars. Moreover, there were fewer side effects with faster resolution in Contractubex®-treated versus corticosteroid-treated scars. [11]

Vitamin A

Vitamin A is known to maintain the integrity of mucosal and epithelial surfaces and has therefore been thought to provide some benefit in the prevention and/or treatment of scars. Studies conducted to investigate this theoretical benefit used vitamin A in the form of 0.5% retinoic acid applied daily. This topical therapy reduced the size of the scar as well as improved scar-associated pruritis, softening, flattening, and color. [12] Side effects of vitamin A therapy include the risks for teratogenicity and vitamin toxicity, which may limit its use for this indication.

Vitamin E

Vitamin E is a fat-soluble antioxidant that primarily exerts its effects within the reticular dermis by preventing oxidative damage to DNA, cell membranes, and lipids. It also stabilizes membranes by altering collagen and glycosaminoglycan production as well as inhibiting cellular membrane lipid peroxidation, thus serving as a potential therapy for improving scar appearance. [12] Baumann et al. looked at the improvement in the appearance of scars after topical vitamin E therapy versus a standard emollient. There was no significant difference in cosmetic outcome of new surgical scars treated with topical vitamin E versus placebo groups. Furthermore, a significant number of patients in the vitamin E treated group developed contact dermatitis. [13] Due to its lack of proven efficacy and potential for irritation and scar worsening, topical vitamin E is not recommended for the treatment of scars.

Vitamin D

Vitamin D has been investigated for use in the treatment and prevention of hypertrophic scars due to its anti-inflammatory properties and ability to influence keratinocytes and Langerhans cells, theoretically offering a benefit in wound maturation. However, a recent randomized controlled trial found no difference in scar thickness or the prevalence of hypertrophic scars after treatment with topical calcipotriol (synthetic derivative of vitamin D) when compared to placebo. [14]

Imiquimod 5%

Imiquimod is a topical immunomodulator that stimulates pro-inflammatory cytokines, in particular interferon-α. Interferon-α promotes collagen breakdown and alters the expression of genes involved in apoptosis, possibly preventing keloid recurrence after scar excision. Preliminary studies investigating the efficacy of topical imiquimod for hypertrophic scars and keloids have shown promising results. [15] Side effects are consistent with a local inflammatory response and are characterized by erythema, pain, and pinpoint bleeding. [15]

Non-Steroidal Anti-Inflammatory Drugs (NSAIDs)

Aptly named, NSAIDs are anti-inflammatory agents that function in a mechanism independent of steroids. Animal models evaluating the effect of topical NSAIDs on scar formation found that acetylsalicylic acid (ASA) resulted in a 73% reduction in scar volume, 41% reduction in total cellularity, and 91% reduction in CD3+ T cells when compared to controls. [16] In another animal model, topical celecoxib, a cyclooxygenase-2 (COX-2) inhibitor reduced scar formation without disrupting epithelialization or reducing tensile strength. [17] While these results are promising, clinical trials are necessary to fully assess the efficacy in humans.

Corticosteroids

Intralesional corticosteroid delivery is widely used in the treatment of mature scars; however, corticosteroids are occasionally applied topically, either with or without occlusion in an attempt to achieve the same effect. While associated with fewer adverse effects when compared to intralesional or systemic therapy, topical steroid use has not been shown to be effective. [18] A recent study found that a combination of 0.5% hydrocortisone, silicone, and vitamin E preparation yielded the highest mean percent improvement in almost all scar parameters when compared to an onion-extract based product and placebo. [8] Topical corticosteroid combination preparations therefore may have a role in the treatment of hypertrophic scars and keloids; however it is not recommended as monotherapy.

Risks and Side Effects

Overall risks and side effects of topical therapies for scars are minor and mostly self-limited. Hypersensitivity or allergic reactions to topical agents are always possible. Furthermore, if topical dressings are not changed as recommending, chafing, maceration and pruritis may occur. Each agent carries its own specific side effect profile and should be considered and discussed with patients prior to treatment.

Cryosurgery

Cryosurgery (or cryotherapy, cryoablation) uses very low temperatures to freeze, and subsequently destroy, tissue. The mechanism of this ablation is considered to be osmotic damage with secondary microvascular destructon, blood stasis, ischemia and necrosis. [19] Due to the excessive tissue characteristic of hypertrophic scars or keloids, it has been considered a potential way to reduce these lesions. It has also thought to be more applicable in younger and smaller lesions and in patients with fair skin, as hypopigmentation is a reported side effect. [20] Several sessions are required to achieve maximum efficacy and these should be spaced at least 3-4 weeks apart. [21]

Topical cryotherapy can also be used in conjunction with other treatment modalities, such as intralesional corticosteroids or following surgical excision of the scar. One study looking at the effect of cryotherapy on 166 keloids cited an approximately 80% response rate. [22] Another study of 30 patients, however, reported an overall average reduction of just over 30%. [20] Unfortunately, most reports evaluating the value of cryosurgery are comprised of small patient populations. Larger controlled studies are needed before blanket statements on efficacy can be made.

Indications

Topical cryotherapy is mostly indicated for scars with features of excessive tissue formation such as hypertrophic scars and keloids, however this may also apply to burn and traumatic scars. The latter may be especially true in children as young skin is more prone to scarring even with minor injury. [21]

Risks and Side Effects

One of the most common side effects of topical cryotherapy is either permanent or temporary hypopigmentation. This is especially more common in darker skinned individuals, the same group most prone to develop hypertrophic scars and keloids. Additional side effects include atrophy, pain, and superficial necrosis.

Intralesional Cryotherapy

Due to clinical improvement seen in some scars following topical cryotherapy, it has been suggested that intralesional cryotherapy may be more efficacious in larger, bulkier scars. Weshahy first attempted an intralesional application of cryosurgery in 1993 with the use of cryosurgery needles. [23] By directly targeting the deeper layers of keloids and hypertrophic scars with extreme cold, intralesional cryotherapy can reduce the number of fibroblasts and mast cells and thus change collagen structure to a more normal organization. [24]

The clinical efficacy of intralesional cryotherapy has ranged from 20 to greater than 75% scar volume reduction. [25-28] Reported side effects include pain, edema, mild epidermolysis and temporary hypopigmentation, however pain may be less than that in contact cryotherapy. [26,29] Due to thermal conductivity, the tissue temperature, as a function of the distance from the cryoneedle, is radially reduced and therefore skin surface is relatively warmer and the end temperature is significantly higher than with the contact cryotechnique, thus sparing melanocyte destruction and explaining the reduced incidence of hypopigmentation. [30]

Cost

Cryotherapy is a very inexpensive treatment modality for scars, even considering the need for multiple treatment sessions. One liter of liquid nitrogen may cost anywhere from $0.06 to $1.50. [31] Furthermore, one refillable cryogen spray device retails for about $700-900.

Microdermabrasion

Dermabrasion is an invasive technique that is aimed at physically removing the epidermis and creating a mid-dermal wound. Originally utilizing wire brushes, sandpaper or diamond fraise, dermabrasion was dangerous to both patient and physician. This process has been refined over the years to reduce bleeding and implantation of foreign particles, however the modality still requires significant healing time and is associated with increased risks. Microdermabrasion was created as an attempt to achieve the same efficacy found with dermabrasion, however without the severe trauma and lengthy recovery period required of its predecessor.

Microdermabrasion works by using inert crystals, typically aluminum oxide or sodium chloride, to exfoliate the skin. A controlled, compressed air source projects the crystals onto the skin causing detachment of the most superficial cells. Prior to treating scars with microdermabrasion, the area should be cleaned with soap and water. Facial units should be treated one at a time and a greater depth of penetration can be achieved by increasing the number of passes, increasing particle size, or increasing particle speed. The amount of exfoliation is similar to that of a chemical peel but not nearly as dramatic as an ablative laser. [32]

Improvement has been attributed to basal cell stimulation, normalization of cell layers, and redistribution of melanosomes. [33]

Indications

Microdermabrasion can be used for acne, trauma, burn, and pox scars yet efficacy is variable. [32,34] It is best for superficial scars, yet can improve the appearance of deep scars. Ice pick scars do not normally show improvement, nor is microdermabrasion effective for keloids. It is generally considered a "no down-time" procedure and can be used in all skin types. [35]

Blome-Eberwein and colleagues used microdermabrasion for split-thickness skin graft scars in an attempt to eliminate the mesh-like pattern characteristic of these lesions. [36] Multiple sessions were administered, with a non-significant improvement in function, thickness and elasticity.

Risks and Side Effects

Erythema, photo and general sensitivity, and pigmentary changes may occur after microdermabrasion, yet side effects in general are not common. Herpes Simplex Virus reactivation may occur in susceptible patients if treating around the mouth. With a history of recurrent herpes infections around the mouth, prophylactic anti-virals should be administered.

Subcision (Subcutaneous Incisionless Surgery)

Subcision is the method of cutting under a depressed scar or wrinkle using a tri-beveled hypodermic needle inserted under the skin through a needle puncture. [53] The effectiveness of subcision for correcting various types of skin depressions depends on two distinct phenomena. First, the act of surgically releasing the skin from its attachment to deeper tissues results in skin elevation. Second, the introduction of a controlled trauma initiates wound healing, with consequent formation of connective tissue that augments the depressed site. [53-57] This procedure also produces a pooling of blood under the defect. The blood acts as a spacer, keeping the scar base from immediately reattaching to the surface layers. The subsequent organization of this blood clot induces a longer-term correction, by the formation of connective tissue. [58,59]

Subcision can be useful when the subdermal tethering precludes treatment from the skin surface and correction of the subdermal component is essential for treatment success. This can be obtained by reaching depths below that reached with conventional skin resurfacing options. [54,59]

Practical Tips

- Extended release cefaclor 375 mg (twice a day for 5 days) can be prescribed on the day of subcision.

- Mark the area of concern and anesthetize with topical anesthetic cream for over 30 minutes before subcutaneous anesthetic (1% lidocaine with epinephrine 1:100,000) administration. [59]
- Use an 18-guage Nokor needle mounted on a 1ml syringe, filled with 1% lidocaine and epinephrine 1:100,000. A 1ml-syringe is preferred to a 3ml-syringe because the slimmer barrel allows the needle to assume a more horizontal position (parallel to the skin) than does a 3ml-syringe. This position is better for avoiding penetration into deeper structures (large blood vessels or nerves) and allows the release of tethers that are more superficially located. [59]
- Needle holders can be used to ensure the horizontal position of the triangular tip of the Norkor needle. [56] However, if you use a syringe filled with lidocaine, additional anesthesia into the spot where the patient feels pain is possible without interrupting the procedure. [59]
- The tip of the Norkor needle can be kept horizontal by mounting it parallel to the finger bars of the syringe. In this way, the position of the triangular tip remains visible, even when the tip is inserted into the tissue, thus avoiding unnecessary pulling out and re-penetration of the skin. The position of the summit of the Norkor needle's triangular tip can also be recalled by remembering on which side the gauges are inscribed on the barrel of the syringe. [59]

Chemical Peels

Chemical peels result in accelerated, yet controlled, exfoliation. In this approach, a caustic chemical solution is applied to the skin, leading release of inflammatory mediators and cytokines. This results in thickening of the epidermis, deposition of collagen, reorganization of structural elements, and increases in dermal volume. [37] Depending on the severity of the scarring, several strengths are available. With stronger peels, there is greater chance for both scar improvement and development of adverse effects. The strength of the peel used is also dependent on the nature of the scar, the type of skin and the desired results. Patients with deep scars who do not wish to undergo the more costly, yet efficacious, modalities may opt for repeated peeling sessions in an attempt to reduce the visibility and depth of the scars.

Chemical peels are classified by their depth of action (superficial, medium, or deep). Specific peeling agents should be selected based on the disorder to be treated and used with an appropriate peel depth, determined by the severity of skin pathology, histological level or to maximize success. [38,39] Chemical peels used to treat scars most commonly comprised of glycolic acid, lactic acid, salicylic acid and trichloroacetic acid (TCA).

Indications

Chemical peels are generally used to improve mild acne scars. Deep scars require several treatments and do not achieve complete resolution. Alpha and beta hydroxy acids have been used to improve acne scarring with associated pigmentation. [40] Certain peels are more appropriate than others for certain skin types. Glycolic and lactic acid peels, for example, have been shown to be safe in fair and ethnic skin. [40] Strong, deep peels such as with phenol or high concentrations of trichloroacetic acid are not recommended for darker skin phenotypes.

Glycolic Acid (Superficial)

Glycolic acid (20-70%) is an alpha hydroxy acid commonly used for the treatment of acne scarring with hyperpigmentation, whether or not there is concomitant active acne present. [41] Generally, glycolic acid is more effective in correcting hyperpigmentation than atrophic or hypertrophic scars themselves. In one study, however, repetitive, short-contact, high strength glycolic acid peels showed significant improvement of atrophic scarring. [42] There is no clinical endpoint for glycolic acid peels; the solution is simply left for a specific amount of time.

Lactic Acid (Superficial)

Lactic acid, a mild alpha hydroxy acid, can range in strength from 10% to 92% and is less irritating than glycolic acid. The chemical structure of lactic acid allows it to penetrate the skin slowly and thus reduce treatment-induced inflammation.

Lactic acid peels work by dissolving intercellular desmosomes and thus promoting exfoliation. They are useful in the treatment of superficial scars, albeit with repeated treatments. [40] This type of peel was also shown to be safe in skin types IV-V, even at high concentrations and with repeated sessions. [40]]

Salicylic Acid (Superficial)

Salicylic acid is a beta-hydroxy acid and thus technically weaker than alpha hydroxy acids, but more able to penetrate the skin. Although available in higher percentages, salicylic acid is typically applied in 20% to 30% formulations. [40] It is a hydroxyl derivative of benzoic acid and is a carboxylic acid attached to an aromatic alcohol, phenol. [40,43] Salicylic acid is a lipophilic keratolytic agent and is useful for the treatment of superficial scars. [40,43] The clinical endpoint for salicylic acid peels is the appearance of pseudofrosting.

Trichloroacetic Acid (Medium-depth)

Trichloroacetic acid (TCA) is a synthetically derived peeling agent made of acetic acid and chlorine. Percentages range from 5 to 100%. The mechanism of action for TCA is considered to be coagulation of proteins and necrosis of the cells. In higher concentrations (50 to 100%), it is considered a good method of chemical reconstruction for skin scars. The use of the chemical reconstruction of skin scars, or "CROSS" technique, has been reported as an effective method for the treatment of acne scars. [44] This method consists in a focal application of TCA using a sharpened wooden applicator. It is pressed down firmly over the entire depressed area of the scar, producing multiple, frosted white spots on each acne scar (frosting is considered the clinical endpoint for TCA peels). The recovery period and healing process are faster when this technique is used as opposed to field treatment. [45,46]

Phenol (Deep)

Although deep peels are more likely to correct scarring, they are associated with high risk of side effects and may cause scars themselves. They have been linked to cardiac and renal dysfunction and toxic shock syndrome. [38] While some may argue that they can safely be used for the treatment of scarring, this indication is controversial. [47]

Risks and Side Effects

Complications such as hyper- or hypopigmentation, erythema, hypertrophic and keloid scars, infections, and milia may occur. [38] Alpha hydroxy acid peels, such as glycolic and lactic acid, may result in mild skin irritation, erythema, and dryness but are generally considered safe when used properly. With stronger peels, however, these risks are greater, and should they occur, are very disabling to patients.

Microneedling

Microneedling, or collagen induction therapy, is a procedure in which several micro needles arranged on a cylindrical instrument are passed over the skin. Penetration of the needles into the dermis effectively stimulates neocollagenesis. It is recommended to wait at least six weeks between treatments to allow new collagen to form. [48] The most common device used by dermatologists is the dermaroller, yet microneedles can be found in a variety of shapes and sizes.

Indications

Microneedling can be used for the treatment of most kinds of scars, including acne, traumatic, burn, and surgical scars. It is not the treatment of choice for hypertrophic scars or keloids, however, as the stimulation of new collagen production is counterproductive for these lesions.

Risks and side effects

Side effects are generally minimal and include erythema, stinging, pruritis, and minor peeling, which usually resolve shortly after treatment. [49,50] Tram-tracking, however, or regular patterned scarring, has been reported. [51]

Cost

Microneedling is a simple and inexpensive office procedure, and is safe in all skin types. [49] This procedure can be used in association with other treatments like chemical peels, subcision and microdermabrasion individualized to maximize the benefits to patients. [48,52] Unfortunately, with the use of repeated or combination therapies, this modality becomes more costly.

Intralesional Agents

The majority of intralesional scar therapies are designed to improve the appearance of hypertrophic scars and keloids. Although often considered the same entity, these lesions vary in both appearance and structure. Keloids, for example, may form in already mature scars. Many forms of intralesional therapy are currently available, including but not limited to: steroids, cryotherapy, chemotherapeutic agents and calcium channel blockers. While mechanisms of action may differ for each of these modalities, the ultimate goal is to alter the abnormal cell signaling and proliferation seen in these scars. While some may consider fillers an intralesional therapy, they will be discussed in detailed later in this chapter.

Indications

Intralesional therapies are typically most effective for hypertrophic scars and keloids as the mechanism of action of these therapies are generally targeted at reducing the hyperproliferative collagen formation associated with these lesions. Due to the risk of side effects such as atrophy, ulceration, pain, and dyspigmentation, careful patient, and agent, selection should occur before treatment. Extra care should be taken in darker-skinned individuals, as previously mentioned this population is typically the one most affected by hypertrophic scars.

Corticosteroids

The most commonly utilized intralesional agent for the treatment of hypertrophic scars and keloids, corticosteroids are thought to function by inhibiting fibroblast growth and promoting collagen degradation. [60] Triamcinolone, the most frequently used corticosteroid for this purpose, can be injected into the mid-dermis to avoid scar atrophy. Unfortunately, treatment typically requires many sessions and it is not unusual for patients to prematurely stop treatment secondary to pain. [61]

Atrophy, pain and dyspigmentation are the most common side effects associated with intralesional triamcinolone therapy. Moreover, although rare, systemic effects such as iatrogenic Cushing's syndrome have also been reported. [62] Careful monitoring of total doses as well as placement of the injection can help to prevent some of these effects. A 1:1 mixture of 2% lidocaine and 0.5% bupivacaine can be injected subcutaneously beneath and around the keloid edge prior to treatment, taking care to avoid piercing normal skin and inducing new lesions may help to minimize pain associated steroid administration. [63] Topical lidocaine applications may be of benefit as well. [64]

5-Fluorouracil (5-FU)

In rabbit cell culture, 5-FU was shown to inhibit fibroblast proliferation. In addition, more recently, 5-FU was demonstrated to induce fibroblast apoptosis via G2/M cell cycle arrest without necrosis, a factor to consider in scar prevention. [65,66] Furthermore, 5-FU is known to inhibit transforming growth factor-beta (TGF-beta) signaling in collagen I production, a pathway considered to be responsible in keloid formation. [67]

Although 5–FU is typically used for scars refractive to triamcinolone therapy, there is a paucity of studies directly comparing the two modalities. Success rates with 5-FU are variable, however greater improvement is typically seen in younger scars. [68] Pain and hyperpigmentation are common side effects. [66,68,69]

Bleomycin

Bodokh and Brun first studied the effects of intralesional bleomycin on keloid or hypertrophic scars in 1996. [70] In this study, 36 scars were treated with 3-5 sessions of intralesional bleomycin with total scar regression in 80% of lesions. Results of this study subsequently led to several studies evaluating the effect of bleomycin for scars. Overall, complete or significant scar flattening has been reported in 66 to 100% of lesions. [71-73] Furthermore, bleomycin was found to be better than combination cryotherapy and intralesional triamcinolone for lesions greater than 100mm^2. [72-74]

Local administration of bleomycin, in low doses, is considered safe in human skin and not associated with systemic effects despite causing DNA damage similar to that following X-irradiation. [75,76] At the cellular level, intralesional bleomycin results in dyskeratosis and reduced collagen synthesis by fibroblasts. [76,77]

Verapamil

Several mechanisms have been implicated for verapamil's role in the improvement of keloid or hypertrophic scars. Calcium antagonists have been shown to reduce extracellular matrix production, induce fibroblast procollagenase synthesis, and inhibit interleukin-6, vascular endothelial growth factor and cellular proliferation of fibroblasts. [78-80] In addition, quantities of decorin may be decreased in hypertrophic and keloid scars. Verapamil, a calcium channel blocker, has been shown in augment decorin expression in animal models. [81] Verapamil was also shown to inhibit proliferation of and TGF-beta1 expression in fibroblasts, as well as induce apoptosis. [82] Clinically, verapamil has shown to be of benefit following surgical excision of hypertrophic and keloidal scars. [83-85] In a head-to-head analysis with triamcinolone, although both improved the appearance of proliferative scars, verapamil resulted in fewer adverse effects. [86]

Other Agents

Intralesional interferon-alpha 2b, mitomycin C, tumor necrosis factor-alpha (TNF-α), and tacrolimus have also been studied for the improvement of keloidal or hypertrophic scars. Interferons are thought to improve hypertrophic or keloidal scars by inhibition of collagen synthesis by fibroblasts, specifically collagen I and III. [87,88] Interferon-alpha 2 is also known to increase collagenase production. [89] Success with this modality varies, however, and side effects may be systemic and severe, such as flu-like symptoms. [90,91]

Although short-contact topical mitomycin C was found to prevent the reoccurrence of hypertrophic scars or keloids after excision, intralesional mitomycin C may not be as promising as it was found to worsen lesions and cause ulcerations. [92]

In addition, while TNF-α was effective in reducing pruritus associated with scars, intralesional triamcinolone was still more efficacious in scar improvement overall. [93]

Tacrolimus, a macrolide, has been shown to decrease the formations of hypertrophic scars on rabbit ears in a dose-dependent manner. [94] No adverse events were noted at the site of treatment. Histologically, both dermal thickness and dermal cell density were decreased in ears treated with intradermal tacrolimus.

Combination Therapy

Several combinations of therapies for the treatment of scars have been studied. Contact cryotherapy, 5-FU, interferon-alpha 2b, and topical steroids have all been considered as adjuvant therapies to intralesional triamcinolone, with varying success. As mechanisms of action differ for each of these modalities, it may be that targeting different aberrant pathways can lead to greater clinical efficacy.

Risks and Side Effects

Like most other treatment modalities, different intralesional therapies carry a wide range of side effect profiles, depending on the agent. Hyperpigmentation, hypopigmentation, atrophy, ulceration, pain, and flu-like symptoms have all been reported.

Cost

Given the requirement for many sessions, the large size of many lesions, and the tendency for these lesions to recur, intralesional therapy for scars may become costly. When evaluating the cost-effectiveness of intralesional corticosteroids for the treatment of hypertrophic scars and keloids, one study showed that by initially starting with low-dose steroids and then advancing to high-dose steroids in later sessions, treatment is most cost effective with the least risk of recurrence. [95] Cost may also vary depending on geographic location. One group of authors report that the cost of bleomycin is actually less than cryotherapy in Iran and possibly other countries. [96]

Fillers

The use of fillers began over a century ago with the development of autologous fat transplantation. Over time, the use of intradermal or subdermal fillers has evolved to include paraffin and silicone, however paraffin has been abandoned due to high incidence of adverse effects such as granulomatous and foreign body reactions. Silicone for soft tissue augmentation remains controversial. Currently, several fillers are available for the restoration of dermal and subcutaneous tissue loss including, but not limited to, bovine and human collagen, hyaluronic acid derivatives, calcium hydroxyapatite, poly-l-lactic acid, and polymethylmethacrylate. Although not without side effects, these agents may provide a successful and safe modality for improving the appearance of scars.

Indications

Fillers are typically used for atrophic or depressed scars since the fundamental idea behind fillers is to replace lost tissue. While many types of scars can be categorized as atrophic or depressed, fillers work best for scars that have rolling edges or are flattened when stretching adjacent skin. Ice-pick and boxcar scars secondary to varicella infection, for example, are not ideal for this method. Fillers can be used in all skin types.

Collagen (Temporary)

Typically derived from either bovine or human collagen, reconstituted injectable collagen can be injected intradermally to help improve the appearance of depressed or atrophic scars. Due to dense fibrotic stroma associated with ice pick scars or scars with sharp borders, intradermal collagen is ineffective for these lesions and is instead preferred for soft or rolling scars. [97] In general, if the scar flattens when surrounding skin is stretched, intradermal collagen may be helpful in improving the appearance of the scar. [97] This technique is also used when determining if a scar may be amenable to intradermal therapy with several other agents as well.

The short duration of collagen serves as both an advantage and disadvantage. Lasting approximately 3 months, collagen implantation is forgiving should there be operator error or an unexpected reaction as the effects will only be evident for a short period of time. This same fact, on the other hand, requires that patients return regularly for augmentation, which is inconvenient and over time may become very costly. Due to the high absorption of water by collagen soon after treatment, overcorrection by 150-200% is also necessary. [98]

Approximately 5% of population is allergic to or will develop a hypersensitivity to bovine collagen. [98] This therefore requires that patients undergo a skin test prior to treatment. The use of autologous or homologous human-derived collagen does not require a skin test, however, as there is reduced immunogenicity. [99,100] Common side effects include bruising and edema, yet additional side effects such as foreign body or palisading granulomas, sterile abscesses, local necrosis and rarely unilateral or bilateral vision loss due to retinal artery occlusion have been reported. Collagen is not recommended in those who have active inflammation or infection, which may be a problem for those concomitantly suffering from acne. [101]

Hyaluronic Acid (Temporary)

Like collagen, hyaluronic acid is preferred for mild, soft atrophic scarring as opposed to sharply dermarcated depressions or ice-pick scars. Efficacy has also been reported in scars secondary to skin cancer reconstruction, as well as trauma. [102,103] While hyaluronic acid is a temporary filler typically lasts 6-9 months, slightly longer than the 3-6 months expected with collagen fillers, one report notes successful correction of atrophic scarring with hyaluronic acid lasting 2 years after a single treatment. [104] Due to similarity of hyaluronic acid in all species, unlike with collagen, a skin test is not necessary prior to use. [98,105]

Despite the similarity of hyaluronic acid between species, however, hypersensitivity reactions may still occur. Rare foreign body granulomas, angioedema, and herpes simplex virus reactivation have all been reported. [105-107] Furthermore, a bluish discoloration in treated areas may be appreciated. This phenomenon, known as the Tyndall effect, occurs as a result of light scattering through clear filler, such as hyaluronic acid. [108] Care should be taken in areas of thin fragile skin, such as around the eyes and in elderly and fair skin. Hyaluronic acid should also not be injected too superficially, although properly placed filler may still migrate. Correction of the bluish discoloration can be made with simple surgical extraction, the use of hyaluronidase, or the 1064 nm Nd: YAG laser. [108-110]

Poly-l-lactic Acid (Semi-Permanent)

Poly-l-lactic acid, the l-isomer of polylactic acid, is currently FDA approved for the treatment of facial lipoatrophy in patients Human Immunodeficiency Virus (HIV) yet can be used for deep dermal scars and tunnels, as well as large atrophic scars and lipoatrophy secondary to acne. [111,112] Like other fillers, the greatest effect can be seen in scars that are corrected when the surrounding skin is stretched; ice-pick and boxcar scars are more resistant to treatment. Considered a semi-permanent filler, poly-l-lactic acid can last approximately 1.5 to 2 years. Although efficacy may be attributed to re-volumization of depressed or atrophic scars, Beer proposes that efficacy may also be secondary to subscision of the scar as well as neocollegenesis. [113] Over-correction is not necessary.

The most common side effect associated with poly-l-lactic acid is the formation of nodules at the site of treatment. These may or may not be visually appreciated, but are almost always palpable. This may be avoided with proper dilution as cases of nodule formation are more common with more concentrated formulations. [114] Even with proper dilution, if nodules do develop, surgical excision is the best option for resolution. [115]

Calcium Hydroxylapatite (Semi-Permanent)

Calcium hydroxylapatite is the heaviest of all dermal fillers and thus can be used for moderate to severe, rolling depressions. Goldberg and colleagues found a moderate improvement of these types of scars with no improvement in ice-pick scars. [116] Injected into the mid to deep dermis, in the subcutaneous fat, or in the dermal-subcutaneous junction, calcium hydroxyapatite does not typically migrate and its synthetic nature lends itself to reduce immunogenicity. [98,116] The use of calcium hydroxylapatite, furthermore, is safe in darker skin types with no keloid formation, hypertrophic scars or dyspigmentation noted. [117]

After initially adding volume to depressed scars, calcium hydroxylapatite is then engulfed by phagocytic cells leading to the formation of new collagen. Care around delicate areas such as the lips and perioral areas as nodules are more likely to develop in these areas. [118] Should nodules develop, however, they may be removed by surgical excision or ameliorated with fractional ablative laser therapy. [119] For scarring, subcision of the scar should be performed first following by filling of the defect; it is not necessary to over-correct. While reported to last up to five years, one may reasonably expect an effect for approximately 2 years. [118,120]

Silicone (Permanent)

Injectable silicone is available in oil or gel form and results in permanent soft tissue augmentation. Due to the high risk of migration and granuloma formation, silicone for the improvement of scars and other cosmetic procedures has fallen out of favor. Many physicians argue, however, that silicone can be a viable option for improvement of depressed and atrophic scars because the adverse events associated with silicone use are due to operator error and inexperience. Silicone, for example, should not be used to augment inflexible scars, such as ice-pick scars, since migration is more likely. Furthermore, patients who suffer multiple allergies or inflammatory/autoimmune syndromes should not be treated with silicone. [121]

A microdroplet, multiple injection approach is recommended when treating broad-based acne scars with silicone. [122] It is important to only inject minimal amounts of filler into the deep dermis at each session to prevent migration; overcorrection should be avoided. While this may require more treatment sessions in order to achieve the desired result, this is preferred over creating permanent, unwanted effects. Sessions should be spaced at least one month apart to allow for stabilization of the scar. [122] Side effects associated with silicone include foreign body granuloma formation, rosacea-like eruptions, pigmentary changes and rare reports of necrosis. [121]

Polymethylmethacrylate (PMMA; Permanent)

PMMA is the most preferred of the permanent soft tissue fillers currently available for the treatment of depressed or atrophic scars. Combined with bovine collagen and lidocaine, PMMA solution corrects defects by first re-volumizing the area and then serving as a scaffold for new collagen production over time. [120] It is theorized that due to the decreased electrostatic charge, PMMA is less prone to cause foreign body granulomas. [123] Skin testing prior to use is required, however, due to the bovine collagen present in the solution.

One pilot study assessing the efficacy of PMMA for the correction of atrophic scars secondary to acne found that nearly all treated scars showed some level of improvement eight months after treatment. [124] Although side effects associated with PMMA include granuloma formation and hypersensitivity reactions, this study did not report any adverse events. Granulomas that do appear after the use of PMMA may appear white under the skin. While it has been reported that these granulomas may disappear spontaneously after 2-3 years, steroids, surgical excision or superficial dermabrasion is generally recommended. [120]

Autologous Fat (Variable)

The use of autologous fat for the correction of atrophic or depressed scars is appealing to physicians and patients due to the fact there is reduced concern for immunogenicity. Patients also are drawn to the fact that fat may be harvested and stored when undergoing a separate cosmetic procedure, such as liposuction. Autologous fat transplantation is the oldest of all the filler modalities and is typically used for severe, diffuse atrophic scarring.

Unfortunately, however, the longevity of autologous fat transplantation is unpredictable. Although attempts have been made to identify the factors that may help physicians better predict duration, there are still no definitive guidelines. It has been proposed that the handling of the fat during harvesting, as well as the quality of the fat, such as whether or not the fat was subjected to a prior cosmetic procedure like liposuction, plays a role in the durability of the transplant. [98] Autologous fat fillers may be permanent or last only 6 months.

Due to the fact that there is reabsorption of the new fat, overcorrection is suggested. Furthermore, fat transplants should be placed in the subdermis. Should the effect be permanent, however, overcorrection and placement may pose a problem. In addition to the side effects with the use of fillers for scars in general, the added risks of using autologous fat include depressions/defects in the donor site, clumping and infection.

Risks and Side Effects

Aside from the possible adverse events listed with each of the therapies listed above, several side effects are known to all fillers, the most dangerous of which is ischemic necrosis. Either secondary to direct injection of fillers into vascular lumen, or outside compression, ischemic necrosis is not as rare as one would like to believe. The glabellar region is the most commonly affected and knowledge of facial vasculature is critical. Also, certain clues may warn a physician that vascular compromise may have occurred. If there is prolonged blanching or duskiness of the skin immediately after injection, the area should be massaged with warm compresses to help restore blood flow. Topical vasodilator therapy may also help. [125] Hyaluronidase may also be used to dissolve hyaluronic acid.

Cost

Due to the temporary nature of most fillers and thus the need for frequent re-treatment, fillers for the treatment of atrophic or depressed scars can become costly. In terms of duration of treatment and cost per session, silicone is the least expensive of all fillers both per session and overall due to its permanency. Patients may opt, however, to pay the additional cost required of temporary fillers such as hyaluronic acid in order to have the security that should an error occur, the effects are reversible. Over time, and with confidence in the expertise of the physician, patients may opt to undergo more permanent options. The most expensive of the fillers currently available is estimated to be autologous fat transplantation, due to the additional processing required, and PMMA, due to its permanency and need for fewer overall treatment sessions.

Techniques to Camouflage Scars

Unfortunately, despite both the patient's and physician's best efforts, certain scars may not fully resolve with non- or minimally invasive treatment options. If patients are not willing to or cannot undergo more invasive options to improve the appearance of their scars, yet still find them unsightly, there are techniques to help camouflage or cover them.

Many people are aware that make-up can be used to help cover scars, yet they do not know the techniques used to help them look natural. Many patients complain that the amount of make-up necessary to cover acne scars, for example, makes the foundation appear caked-on or just causes more break-outs leading to more scarring. It is important to pick a high quality foundation, therefore, that is non-comedogenic. Unfortunately, these may be a little more costly than brands found in local drug stores. The investment, however, is worthwhile. Clinique™ (Clinique Laboratories LLC) carries a line "Acne Solutions" that is not only comedogenic, but also contains salicylic acid to help treat and prevent breakouts. It is also important to understand the differences in types of make-up and what they are most appropriate for. These steps may help when applying make-up to cover diffuse mild scarring on the face, such as with acne:

- Wash and dry both face and hands
- Apply moisturizer with sunscreen
- Apply foundation to the entire face. The color of the foundation should either match the skin or be one shade *lighter*. Make-up salespeople can help with this. Be sure to blend into hairline and down neck.

- Apply concealer under the eyes to help re-create the natural contrast in skin tones that may have been lost after application of foundation. This concealer should be one or two shades *lighter* than the foundation.
- Apply concealer to specific scars or discoloration, being careful to blend into foundation. This should be the *same* shade as the foundation.
- Brushing some setting powder can help cover specific areas and make it easier to blend with the foundation. If your skin is dry or the make-up is thick, avoid applying powder to the entire face.
- If desired, blush and bronzer can be lightly applied to help further re-create the natural contrasts in skin tone. Bronzer should be lightly applied just above the eyebrows, on the cheekbones, and lightly on the chin. This technique is good for those trying to avoiding a monochrome caked-on appearance.

For more severe scarring, or scarring on other areas of the body, professional make-up may be useful. Dermablend™ (L'Oral USA S/D, Inc) offers several products with the goal of achieving coverage for a wide variety of dermatologic conditions. Their Cover Creme products are recommended for scars on the face, neck, and hands as well as for legs and body. The company's website offers tips and instructions for several products.

Lastly, clothing can be utilized to strategically cover certain scarred areas. This simple tip is often forgotten, and while not ideal for every situation, may be an option on certain occasions.

Future Directions

In order to reach FDA approval, investigational agents must prove efficacy and safety in several phases of research. While far from use in everyday clinical practice, several agents in addition to those discussed above are currently being investigated.

Topical Pirfenidone

Pirfenidone is a pyridine currently used for the treatment of idiopathic pulmonary fibrosis. It functions as an anti-fibrotic and anti-inflammatory agent, inhibiting fibroblast production and collagen formation. One study evaluated the effects of 8% pirfenidone gel applied three times per day on pediatric hypertrophic scars caused by burns. [126] Authors report significantly greater reduction in scar formation when compared to standard pressure therapy control with no serious adverse events. Cutaneous side effects of systemic pirfenidone include photosensitivity, rash, and pruritis, however. While this is far from being used in everyday practice, further studies are warranted.

Intralesional Agents

It is important to note that the intralesional agents discussed previously are only some of the intralesional therapies investigated for hypertrophic scars and keloids. Botulinum toxin A, for example, has been shown to minimize scar tension and improve erythema, pruritus and pliability ultimately helping to prevent the development of keloids and hypertrophic scars in predisposed patients. [127,128] Pentoxifylline, a methylxanthine derivative, has also been shown to improve the elasticity of hypertrophic scars. [129] In animal models, minocycline reduced hypertrophy by 85% and collagen-glycosaminoglycan copolymers have been used as adjuvant therapy in human chest keloids with success. [90,130,131] Lastly, due to its success in treating cutaneous hemangiomas, even intralesional propranolol has been hypothesized as a playing a role in the armamentarium of intralesional agents for the treatment of scars as well. [132]

Preserved Particulate Fascia Lata

Preserved particulate fasica lata is used for reconstruction in many other medical specialties, including ophthalmology and orthopedics surgery. After being harvested from cadavers, fascia lata is irradiated to allow for transplantation. One study used preserved particulate fascia lata to help correct acne scars, particularly ice pick acne scars. [133] After the creation of a pocket underneath the scar via subcision, the pocket was filled with the transplanted agent. Improvement in the appearance of the scar lasted approximately 3-4 months with no major adverse events, aside from temporary dyspigmentation in darker skin types. While this is not a new modality, this agent warrants re-exploration given the favorable side effect profile and positive outcome with ice pick scars.

Negative Pressure

The application of negative pressure system to keloids has been shown to improve pruritis, vessel appearance and thickness. [134] Comprised of a silicone dressing that distributes 80-mmHg negative pressure, this system was applied for a one month period being changed once a week. The effect remained at 2 months follow-up.

Electrical Stimulation

One study evaluated the effect of biofeedback electrical stimulation on symptomatic scars (painful and/or pruritic). [135] Both patient-reported subjective ratings, as well as objective measurements using the Manchester scar scale score improved after treatment. Larger, controlled trials are warranted to help fully understand the mechanism and effectiveness of this non-invasive modality.

References

[1] Tolhurst DE. Hypertrophic scarring prevented by pressure: a case report. *British journal of plastic surgery* 1977;30:218-9.

[2] Kischer CW, Shetlar MR, Shetlar CL. Alteration of hypertrophic scars induced by mechanical pressure. *Archives of dermatology* 1975;111:60-4.

[3] Staley MJ, Richard RL. Use of pressure to treat hypertrophic burn scars. Advances in wound care: *The journal for prevention and healing* 1997;10:44-6.

[4] Ward RS. Pressure therapy for the control of hypertrophic scar formation after burn injury. A history and review. *The Journal of burn care & rehabilitation* 1991;12:257-62.

[5] Perkins K, Davey RB, Wallis KA. Silicone gel: a new treatment for burn scars and contractures. *Burns, including thermal injury* 1983;9:201-4.

[6] Quinn KJ, Evans JH, Courtney JM, Gaylor JD, Reid WH. Non-pressure treatment of hypertrophic scars. *Burns, including thermal injury* 1985;12:102-8.

[7] Fette A. Influence of silicone on abnormal scarring. Plastic surgical nursing: *Official Journal of the American Society of Plastic and Reconstructive Surgical Nurses* 2006;26:87-92.

[8] Perez OA, Viera MH, Patel JK, et al. A comparative study evaluating the tolerability and efficacy of two topical therapies for the treatment of keloids and hypertrophic scars. *Journal of drugs in dermatology: JDD* 2010;9:514-8.

[9] Augusti KT. Therapeutic values of onion (Allium cepa L.) and garlic (Allium sativum L.). *Indian journal of experimental biology* 1996;34:634-40.

[10] Willital GH, Heine H. Efficacy of Contractubex gel in the treatment of fresh scars after thoracic surgery in children and adolescents. *International journal of clinical pharmacology research* 1994;14:193-202.

[11] Beuth J, Hunzelmann N, Van Leendert R, Basten R, Noehle M, Schneider B. Safety and efficacy of local administration of contractubex to hypertrophic scars in comparison to corticosteroid treatment. Results of a multicenter, comparative epidemiological cohort study in Germany. *In Vivo* 2006;20:277-83.

[12] Zurada JM, Kriegel D, Davis IC. Topical treatments for hypertrophic scars. *Journal of the American Academy of Dermatology* 2006;55:1024-31.

[13] Baumann LS, Spencer J. The effects of topical vitamin E on the cosmetic appearance of scars. *Dermatologic surgery: official publication for American Society for Dermatologic Surgery [et al]* 1999;25:311-5.

[14] van der Veer WM, Jacobs XE, Waardenburg IE, Ulrich MM, Niessen FB. Topical calcipotriol for preventive treatment of hypertrophic scars: a randomized, double-blind, placebo-controlled trial. *Archives of dermatology* 2009;145:1269-75.

[15] Prado A, Andrades P, Benitez S, Umana M. Scar management after breast surgery: preliminary results of a prospective, randomized, and double-blind clinical study with aldara cream 5% (imiquimod). *Plastic and reconstructive surgery* 2005;115:966-72.

[16] Rahmani-Neishaboor E, Yau FM, Jalili R, Kilani RT, Ghahary A. Improvement of hypertrophic scarring by using topical anti-fibrogenic/anti-inflammatory factors in a rabbit ear model. *Wound repair and regeneration: official publication of the Wound Healing Society [and] the European Tissue Repair Society* 2010;18:401-8.

[17] Wilgus TA, Vodovotz Y, Vittadini E, Clubbs EA, Oberyszyn TM. Reduction of scar formation in full-thickness wounds with topical celecoxib treatment. Wound repair and regeneration: *Official publication of the Wound Healing Society [and] the European Tissue Repair Society* 2003;11:25-34.

[18] Jenkins M, Alexander JW, MacMillan BG, Waymack JP, Kopcha R. Failure of topical steroids and vitamin E to reduce postoperative scar formation following reconstructive surgery. *The Journal of burn care & rehabilitation* 1986;7:309-12.

[19] Whittaker DK. Mechanisms of tissue destruction following cryosurgery. Annals of the Royal College of Surgeons of England 1984;66:313-8.

[20] Barara M, Mendiratta V, Chander R. Cryotherapy in treatment of keloids: evaluation of factors affecting treatment outcome. *Journal of cutaneous and aesthetic surgery* 2012;5:185-9.

[21] Berman B, Viera MH, Amini S, Huo R, Jones IS. Prevention and management of hypertrophic scars and keloids after burns in children. *The Journal of craniofacial surgery* 2008;19:989-1006.

[22] Rusciani L, Paradisi A, Alfano C, Chiummariello S, Rusciani A. Cryotherapy in the treatment of keloids. *Journal of drugs in dermatology: JDD* 2006;5:591-5.

[23] Weshahy AH. Intralesional cryosurgery. A new technique using cryoneedles. *The Journal of dermatologic surgery and oncology* 1993;19:123-6.

[24] Har-Shai Y, Brown W, Labbe D, et al. Intralesional cryosurgery for the treatment of hypertrophic scars and keloids following aesthetic surgery: the results of a prospective observational study. *The international journal of lower extremity wounds* 2008;7:169-75.

[25] Zouboulis CC, Rosenberger AD, Forster T, Beller G, Kratzsch M, Felsenberg D. Modification of a device and its application for intralesional cryosurgery of old recalcitrant keloids. *Archives of dermatology* 2004;140:1293-4.

[26] Har-Shai Y, Amar M, Sabo E. Intralesional cryotherapy for enhancing the involution of hypertrophic scars and keloids. *Plastic and reconstructive surgery* 2003;111:1841-52.

[27] Har-Shai Y, Sabo E, Rohde E, Hyams M, Assaf C, Zouboulis CC. Intralesional cryosurgery enhances the involution of recalcitrant auricular keloids: a new clinical approach supported by experimental studies. *Wound repair and regeneration: Official publication of the Wound Healing Society* [and] the European Tissue Repair Society 2006;14:18-27.

[28] Gupta S, Kumar B. Intralesional cryosurgery using lumbar puncture and/or hypodermic needles for large, bulky, recalcitrant keloids. *International journal of dermatology* 2001;40:349-53.

[29] Mirmovich O, Gil T, Goldin I, Lavi I, Mettanes I, Har-Shai Y. Pain evaluation and control during and following the treatment of hypertrophic scars and keloids by contact and intralesional cryosurgery--a preliminary study. *Journal of the European Academy of Dermatology and Venereology: JEADV* 2012;26:440-7.

[30] Har-Shai Y, Dujovny E, Rohde E, Zouboulis CC. Effect of skin surface temperature on skin pigmentation during contact and intralesional cryosurgery of keloids. *Journal of the European Academy of Dermatology and Venereology: JEADV* 2007;21:191-8.

[31] . (Accessed at http://hypertextbook.com/facts/2007/KarenFan.shtml.)

[32] Bhalla M, Thami GP. Microdermabrasion: Reappraisal and brief review of literature. *Dermatologic surgery: official publication for American Society for Dermatologic Surgery [et al]* 2006;32:809-14.

[33] Freedman BM, Rueda-Pedraza E, Waddell SP. The epidermal and dermal changes associated with microdermabrasion. *Dermatologic surgery: official publication for American Society for Dermatologic Surgery* [et al] 2001;27:1031-3; discussion 3-4.

[34] Tsai RY, Wang CN, Chan HL. Aluminum oxide crystal microdermabrasion. A new technique for treating facial scarring. *Dermatologic surgery: official publication for American Society for Dermatologic Surgery* [et al] 1995;21:539-42.

[35] Bernard RW, Beran SJ, Rusin L. Microdermabrasion in clinical practice. *Clinics in plastic surgery* 2000;27:571-7.

[36] Blome-Eberwein SA, Roarabaugh C, Gogal C, Eid S. Exploration of nonsurgical scar modification options: can the irregular surface of matured mesh graft scars be smoothed with microdermabrasion? *Journal of burn care & research: official publication of the American Burn Association* 2012;33:e133-40.

[37] Fabbrocini G. *Chemical peels.* Medscape 2012.

[38] Camacho FM. Medium-depth and deep chemical peels. *Journal of cosmetic dermatology* 2005;4:117-28.

[39] Rendon MI, Berson DS, Cohen JL, Roberts WE, Starker I, Wang B. Evidence and considerations in the application of chemical peels in skin disorders and aesthetic resurfacing. *The Journal of clinical and aesthetic dermatology* 2010;3:32-43.

[40] Sachdeva S. Lactic acid peeling in superficial acne scarring in Indian skin. *Journal of cosmetic dermatology* 2010;9:246-8.

[41] Garg VK, Sinha S, Sarkar R. Glycolic acid peels versus salicylic-mandelic acid peels in active acne vulgaris and post-acne scarring and hyperpigmentation: a comparative study. *Dermatologic surgery: official publication for American Society for Dermatologic Surgery* [et al] 2009;35:59-65.

[42] Erbagci Z, Akcali C. Biweekly serial glycolic acid peels vs. long-term daily use of topical low-strength glycolic acid in the treatment of atrophic acne scars. *International journal of dermatology* 2000;39:789-94.

[43] Fung W, Orak D, Re TA, Haughey DB. Relative bioavailability of salicylic acid following dermal application of a 30% salicylic acid skin peel preparation. *Journal of pharmaceutical sciences* 2008;97:1325-8.

[44] Lee JB, Chung WG, Kwahck H, Lee KH. Focal treatment of acne scars with trichloroacetic acid: chemical reconstruction of skin scars method. *Dermatologic surgery: official publication for American Society for Dermatologic Surgery* [et al] 2002;28:1017-21; discussion 21.

[45] Fabbrocini G, Cacciapuoti S, Fardella N, Pastore F, Monfrecola G. CROSS technique: chemical reconstruction of skin scars method. *Dermatol Ther* 2008;21 Suppl 3:S29-32.

[46] Bhardwaj D, Khunger N. An Assessment of the Efficacy and Safety of CROSS Technique with 100% TCA in the Management of Ice Pick Acne Scars. *Journal of cutaneous and aesthetic surgery* 2010;3:93-6.

[47] Landau M. Advances in deep chemical peels. *Dermatology nursing / Dermatology Nurses' Association* 2005;17:438-41.

[48] Doddaballapur S. Microneedling with dermaroller. *Journal of cutaneous and aesthetic surgery* 2009;2:110-1.

[49] Sharad J. Combination of microneedling and glycolic acid peels for the treatment of acne scars in dark skin. *Journal of cosmetic dermatology* 2011;10:317-23.

[50] Majid I. Microneedling therapy in atrophic facial scars: an objective assessment. *Journal of cutaneous and aesthetic surgery* 2009;2:26-30.

[51] Pahwa M, Pahwa P, Zaheer A. "Tram track effect" after treatment of acne scars using a microneedling device. *Dermatologic surgery: official publication for American Society for Dermatologic Surgery* [et al] 2012;38:1107-8.

[52] Badran MM, Kuntsche J, Fahr A. Skin penetration enhancement by a microneedle device (Dermaroller) in vitro: dependency on needle size and applied formulation. *European journal of pharmaceutical sciences: official journal of the European Federation for Pharmaceutical Sciences* 2009;36:511-23.

[53] Orentreich DS, Orentreich N. Subcutaneous incisionless (subcision) surgery for the correction of depressed scars and wrinkles. *Dermatol Surg* 1995;21:543-9.

[54] Jacob CI, Dover JS, Kaminer MS. Acne scarring: a classification system and review of treatment options. *Journal of the American Academy of Dermatology* 2001;45:109-17.

[55] Alam M, Omura N, Kaminer MS. Subcision for acne scarring: technique and outcomes in 40 patients. *Dermatol Surg* 2005;31:310-7; discussion 7.

[56] AlGhamdi KM. A better way to hold a Nokor needle during subcision. *Dermatol Surg* 2008;34:378-9.

[57] Al-Khenaizan S. Nokor needle marking: a simple method to maintain orientation during subcision. *J Drugs Dermatol* 2007;6:343-4.

[58] Goodman GJ. Postacne scarring: a review of its pathophysiology and treatment. *Dermatol Surg* 2000;26:857-71.

[59] Lee Y. Combination Treatments of Facial Atrophic Post-Acne Scars in Asians: Retrospective Analysis of 248 pairs of Pre- and Post-Treatment Photographs. In: *Awarded with Antonie de Gimbernat International Prize*. Cambrils, Spain: Antoni de Gimbernat Foundation; 2010.

[60] McCoy BJ, Diegelmann RF, Cohen IK. In vitro inhibition of cell growth, collagen synthesis, and prolyl hydroxylase activity by triamcinolone acetonide. *Proc Soc Exp Biol Med* 1980;163:216-22.

[61] Muneuchi G, Suzuki S, Onodera M, Ito O, Hata Y, Igawa HH. Long-term outcome of intralesional injection of triamcinolone acetonide for the treatment of keloid scars in Asian patients. *Scandinavian journal of plastic and reconstructive surgery and hand surgery / Nordisk plastikkirurgisk forening [and] Nordisk klubb for handkirurgi* 2006;40:111-6.

[62] Liu MF, Yencha M. Cushing's syndrome secondary to intralesional steroid injections of multiple keloid scars. *Otolaryngology--head and neck surgery: official journal of American Academy of Otolaryngology-Head and Neck Surgery* 2006;135:960-1.

[63] Mishra S. Safe and less painful injection of triamcenolone acetonide into a keloid--a technique. *Journal of plastic, reconstructive & aesthetic surgery: JPRAS* 2010;63:e205.

[64] Tosa M, Murakami M, Hyakusoku H. Effect of lidocaine tape on pain during intralesional injection of triamcinolone acetonide for the treatment of keloid. *Journal of Nihon Medical School = Nihon Ika Daigaku zasshi* 2009;76:9-12.

[65] Blumenkranz MS, Claflin A, Hajek AS. Selection of therapeutic agents for intraocular proliferative disease. Cell culture evaluation. *Archives of ophthalmology* 1984;102:598-604.

[66] Huang L, Wong YP, Cai YJ, Lung I, Leung CS, Burd A. Low-dose 5-fluorouracil induces cell cycle G2 arrest and apoptosis in keloid fibroblasts. *The British journal of dermatology* 2010;163:1181-5.

[67] Wendling J, Marchand A, Mauviel A, Verrecchia F. 5-fluorouracil blocks transforming growth factor-beta-induced alpha 2 type I collagen gene (COL1A2) expression in human fibroblasts via c-Jun NH2-terminal kinase/activator protein-1 activation. *Molecular pharmacology* 2003;64:707-13.

[68] Gupta S, Kalra A. Efficacy and safety of intralesional 5-fluorouracil in the treatment of keloids. *Dermatology* 2002;204:130-2.

[69] Kontochristopoulos G, Stefanaki C, Panagiotopoulos A, et al. Intralesional 5-fluorouracil in the treatment of keloids: an open clinical and histopathologic study. *Journal of the American Academy of Dermatology* 2005;52:474-9.

[70] Bodokh I, Brun P. [Treatment of keloid with intralesional bleomycin]. *Annales de dermatologie et de venereologie* 1996;123:791-4.

[71] Aggarwal H, Saxena A, Lubana PS, Mathur RK, Jain DK. Treatment of keloids and hypertrophic scars using bleom. *Journal of cosmetic dermatology* 2008;7:43-9.

[72] Saray Y, Gulec AT. Treatment of keloids and hypertrophic scars with dermojet injections of bleomycin: a preliminary study. *International journal of dermatology* 2005;44:777-84.

[73] Espana A, Solano T, Quintanilla E. Bleomycin in the treatment of keloids and hypertrophic scars by multiple needle punctures. *Dermatologic surgery: official publication for American Society for Dermatologic Surgery [et al]* 2001;27:23-7.

[74] Naeini FF, Najafian J, Ahmadpour K. Bleomycin tattooing as a promising therapeutic modality in large keloids and hypertrophic scars. *Dermatologic surgery: official publication for American Society for Dermatologic Surgery* [et al] 2006;32:1023-9; discussion 9-30.

[75] Kuo MT, Haidle CW. Characterization of chain breakage in DNA induced by bleomycin. Biochimica et Biophysica Acta (BBA) - *Nucleic Acids and Protein Synthesis* 1974;335:109-14.

[76] Templeton SF, Solomon AR, Swerlick RA. Intradermal bleomycin injections into normal human skin. A histopathologic and immunopathologic study. *Archives of dermatology* 1994;130:577-83.

[77] Hendricks T, Martens MF, Huyben CM, Wobbes T. Inhibition of basal and TGF beta-induced fibroblast collagen synthesis by antineoplastic agents. Implications for wound healing. *British journal of cancer* 1993;67:545-50.

[78] Lee RC, Ping JA. Calcium antagonists retard extracellular matrix production in connective tissue equivalent. *The Journal of surgical research* 1990;49:463-6.

[79] Doong H, Dissanayake S, Gowrishankar TR, LaBarbera MC, Lee RC. The 1996 Lindberg Award. Calcium antagonists alter cell shape and induce procollagenase synthesis in keloid and normal human dermal fibroblasts. *The Journal of burn care & rehabilitation* 1996;17:497-514.

[80] Giugliano G, Pasquali D, Notaro A, et al. Verapamil inhibits interleukin-6 and vascular endothelial growth factor production in primary cultures of keloid fibroblasts. *British journal of plastic surgery* 2003;56:804-9.

[81] Yang JY, Huang CY. The effect of combined steroid and calcium channel blocker injection on human hypertrophic scars in animal model: a new strategy for the treatment of hypertrophic scars. *Dermatologic surgery: official publication for American Society for Dermatologic Surgery* [et al] 2010;36:1942-9.

[82] Xu SJ, Teng JY, Xie J, Shen MQ, Chen DM. [Comparison of the mechanisms of intralesional steroid, interferon or verapamil injection in the treatment of proliferative scars]. Zhonghua zheng xing wai ke za zhi = Zhonghua zhengxing waike zazhi = *Chinese journal of plastic surgery* 2009;25:37-40.

[83] D'Andrea F, Brongo S, Ferraro G, Baroni A. Prevention and treatment of keloids with intralesional verapamil. *Dermatology* 2002;204:60-2.

[84] Skaria AM. Prevention and treatment of keloids with intralesional verapamil. *Dermatology* 2004;209:71.

[85] Lawrence WT. Treatment of earlobe keloids with surgery plus adjuvant intralesional verapamil and pressure earrings. *Annals of plastic surgery* 1996;37:167-9.

[86] Margaret Shanthi FX, Ernest K, Dhanraj P. Comparison of intralesional verapamil with intralesional triamcinolone in the treatment of hypertrophic scars and keloids. *Indian journal of dermatology, venereology and leprology* 2008;74:343-8.

[87] Jimenez SA, Freundlich B, Rosenbloom J. Selective inhibition of human diploid fibroblast collagen synthesis by interferons. *The Journal of clinical investigation* 1984;74:1112-6.

[88] Granstein RD, Flotte TJ, Amento EP. Interferons and collagen production. *J Invest Dermatol* 1990;95:75S-80S.

[89] Duncan MR, Berman B. Differential regulation of glycosaminoglycan, fibronectin, and collagenase production in cultured human dermal fibroblasts by interferon-alpha, -beta, and -gamma. *Archives of dermatological research* 1989;281:11-8.

[90] Davison SP, Mess S, Kauffman LC, Al-Attar A. Ineffective treatment of keloids with interferon alpha-2b. *Plastic and reconstructive surgery* 2006;117:247-52.

[91] Lee JH, Kim SE, Lee AY. Effects of interferon-alpha2b on keloid treatment with triamcinolone acetonide intralesional injection. *International journal of dermatology* 2008;47:183-6.

[92] Seo SH, Sung HW. Treatment of keloids and hypertrophic scars using topical and intralesional mitomycin C. *Journal of the European Academy of Dermatology and Venereology: JEADV* 2012;26:634-8.

[93] Berman B, Patel JK, Perez OA, et al. Evaluating the tolerability and efficacy of etanercept compared to triamcinolone acetonide for the intralesional treatment of keloids. *Journal of drugs in dermatology: JDD* 2008;7:757-61.

[94] Gisquet H, Liu H, Blondel WC, et al. Intradermal tacrolimus prevent scar hypertrophy in a rabbit ear model: a clinical, histological and spectroscopical analysis. *Skin Res Technol* 2011;17:160-6.

[95] Anthony ET, Lemonas P, Navsaria HA, Moir GC. The cost effectiveness of intralesional steroid therapy for keloids. *Dermatologic surgery: official publication for American Society for Dermatologic Surgery [et al]* 2010;36:1624-6.

[96] Adalatkhah H, Khalilollahi H, Amini N, Sadeghi-Bazargani H. Compared therapeutic efficacy between intralesional bleomycin and cryotherapy for common warts: a randomized clinical trial. *Dermatology online journal* 2007;13:4.

[97] Varnavides CK, Forster RA, Cunliffe WJ. The role of bovine collagen in the treatment of acne scars. *The British journal of dermatology* 1987;116:199-206.

[98] Cheng JT, Perkins SW, Hamilton MM. Collagen and injectable fillers. *Otolaryngologic clinics of North America* 2002;35:73-85, vi.

[99] Sclafani AP, Romo T, 3rd, Parker A, McCormick SA, Cocker R, Jacono A. Autologous collagen dispersion (Autologen) as a dermal filler: clinical observations and histologic findings. *Archives of facial plastic surgery* 2000;2:48-52.

[100] Sclafani AP, Romo T, 3rd, Parker A, McCormick SA, Cocker R, Jacono A. Homologous collagen dispersion (dermalogen) as a dermal filler: persistence and histology compared with bovine collagen. *Annals of plastic surgery* 2002;49:181-8.

[101] Burgess LP, Goode RL. Injectable collagen. *Facial plastic surgery: FPS* 1992;8:176-82.

[102] Kasper DA, Cohen JL, Saxena A, Morganroth GS. Fillers for postsurgical depressed scars after skin cancer reconstruction. *Journal of drugs in dermatology: JDD* 2008;7:486-7.

[103] Khan F, Richards K, Rashid RM. Hyaluronic acid filler for a depressed scar. *Dermatology online journal* 2012;18:15.

[104] Richards KN, Rashid RM. Twenty-four-month persistence of hyaluronic acid filler for an atrophic scar. *Journal of cosmetic dermatology* 2011;10:311-2.

[105] Dougherty AL, Rashid RM, Bangert CA. Angioedema-type swelling and herpes simplex virus reactivation following hyaluronic acid injection for lip augmentation. *Journal of the American Academy of Dermatology* 2011;65:e21-2.

[106] Pinheiro MV, Bagatin E, Hassun KM, Talarico S. Adverse effect of soft tissue augmentation with hyaluronic acid. *Journal of cosmetic dermatology* 2005;4:184-6.

[107] Micheels P. Human anti-hyaluronic acid antibodies: is it possible? *Dermatologic surgery: official publication for American Society for Dermatologic Surgery [et al]* 2001;27:185-91.

[108] Hirsch RJ, Narurkar V, Carruthers J. Management of injected hyaluronic acid induced Tyndall effects. *Lasers in surgery and medicine* 2006;38:202-4.

[109] Douse-Dean T, Jacob CI. Fast and easy treatment for reduction of the Tyndall effect secondary to cosmetic use of hyaluronic acid. *Journal of drugs in dermatology: JDD* 2008;7:281-3.

[110] Cho SB, Lee SJ, Kang JM, Kim YK, Ryu DJ, Lee JH. Effective treatment of a injected hyaluronic acid-induced Tyndall effect with a 1064-nm Q-switched Nd:YAG laser. *Clinical and experimental dermatology* 2009;34:637-8.

[111] Sadick NS, Palmisano L. Case study involving use of injectable poly-L-lactic acid (PLLA) for acne scars. *The Journal of dermatological treatment* 2009;20:302-7.

[112] Sadove R. Injectable poly-L: -lactic acid: a novel sculpting agent for the treatment of dermal fat atrophy after severe acne. *Aesthetic plastic surgery* 2009;33:113-6.

[113] Beer K. A single-center, open-label study on the use of injectable poly-L-lactic acid for the treatment of moderate to severe scarring from acne or varicella. *Dermatologic surgery: official publication for American Society for Dermatologic Surgery [et al]* 2007;33 Suppl 2:S159-67.

[114] Rossner F, Rossner M, Hartmann V, Erdmann R, Wiest LG, Rzany B. Decrease of reported adverse events to injectable polylactic acid after recommending an increased dilution: 8-year results from the Injectable Filler Safety study. *Journal of cosmetic dermatology* 2009;8:14-8.

[115] Beljaards RC, de Roos KP, Bruins FG. NewFill for skin augmentation: a new filler or failure? *Dermatologic surgery: official publication for American Society for Dermatologic Surgery [et al]* 2005;31:772-6; discussion 6.

[116] Goldberg DJ, Amin S, Hussain M. Acne scar correction using calcium hydroxylapatite in a carrier-based gel. *Journal of cosmetic and laser therapy: official publication of the European Society for Laser Dermatology* 2006;8:134-6.

[117] Marmur ES, Taylor SC, Grimes PE, Boyd CM, Porter JP, Yoo JY. Six-month safety results of calcium hydroxylapatite for treatment of nasolabial folds in Fitzpatrick skin types IV to VI. *Dermatologic surgery: official publication for American Society for Dermatologic Surgery [et al]* 2009;35 Suppl 2:1641-5.

[118] Redbord KP, Busso M, Hanke CW. Soft-tissue augmentation with hyaluronic acid and calcium hydroxyl apatite fillers. *Dermatologic therapy* 2011;24:71-81.

[119] Reddy KK, Brauer JA, Anolik R, et al. Calcium hydroxylapatite nodule resolution after fractional carbon dioxide laser therapy. *Archives of dermatology* 2012;148:634-6.

[120] Broder KW, Cohen SR. ArteFill: a permanent skin filler. *Expert review of medical devices* 2006;3:281-9.

[121] Duffy DM. Liquid silicone for soft tissue augmentation. *Dermatologic surgery: official publication for American Society for Dermatologic Surgery [et al]* 2005;31:1530-41.

[122] Barnett JG, Barnett CR. Treatment of acne scars with liquid silicone injections: 30-year perspective. *Dermatologic surgery: official publication for American Society for Dermatologic Surgery [et al]* 2005;31:1542-9.

[123] Haneke E. Polymethyl methacrylate microspheres in collagen. *Semin Cutan Med Surg* 2004;23:227-32.

[124] Epstein RE, Spencer JM. Correction of atrophic scars with artefill: an open-label pilot study. *Journal of drugs in dermatology: JDD* 2010;9:1062-4.

[125] Cox SE. Clinical experience with filler complications. *Dermatologic surgery: official publication for American Society for Dermatologic Surgery [et al]* 2009;35 Suppl 2:1661-6.

[126] Armendariz-Borunda J, Lyra-Gonzalez I, Medina-Preciado D, et al. A controlled clinical trial with pirfenidone in the treatment of pathological skin scarring caused by burns in pediatric patients. *Annals of plastic surgery* 2012;68:22-8.

[127] Liu RK, Li CH, Zou SJ. Reducing scar formation after lip repair by injecting botulinum toxin. *Plastic and reconstructive surgery* 2010;125:1573-4; author reply 5.

[128] Xiao Z, Zhang F, Cui Z. Treatment of hypertrophic scars with intralesional botulinum toxin type A injections: a preliminary report. *Aesthetic plastic surgery* 2009;33:409-12.

[129] Isaac C, Carvalho VF, Paggiaro AO, de Maio M, Ferreira MC. Intralesional pentoxifylline as an adjuvant treatment for perioral post-burn hypertrophic scars. Burns: *Journal of the International Society for Burn Injuries* 2010;36:831-5.

[130] Henry SL, Concannon MJ, Kaplan PA, Diaz-Arias AA. The inhibitory effect of minocycline on hypertrophic scarring. *Plastic and reconstructive surgery* 2007;120:80-8; discussion 9-90.

[131] Davison SP, Sobanko JF, Clemens MW. Use of a collagen-glycosaminoglycan copolymer (Integra) in combination with adjuvant treatments for reconstruction of severe chest keloids. *Journal of drugs in dermatology:* JDD 2010;9:542-8.
[132] de Mesquita CJ. About strawberry, crab claws, and the Sir James Black's invention. Hypothesis: can we battle keloids with propranolol? *Medical hypotheses* 2010;74:353-9.
[133] Burres SA. Recollagenation of acne scars. Dermatologic surgery: *Official publication for American Society for Dermatologic Surgery [et al]* 1996;22:364-7.
[134] Fraccalvieri M, Sarno A, Gasperini S, et al. Can 'single use negative pressure wound therapy' be an alternative method to manage keloid scarring? A preliminary report of a clinical and ultrasound/colour-power-doppler study. *International wound journal* 2012.
[135] Perry D, Colthurst J, Giddings P, McGrouther DA, Morris J, Bayat A. Treatment of symptomatic abnormal skin scars with electrical stimulation. *Journal of wound care* 2010;19:447-53.

New Treatment Options and New Classification of Scars

In: Scars and Scarring
Editor: Yongsoo Lee

ISBN: 978-1-62808-005-6
© 2013 Nova Science Publishers, Inc.

Chapter 10

Lasers: Physics and Principles

Yongsoo Lee[1] and Inja Bogdan Allemann[2,†]*
[1]Oracle Dermatology Clinic, Daejeon, South Korea
[2]Clinic for Plastic Surgery and Hand Surgery,
University Hospital Zurich,
Zurich, Switzerland

Abstract

This chapter provides essential information on lasers as new options for scar treatments. The physical characteristics of lasers such as coherence, collimation, monochromaticity are described as well as how these characteristics differentiate lasers from lights. Principles of laser-tissue interaction and parameters that can modulate these interactions, in addition to how these principles of interactions practically apply to ablative, non-ablative, and fractional lasers, as well as pulsed dye laser are concisely described.

After reading this chapter, readers will understand how, why and what kind of lasers are used in a wide variety of scar treatments.

LASER is an acronym for 'Light Amplification by Stimulated Emission of Radiation'. Atoms can be in an excited, unstable state by absorbing energy in the form of a photon.

They can only stay in an excited state for a short time, releasing the energy previously absorbed in form of photons when returning to their resting state. This process is called spontaneous emission of radiation. When an already excited electron absorbs yet another photon of equal energy and then returns back to its resting orbit, two photons of the same energy, frequency and direction are released, which is called stimulated emission. In the laser chamber, a number of photons are augmented by repetition of this process. When the majority of the electrons are in an excited state, this is called population inversion. Consequently,

---

[*] Email: exusia@naver.com; Fax: +82-42-825-0289; Office: +82-42-488-8975; Mobile: +82-10-8824-0026.
[†] Inja.bogdan@usz.ch.

stimulated emission becomes more probable and light amplification increases significantly. [1]

Laser differs from lights in the following characteristics:

- *Coherence:* As light can be considered a sine wave, the waves of laser light are temporally and spatially coherent, i.e. the waves are in phase in time and space. [1]
- *Collimation:* The coherence makes the light parallel and non-divergent so that the diameter of the beam changes minimally over distance.
- *Monochromaticity:* Lasers are monochromatic. [2] Monochromatic radiation is radiation of a single wavelength [2], while lights and IPL (intense pulsed light) have a broad range of wavelengths. The atom or molecule being excited determines the wave length of the radiation produced. The lasers are named after the excited molecules (medium) (e.g., Argon laser, carbon dioxide laser). Depending on the wavelength, the laser energy is better absorbed by different targets, called chromophores. Typical chromophores in our skin are melanin, hemoglobin, water and collagen. [1] In cases of scar treatments the chromophores targeted are water and collagen. Oxy-hemoglobin is targeted to correct erythema of scars or to reduce volume of scars by different settings of parameters. [3] Melanin is the target chromophore in hyperpigmented scars and in post-inflammatory hyperpigmentation (PIH) caused by laser scar treatments, especially, in certain ethnic groups.

Parameters Modulating Laser Tissue Interaction

Desired laser-tissue interaction can be achieved by manipulating the following factors:

1. Temporal mode of output
   A. Continuous-Wave (CW) [2]
      i. An uninterrupted beam of irradiation.
      ii. Energy is delivered continuously for as long as the operator desires.
   B. Pulsed [1,2]
      i. Long pulse
         1. Pulse width in the order of 0.1 msec ~ 0.1 seconds.
         2. same peak power as the ungated CW laser's mean power
      ii. Q-switched
         1. pulse width in the order of tens of nanoseconds
         2. high peak powers in the order of megawatts
2. Energy delivery
   A. Fluence (Energy density)
      i. The total energy of the beam divided by its cross-sectional area (joules per square centimeter) [2]
      ii. It reflects the total energy delivered to the tissue, which is directly related to

the volume of tissue that will be treated. [2]
- B. Irradiance (Power density)
  - i. Rate of energy delivery (power) divided by the cross-sectional area of the beam (watts per square centimeter) [2]
  - ii. The primary determinant of the rate of tissue treatment. [2]
- C. Cross sectional power density
  - i. The beam is not usually uniform across the transverse diameter but is made up of transverse electric modes (TEMs)
  - ii. Careful cavity alignment and maintenance of the laser eliminate most higher-order TEMs and most lasers produce at least the lower two or three modes when operating. The lowest order mode TEM00 has Gaussian cross-sectional power density pattern which is relatively uniform. [2]
- D. Spot size
  - i. The fluence and irradiance depend on spot size and on beam divergence. [2]
  - ii. The larger spot size, the deeper penetration as the penetration depth depends on the irradiated area [4] due to less scattering and less loss of energy. [5]
- E. Operating distance
  - i. Operating distances are provided by manufactures and usually are focal length of the lens if present. [2] Away from the manufacturers' specified operating distances, the allowable energy delivery parameters are not known [2] and a beam can produce different tissue responses varying the distance to the treatment site [1], so care must be taken. [2] However, experienced operators can take advantage of pre-focusing and defocusing as the diameter of the beam changes [1] if focused by a lens.
    1. prefocused: the distance to the treatment site is closer than the focal length of the lens
    2. defocused: the distance to the treatment site is farther than the focal length of the lens

Thermal Relaxation Time (TRT)

The time it takes for a tissue to cool to 50% of its maximal temperature, immediately after exposure. [2] TRT is only related to the size of the target chromophore, being proportional to the square of the target diameter squared, and varies from a few nanoseconds through several hundred milliseconds or more. [1]

Selective Photothermolysis [6]

Target chromophores can be damaged or destroyed selectively, minimizing collateral thermal damage to the surrounding non-targeted tissue. The three principles of selective photothermolysis are:

The *wavelength* has to be preferentially absorbed by target chromophores
The *pulse width* has to be shorter than TRT of target chromophores

The *fluence* has to be high enough to destroy target chromophores [1]

Ablative Lasers

The main goal for these lasers is to re-contour scars into a favorable shape. However, human tissue cannot be sculpted like wood or rock, as it reacts to insults or injuries. Laser irradiation causes thermal damage, which then enables the wound to heal thereby changing the contour of the tissue. This makes it more challenging to sculpt human tissue into a desirable contour and, in addition, we need to wait for a certain period of time to see the final out-come. However, we can take advantage of these properties of human tissue by understanding the laser itself and applying the principles of laser-tissue interaction.

The complex wound repair mechanism is initiated by cells sensing the loss of neighboring cells. [7,8] Though we still need to understand more about the signals influencing the recruitment of keratinocytes from the epidermis and follicles [7,8], the initial signal should be considered as 'residual thermal injury' in cases of sculpting scars down into a favorable contour. [9,10]

If we could control the depth of residual thermal damage, it would be possible to control the degree of collagen regeneration and remodeling to a certain degree [3,9,10] as the regenerative process is positively related to the depth of residual thermal damage. [11]

Ablation (or vaporization) of epidermis and dermis is caused by the laser energy absorbed by intracellular water. Carbon dioxide (CO_2) lasers and Erbium:yttrium-aluminum-garnet (Er:YAG) lasers, which have a high absorption rate in water, are typical ablative lasers used for scar treatments. The Er:YAG (2940nm, absorption coefficient 12000 cm^{-1}) laser is more strongly absorbed by intracellular water than the CO_2 laser (10600nm, absorption coefficient 800cm^{-1}) [9,11,12]. The Er:YAG laser evaporates scar tissues, leaving less residual thermal damage than the carbon dioxide laser. [9,11,12] Therefore, Er:YAG laser gives less signal or stimuli to the adjacent cells [7,8,11] and leaves the treated region looking almost the same as it was right after sculpting, even after completion of re-epithelialization, [9] especially, when the pulse duration is set short. [13] When used appropriately, these two lasers are good tools to redefine a scar tissue into more desirable contours. [9]

Non-ablative Lasers

Non-ablative lasers are designed to cause thermal damage to the skin, ideally to structures underneath the epidermis, protecting and thus sparing the epidermis with a proper cooling device [14-28] or other epidermal protection systems. [9] This type of laser treatment provides a safe alternative to the ablative technology and allows the creation of a controlled thermal injury to the dermis with subsequent neocollagenesis and remodeling of scarred skin [29]. The absence of epidermal damage significantly decreases the severity and duration of treatment-related side effects and downtime [9,12,16-18]. Although the wound response in the thermally injured dermis produces new collagen, non-ablative laser techniques have less, or unpredictable, efficacy when compared with ablative laser techniques [9,12,16-19,30,31]. The 1450nm laser is typically used for scar treatments.

Fractional Lasers

Fractional lasers were developed to compensate for the short comings of ablative lasers and non-ablative lasers by treating only a fraction of the skin – thus the name 'fractional'. [12,32] Ablative lasers exert excellent outcomes with experienced operators but accompanied by a high chance of serious complication profiles, while non-ablative lasers guarantee safer treatments with inconsistent outcomes. [9,12,16-19,30,31]

Fractional lasers emit micro arrays of laser beams of ablative wavelength (2790, 2940, 10600 nm) or non-ablative wavelength (1410, 1440, 1540, 1550, 1927nm). [32] Because these laser beams of fractional lasers are absorbed strongly by water, a multitude of water-containing structures can be targeted. Hence, fractional lasers create multiple microscopic treatment zones (MTZs) on treated areas. The MTZs are sharply defined columns like areas of thermally damaged tissue surrounded by unharmed tissue. This unharmed tissue allows rapid epidermal repair as well as decreased complication rates and deeper thermal damage than ablative lasers without compromising safety. [32]

The differences between ablative and non-ablative fractional photothermolysis are:

The stratum corneum is intact with non-ablative FP (NAFP), while disrupted with ablative FP (AFP). [32]

MTZs with NAFP are columns of denatured epidermis and dermis, while MTZs with AFP represent a central ablation zone, which is lined with a thin eschar layer followed by a coagulation zone and then unharmed tissue. [32,33]

Even though, compared to ablative laser surgery [30], length of downtime was significantly shortened with this method, erythema, edema [12], and/or sometimes post inflammatory hyperpigmentation (PIH), especially in Asians, can occur [34,35].

Fractional laser has a unique benefit of proportional re-epithelialization which is completed, with every treatment, within one day. [9,30] This property facilitates epidermal turn over with less side effects and down time. [36]

Thus, fractional lasers are effective in the textural improvement [3,9,10,37] as well as the upward growth of the depressed part of the scar by reorganization of new collagen fibers [36,38], consequently, reducing the scar depth. [39] However, a shortcoming of this device is its limited efficacy in sculpting the contour of the scar, especially when the margin of the scar is sharply angled or the scar surface is highly irregular. [3,9,10]

Since the fractional laser was first introduced, several types of fractional lasers have been utilized in clinical practice. These lasers need further investigation in regards to their comparative efficacy and possible side effects in comparison. [40-47]

Pulsed Dye Laser

Pulsed dye laser (595nm, PDL) can also be utilized to treat certain types of scars. [3] This device spares the epidermis along with other types of non-ablative lasers, however, the target chromophores is oxy-hemoglobin affecting blood vessels. The parameters can be set flexibly depending on the purpose of the treatment. With this versatile device, you can reduce the vascularity to remove excessive redness of facial skin, to improve symptoms of keloids (pain and itch), to soften scar tissue, and/or to reduce the volume of the scar with minor or temporary side effects by down regulating connective tissue growth factor (CTGF) [48].

References

[1] Goldberg DJ. *Laser and LIghts.* Dover JS, editor: Elsivier Saunders. 2005.

[2] Gary P. Lask NJL. *Lasers in Cutaneous and Cosmetic Surgery.* Philadelphia: Churchil Livingstone. 2000.

[3] Lee Y. Combination Treatments and Classification of Scars. *US-China Medical Science* 2011; 8(6):321-334.

[4] Berlien HP, Mu Ller GJ. Applied Laser Medicine. *Journal of biomedical optics* 2004; 9(4):844-845.

[5] Bogdan Allemann I, Kaufman J. Laser principles. *Current problems in dermatology;* 42:7-23.

[6] Anderson RR, Parrish JA. Selective photothermolysis: precise microsurgery by selective absorption of pulsed radiation. *Science* (New York, NY 1983; 220(4596):524-527.

[7] Ito M, Cotsarelis G. Is the hair follicle necessary for normal wound healing? *J Invest Dermatol* 2008; 128(5):1059-1061.

[8] Langton AK, Herrick SE, Headon DJ. An extended epidermal response heals cutaneous wounds in the absence of a hair follicle stem cell contribution. *J Invest Dermatol* 2008; 128(5):1311-1318.

[9] Lee Y. Combination treatment of surgical, post-traumatic and post-herpetic scars with ablative lasers followed by fractional laser and non-ablative laser in Asians. *Lasers in surgery and medicine* 2009; 41(2):131-140.

[10] Lee Y. *Combination Treatments of Facial Atrophic Post-Acne Scars in Asians: Retrospective Analysis of 248 pairs of Pre- and Post-Treatment Photographs.* Awarded with Antonie de Gimbernat International Prize. Cambrils, Spain: Antoni de Gimbernat Foundation; 2010.

[11] Khatri KA, Ross V, Grevelink JM, Magro CM, Anderson RR. Comparison of Erbium:YAG and Carbon Dioxide Lasers in Resurfacing of Facial Rhytides. *Arch Dermatol* 1999; 135(4):391-397.

[12] Manstein D, Herron GS, Sink RK, Tanner H, Anderson RR. Fractional photothermolysis: a new concept for cutaneous remodeling using microscopic patterns of thermal injury. *Lasers Surg Med* 2004; 34(5):426-438.

[13] Ross EV, McKinlay JR, Sajben FP, Miller CH, Barnette DJ, Meehan KJ, Chhieng NP, Deavers MJ, Zelickson BD. Use of a novel erbium laser in a Yucatan minipig: a study of residual thermal damage, ablation, and wound healing as a function of pulse duration. *Lasers Surg Med* 2002; 30(2):93-100.

[14] Herne KB, Zachary CB. New facial rejuvenation techniques. *Semin Cutan Med Surg* 2000; 19(4):221-231.

[15] Bjerring P, Clement M, Heickendorff L, Egevist H, Kiernan M. Selective non-ablative wrinkle reduction by laser. *J Cutan Laser Ther* 2000; 2(1):9-15.

[16] Ross EV, Sajben FP, Hsia J, Barnette D, Miller CH, McKinlay JR. Nonablative skin remodeling: selective dermal heating with a mid-infrared laser and contact cooling combination. *Lasers Surg Med* 2000; 26(2):186-195.

[17] Menaker GM, Wrone DA, Williams RM, Moy RL. Treatment of facial rhytids with a nonablative laser: a clinical and histologic study. *Dermatol Surg* 1999; 25(6):440-444.

[18] Kelly KM, Nelson JS, Lask GP, Geronemus RG, Bernstein LJ. Cryogen spray cooling in combination with nonablative laser treatment of facial rhytides. *Arch Dermatol* 1999; 135(6):691-694.

[19] Grema H, Greve B, Raulin C. Facial rhytides--subsurfacing or resurfacing? A review. *Lasers in surgery and medicine* 2003; 32(5):405-412.

[20] Goldberg DJ, Whitworth J. Laser skin resurfacing with the Q-switched Nd:YAG laser. *Dermatol Surg* 1997; 23(10):903-906; discussion 906-907.

[21] Goldberg DJ. Full-face nonablative dermal remodeling with a 1320 nm Nd:YAG laser. *Dermatol Surg* 2000; 26(10):915-918.

[22] Trelles MA, Allones I, Luna R. Facial rejuvenation with a nonablative 1320 nm Nd:YAG laser: a preliminary clinical and histologic evaluation. *Dermatol Surg* 2001; 27(2):111-116.

[23] Levy JL, Trelles M, Lagarde JM, Borrel MT, Mordon S. Treatment of wrinkles with the nonablative 1,320-nm Nd:YAG laser. *Ann Plast Surg* 2001; 47(5):482-488.

[24] Lupton JR, Williams CM, Alster TS. Nonablative laser skin resurfacing using a 1540 nm erbium glass laser: a clinical and histologic analysis. *Dermatol Surg* 2002; 28(9):833-835.

[25] Fournier N, Dahan S, Barneon G, Rouvrais C, Diridollou S, Lagarde JM, Mordon S. Nonablative remodeling: a 14-month clinical ultrasound imaging and profilometric evaluation of a 1540 nm Er:Glass laser. *Dermatol Surg* 2002; 28(10):926-931.

[26] Mordon S, Capon A, Creusy C, Fleurisse L, Buys B, Faucheux M, Servell P. In vivo experimental evaluation of skin remodeling by using an Er:Glass laser with contact cooling. *Lasers Surg Med* 2000; 27(1):1-9.

[27] Fournier N, Dahan S, Barneon G, Diridollou S, Lagarde JM, Gall Y, Mordon S. Nonablative remodeling: clinical, histologic, ultrasound imaging, and profilometric evaluation of a 1540 nm Er:glass laser. *Dermatol Surg* 2001; 27(9):799-806.

[28] Muccini JA, Jr., O'Donnell FE, Jr., Fuller T, Reinisch L. Laser treatment of solar elastosis with epithelial preservation. *Lasers Surg Med* 1998; 23(3):121-127.

[29] Tanzi EL, Alster TS. Comparison of a 1450-nm diode laser and a 1320-nm Nd:YAG laser in the treatment of atrophic facial scars: a prospective clinical and histologic study. *Dermatol Surg* 2004; 30(2 Pt 1):152-157.

[30] Geronemus RG. Fractional photothermolysis: current and future applications. *Lasers Surg Med* 2006; 38(3):169-176.

[31] Khan MH, Sink RK, Manstein D, Eimerl D, Anderson RR. Intradermally focused infrared laser pulses: thermal effects at defined tissue depths. *Lasers Surg Med* 2005; 36(4):270-280.

[32] Bogdan Allemann I, Kaufman J. Fractional photothermolysis. *Current problems in dermatology;* 42:56-66.

[33] Alster TS, Tanzi EL, Lazarus M. The use of fractional laser photothermolysis for the treatment of atrophic scars. *Dermatol Surg* 2007; 33(3):295-299.

[34] Jeong JT, Kye YC. Resurfacing of pitted facial acne scars with a long-pulsed Er:YAG laser. *Dermatol Surg* 2001; 27(2):107-110.

[35] Chan HH, Manstein D, Yu CS, Shek S, Kono T, Wei WI. The prevalence and risk factors of post-inflammatory hyperpigmentation after fractional resurfacing in Asians. *Lasers Surg Med* 2007; 39(5):381-385.

[36] Mario A. Trelles MV, Serge Mordon. Correlation of Histological Findings of Single session Er:YAG Skin Fractional Resurfacing with Various Passes and Energies and the Possible Clinical Implications. *Lasers Surg Med* 2008; 40:174-177.

[37] Cameron K. Rokhsar YT, and Richard Fitzpatrick. Fractional Photothermolysis in the Treatment of Scars. *Lasers Surg Med* 2005; 36(S17):30.

[38] Karen H. Kim GHF, Leonard J. Bernstein, Suleman Bangesh, Greg Skover, and Roy G. Geronemus. Treatment of Acneiform Scars with Fractional Photothermolysis. *Lasers Surg Med* 2005; S17(36):31.

[39] Lee HS, Lee JH, Ahn GY, Lee DH, Shin JW, Kim DH, Chung JH. Fractional photothermolysis for the treatment of acne scars: a report of 27 Korean patients. *The Journal of dermatological treatment* 2008; 19(1):45-49.

[40] Kim HS, Lee JH, Park YM, Lee JY. Comparison of the effectiveness of nonablative fractional laser versus ablative fractional laser in thyroidectomy scar prevention: A pilot study. *J Cosmet Laser Ther;* 14(2):89-93.

[41] Khatri KA, Mahoney DL, McCartney MJ. Laser scar revision: A review. *J Cosmet Laser Ther;* 13(2):54-62.

[42] Brightman LA, Brauer JA, Anolik R, Weiss ET, Karen J, Chapas A, Hale E, Bernstein L, Geronemus RG. Reduction of thickened flap using fractional carbon dioxide laser. *Lasers in surgery and medicine*; 43(9):873-874.

[43] Chan NP, Ho SG, Yeung CK, Shek SY, Chan HH. Fractional ablative carbon dioxide laser resurfacing for skin rejuvenation and acne scars in Asians. *Lasers in surgery and medicine;* 42(9):615-623.

[44] Goel A, Krupashankar DS, Aurangabadkar S, Nischal KC, Omprakash HM, Mysore V. Fractional lasers in dermatology--current status and recommendations. *Indian journal of dermatology, venereology and leprology;* 77(3):369-379.

[45] Tierney EP, Eisen RF, Hanke CW. Fractionated CO2 laser skin rejuvenation. *Dermatologic therapy;* 24(1):41-53.

[46] Verhaeghe E, Ongenae K, Dierckxsens L, Bostoen J, Lambert J. Nonablative fractional laser resurfacing for the treatment of scars and grafts after Mohs micrographic surgery: a randomized controlled trial. *J Eur Acad Dermatol Venereol.*

[47] Zelickson B, Walgrave S, Al-Arashi M, Yaroslavsky I, Altshuler G, Childs J, Smirnov M, Tabatadze D. Evaluation of a fractional laser with optical compression pins. *Lasers in surgery and medicine;* 43(2):137-142.

[48] Yang Q, Ma Y, Zhu R, Huang G, Guan M, Avram MM, Lu Z. The effect of flashlamp pulsed dye laser on the expression of connective tissue growth factor in keloids. *Lasers in surgery and medicine;* 44(5):377-383.

Chapter 11

Classification of Scars: Conventional and New

Yongsoo Lee[*]
Oracle Dermatology Clinic, Soe-gu, Daejeon, South Korea

Abstract

As new options in scar treatments (lasers) have become widely available, discordance between conventional scar classification and responses of each class of scars to the newly available treatment options have been demonstrated in published articles. Though the conventional scar classification system has contributed much to the research and treatments of scars a great deal, so far, a new scar classification system became necessary due to the discordance between conventional scar classification and reactions of scars to laser treatments.

The new classification system needs to be based on responses of scars to treatments as well as their morphology and natural behavior. This new classification system will help treatment plans to become more successful. Consequently more accurate prognoses will be developed so that each scar class will undergo the same treatment protocols, which can be updated more consistently.

Human beings started describing unknown objects by classifying them, probably, from the beginning, as Adam named all the beasts of the field and all the birds in the air. [1] This must be the beginning and basis of understanding the nature. Just as Adam likely named animals by their appearances, criteria are prerequisites for classifications. In Adam's case, the criterion was morphology.

The first and basic step of classification is to name the objects by their gross morphologies. After microscopes became available, scientists classified microorganisms by microscopic morphologies and as science progressed, they classified them by metabolic pathways i.e., aerobic or anaerobic bacteria. In the same manner, classifications of objects can

---

[*] Email: exusia@naver.com; Fax: +82-42-825-0289; Office: +82-42-488-8975; Mobile:+82-10-8824-0026.

vary depending on criteria as a bacterium can be bacillus and anaerobic at the same time. Criteria should be determined according to the purpose of the classification system.

The existing scar classifications were determined by the morphologies and natural behaviors, primarily as atrophic scars, hypertrophic scars and keloids. Current classifications have greatly contributed to research and treatments of scars up to this point. However, a new scar classification has become necessary due to the discordance between conventional scar classification and the responses of the scars to the newly available treatment options. [2-5]

In order to enable the new classification system to improve treatment plans by making consistent prognoses so that each scar class would undergo the same treatment protocols, which could be consistently updated. The new classification system must be based on scars responses to treatments as well as their morphology and the natural behavior. (Table 1) [2-5].

Table 1. As new treatment options have become available, a new classification system based on the responses of scars to the treatments as well as the morphology and the natural behavior has proven necessary, in order for each class to undergo the same treatment protocols as the same prognosis is expected. Source: Journal of US-China Medical Science (ISSN 1548-6648), Vol. 8, Issue 6, June 2011, pp.321–334, David Publishing Company, USA. Reprinted with permission

Y. Lee Classification of Cutaneous Scars

	NEW CLASS	SUBCLASS (=CONVENTIONAL CLASS)	MORPHOLOGY
Cutaneous SCARS	non-hypertrophic	Atrophic	depressed
		Textural	flat or minimally elevated
	Fibroproliferative*	hypertrophic	elevated
		Keloids	*Include protruding scars caused by acne
	FAPS =facial atrophic post-acne scars		- cluster of small pleomorphic atrophic scars congregated closely - the openings are narrow in comparison to the depth
	burn scars		

As connective tissue, pigments and vascularity have different tissue properties. When lasers are factored into possible treatment options, this issue becomes much more important because connective tissues, pigments and blood vessels are distinctively different target chromophores. Consequently, treatments of dyschromia (disorder of pigments and vascularity) need to be discussed under a separate heading.

Non-hypertrophic Scars (NHS) [3-5]

Non-hypertrophic scars include the scars that are not protruding, which include atrophic scars and textural scars. Textural scars are literally flat or protrude minimally above the level of the surrounding normal skin. [3-5] (Figure 1)(Figure 2)

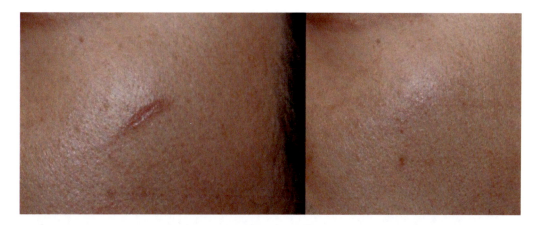

Figure 1. Pre- and Post-Treatment Photographs, 34 year old male, NHS (post-traumatic).

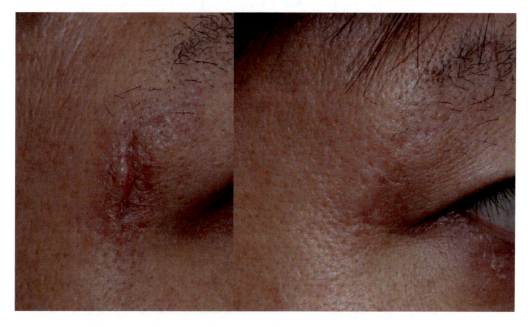

Figure 2. Pre- and Post-Treatment Photographs, 41 year old male, NHS (post-surgical).

Fibroproliferative Scars (FPS) [3-5]

Protruding scars would better be classified into a single class of fibroproliferative scars which includes keloids and hypertrophic scars. Even though keloids and hypertrophic scars are different in natural behavior, gross morphology and histopathology, [6] they respond to similar treatment protocols; sometimes, it is difficult to distinguish one from the other; there are even cases in which keloids and hypertrophic scars are combined. [7] Also, there are scars with growth and histologic features of both hypertrophic scars and keloids. [8] Furthermore, there is a possibility that these two subclasses of FPS are manifestations of the same fibroproliferative disorder of the skin that is expressed by a continuum of features. [9] (Figure 3)(Figure 4)

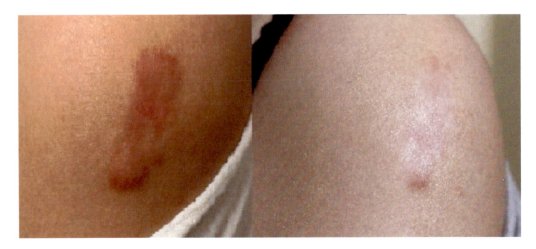

Figure 3. Pre- and Post-Treatment Photograph, 28 year old female, FPS (Keloid), Left Shoulder.

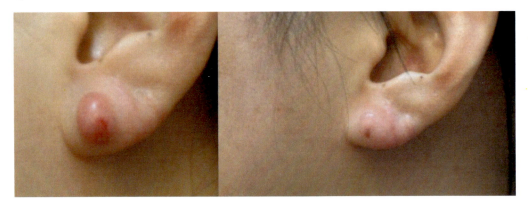

Figure 4. Pre- and Post-Treatment Photograph, 31 year old female, FPS (Keloid), Left Ear Lobe.

Facial Atrophic Post-acne Scars (FAPS) [3-5]

This class of scars has unique characteristics that require a separate entity. FAPS are a cluster or clusters of small pleomorphic atrophic scars congregated close to each other. The openings are frequently narrow in comparison to the depth of the scar. The rationale to this classification would be provided in the treatment section of FAPS. (Figure 5) However, protruding scars caused by acne, wherever they are located, will be classified as FPS.

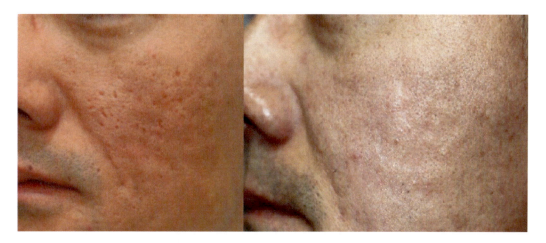

Figure 5. Pre- and Post-Treatment Photograph, 45 year old male, FAPS (post-acne scar).

Even though FAPS seems to be named by its cause, acne, it follows the criteria of morphology, natural behavior and the same responses of the scars to treatments. Therefore, regardless of the cause, if the depressed scars are multiple and congregated close to each other, they can be classified as FAPS and follow the treatment protocols for FAPS, for example, pockmarks. (Figure 6)

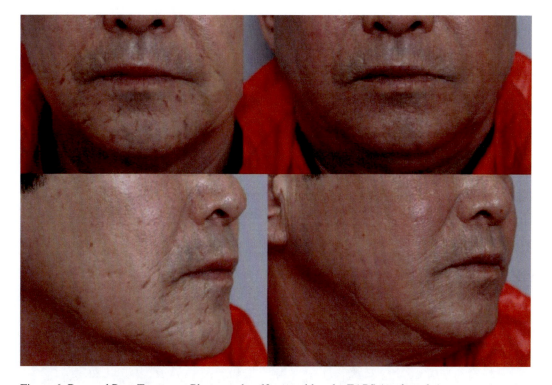

Figure 6. Pre- and Post-Treatment Photographs, 62 year old male, FAPS (pockmarks).

Burn Scars [3-5]

Burn scars are a heterogeneous group, of which criterion of classification is the 'cause', not morphology, natural behavior, pathologic findings nor responses to treatments. The heterogeneity comes from the potency of the burn injury, i.e., the wide range of severity of burn injuries, which is roughly classified into three categories of first to third degree burns. Burns can affect not only the skin but also other organs of proximity simultaneously. This gives burn scars unique characteristics of their own requiring a separate class of "burn scars".

1. There are significantly different depths and areas of burns from one scar to another.
   A) This makes the number of viable pilosebaceous units different from one burn scar to another [2,4,10,11], and
   B) Also makes the distance between the margins of the burn wound significantly different [2,4,10,11].
2. Differentiation of burn scars is also evidenced by the depth of the burn injury and the involvement of adjacent organs such as subcutaneous fat, cartilages, muscles, tendons, nerves and/or major blood vessels. Depending on the involved organs, the properties of the resultant scars could be significantly different from other types of scars. [4,12,13]
3. Properties of burn scars also can vary depending on their locations as well, for example, mouth, eyelids, genitalia, anal area, nose, ears and/or joints. In such cases, different specialties need to be collaborate together. [4]

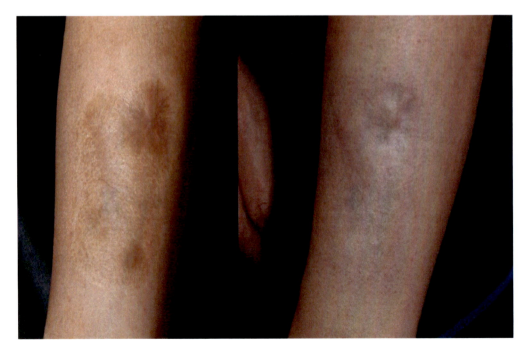

Figure 7. Pre- and Post-Treatment Photograph, 51 year old male, Burn Scar.

These different properties necessitate having a separate system of subclassification of burn scars depending on the area, depth, involved organs, location of the scar, and responses to newly available treatment options in order to be helpful in establishing treatment plans, predicting prognosis and improving research. [4]

However, some burn scars could be classed as either NHS or FPS if their area and depth would be relatively minor. The critical subjects of area and depth of such scars require further burn research. (Figure 7)

For this purpose, the extensiveness, depth [14,15], involved organs and the locations [16] of the burn, need to be documented meticulously during the first examination and reflected on the planning of burn scar treatments. The burn treatments should always include preventive measures for scars. [4,17-19]

Research to further establish subclassifications of burn scars and treatment protocols for each subclass are needed.

Acknowledgments

Some of the figures, tables and descriptions presented in this chapter were used under the generous permission from David Publishing Company (EL Monte, CA, USA) and Edition MF (Paris, France).

References

[1] The Holy Bible, *New International Version.* Grand Rapids, Michigan: Zondervan Publishing House. 1984.

[2] Lee Y. Combination treatment of surgical, post-traumatic and post-herpetic scars with ablative lasers followed by fractional laser and non-ablative laser in Asians. *Lasers in surgery and medicine* 2009; 41(2):131-140.

[3] Lee Y. *Combination Laser Treatments and Classification of Scars.* International Scar Meeting in Tokyo 2010. Tokyo, Japan; 2010.

[4] Lee Y. Combination Treatments and Classification of Scars. US-China Medical Science 2011; 8(6):321-334.

[5] Lee Y. Combination Laser Treatments and Classification of Cutaneous Scars. *Journal of Wound Technology* 2012; 15:45-46.

[6] Ehrlich HP, Desmouliere A, Diegelmann RF, Cohen IK, Compton CC, Garner WL, Kapanci Y, Gabbiani G. Morphological and immunochemical differences between keloid and hypertrophic scar. *Am J Pathol* 1994; 145(1):105-113.

[7] Ogawa R, Miyashita T, Hyakusoku H, Akaishi S, Kuribayashi S, Tateno A. Postoperative radiation protocol for keloids and hypertrophic scars: statistical analysis of 370 sites followed for over 18 months. *Ann Plast Surg* 2007; 59(6):688-691.

[8] Ogawa R, Akaishi S, Izumi M. Histologic analysis of keloids and hypertrophic scars. *Ann Plast Surg* 2009; 62(1):104-105.

[9] Tredget EE. The molecular biology of fibroproliferative disorders of the skin: potential cytokine therapeutics. *Ann Plast Surg* 1994; 33(2):152-154.

[10] Langton AK, Herrick SE, Headon DJ. An extended epidermal response heals cutaneous wounds in the absence of a hair follicle stem cell contribution. *J Invest Dermatol* 2008; 128(5):1311-1318.

[11] Ito M, Cotsarelis G. Is the hair follicle necessary for normal wound healing? *J Invest Dermatol* 2008; 128(5):1059-1061.

[12] Kwan P, Hori K, Ding J, Tredget EE. Scar and contracture: biological principles. *Hand Clin* 2009; 25(4):511-528.

[13] Aarabi S, Longaker MT, Gurtner GC. Hypertrophic scar formation following burns and trauma: new approaches to treatment. *PLoS Med* 2007; 4(9):e234.

[14] Jaskille AD, Ramella-Roman JC, Shupp JW, Jordan MH, Jeng JC. Critical review of burn depth assessment techniques: part II. Review of laser doppler technology. *J Burn Care Res;* 31(1):151-157.

[15] Jaskille AD, Shupp JW, Jordan MH, Jeng JC. Critical review of burn depth assessment techniques: Part I. Historical review. *J Burn Care Res* 2009; 30(6):937-947.

[16] Ogawa R. The most current algorithms for the treatment and prevention of hypertrophic scars and keloids. *Plast Reconstr Surg* 2010; 125(2):557-568.

[17] Anzarut A, Olson J, Singh P, Rowe BH, Tredget EE. The effectiveness of pressure garment therapy for the prevention of abnormal scarring after burn injury: a meta-analysis. *J Plast Reconstr Aesthet Surg* 2009; 62(1):77-84.

[18] Berman B, Viera MH, Amini S, Huo R, Jones IS. Prevention and management of hypertrophic scars and keloids after burns in children. *J Craniofac Surg* 2008; 19(4):989-1006.

[19] Harte D, Gordon J, Shaw M, Stinson M, Porter-Armstrong A. The use of pressure and silicone in hypertrophic scar management in burns patients: a pilot randomized controlled trial. *J Burn Care Res* 2009; 30(4):632-642.

In: Scars and Scarring
Editor: Yongsoo Lee

ISBN: 978-1-62808-005-6
© 2013 Nova Science Publishers, Inc.

Chapter 12

Treatment Options - Combination Treatments: Combination of Lasers / Combination of Lasers and Surgical Scar Revision

Yongsoo Lee[*]
Oracle Dermatology Clinic, Soe-gu, Daejeon, South Korea

Abstract

As mentioned in previous chapters, there are now many different types of lasers available for scar treatments. These lasers have their own distinctive characteristics. The unique characteristics of different types of lasers need to be combined to provide better treatment and better outcomes with less chance of side effects and down time.

Conventional scar treatments such as surgical scar revisions, subscision, CROSS, etc., do not need to be abandoned even though the lasers can bring about many effects that can not be accomplished by conventional treatments. Rather, it is best to take advantage of conventional treatment options that cannot be effected by laser treatments and combine them.

This chapter provides the means of combining treatment options to take advantage of unique characteristics of each treatment modality to get closer to ideal treatment plans which could remove scars instantly in one session of treatment without downtime and adverse effects. Even though such an ideal treatment does not exist, we need to pursue the five components of best treatment practice: complete removal (efficacy), period of time for treatments (effectiveness), downtime, discomfort and possible adverse effects.

The ideal scar treatment would remove scars completely and instantly with single treatment without downtime, discomfort or any adverse effects. Such an ideal scar treatment does not exist yet. However, the above-mentioned five components of an ideal treatment must

---

[*] Email: exusia@naver.com. Fax: +82-42-825-0289; Office: +82-42-488-8975; Mobile: +82-10-8824-0026.

be remembered and pursued: complete removal (efficacy), period of time for treatments (effectiveness), downtime, discomfort and possible adverse effects.

Attributes of the above mentioned components of scar treatment devices or modalities are well described in many publications. Until the ideal device is developed, we need to combine available modalities based on their well-known characteristics to achieve better outcomes within shorter periods of time with less downtime and discomfort as well as less chance of adverse effects.

Successful combination treatments were demonstrated by analyzing pre- and post-treatment photographs statistically in recent articles. [1-5] These articles have more closely focused upon each class of scars through Y. Lee's classification of cutaneous scars. [2,4,5]

Combination Lasers Treatments (CLT)

Non-Hypertrophic Scars (NHS)

Atrophic Scars

Atrophic scars are depressed by definition. These scars need first to be flattened and then the texture normalized to make them indistinguishable from adjacent skin. The causes of depression are dermal deformity (depression), tethering scar tissue under the dermis or both.

In cases of dermal depression without an acute angled margin, sculpting may be unnecessary in a small number of cases. Although the margin is not acutely angled, sculpting is indispensable if the bottom of the depressed area is irregular. Without sculpting, the acute angled margin and/or irregular bottom of the atrophic scar could become shallower than the level of surrounding unaffected skin but still easily noticeable by the irregularity of the surface due to the accumulation of make-up or sunscreen lotion and the projection of their margins casts a dark shadow on the bottom. [6]

Tethering scar tissue under the skin can be detected by making the patient smile or frown. The depressed scar will look more depressed than without frowning or smiling if there is a tethering scar tissue underneath. Subcision is a good treatment option for this condition.

1. Sculpting: The main goal of this stage of treatment is to make a new wound, which would result in less scar tissue and less disfigurement than the original wound that has resulted in the current scar, as well as to smooth off the surface of the scar. [1]
    A) Pre-Operative Care: Acyclovir (400mg) tablet three times a day and extended release tablet of Cefaclor 375mg twice a day for 5 days should be prescribed on the day of ablative laser treatment. Before beginning treatments, photographs are taken with the consent of the patient and the patient warned about possible prolonged erythema and/or post inflammatory hyperpigmentation. Sun avoidance and sun protection are advised. The scar is anesthetized with topical anesthetic cream (EMLA) and occluded with plastic wrap for over 30 minutes. [1]
    B) Procedures with Ablative Lasers
        i. Er:YAG laser: The purpose of this procedure is to redefine the contour. A desirable resultant contour after Er:YAG sculpting is a smooth concave

wound that has no angle formed on the margins. To prevent the irregular contour of pre-treatment after re-epithelialization, residual thermal damage to the remaining tissue needs to be minimalized as the regenerative process is positively related to the depth of residual thermal damage. [7] Er:YAG laser leaves less residual thermal damage than the CO_2 laser, especially when the pulse duration is set short. Less residual thermal damage means less signal of loss of adjacent cells to the remaining tissue. Consequently, the resultant contour would remain almost the same as the contour right after being sculpted down, even after re-epithelialization. [1]

ii. CO_2 laser: The next step is to cause non-fatal thermal damage to the surface of the newly created contour. This smoothly concave contour needs to be raised by regeneration up to the level of the surrounding unaffected skin. This procedure needs to create deeper residual thermal damage as the regenerative process is positively related to the depth of residual thermal damage. [7] This step is performed with a pulsed CO_2 laser at the setting of 1mm spot size, 800W, and 0.1msec pulse duration and 100Hz frequency. The strokes of pulsed CO_2 laser beam are made from the center of concavity toward the outside or vice versa, which makes linear patterns rectangular to the circumference of the concavity made by Er:YAG laser. These strokes smooth out the strata made by circumferential movement of the Er:YAG laser beam. The resultant pattern, after multiple passes of pulsed CO_2 laser exposure, looks like a flower. In cases where the white scar tissue, exposed after the above-mentioned procedure is too dense, a certain portion, but not all of the scar tissue need to be removed with a pulsed CO_2 laser by making holes close together. If the exposed white scar tissue is removed completely, this would recreate the same wound as the original wound that has resulted in the current scar. The final shape of the newly formed wound is smoothly concave with smooth margins, the center of which looks like a honeycomb surrounded by flower petals, if the original scar were round. [1] (Figure 1)

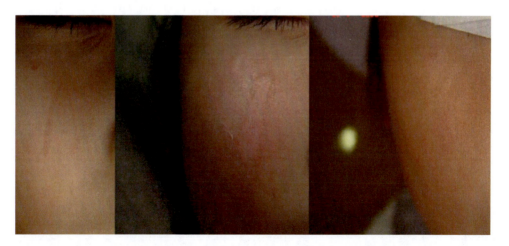

Figure 1. Ten year old female, NHS. Left: Pre-treatment, Middle: Immediate after sculpting, Right: After alternate sessions of non-ablative and fractional laser treatments.

C) Post-Operative Care: The final step is to place the occlusive dressing: the newly made wound is cleansed gently with a cotton ball soaked with normal saline, which is then dried with dry gauze by gentle patting. Rubbing or stroking with gauze, which would affect the survival of the thermally damaged but still viable tissues, is prohibited. In addition, H_2O_2 or Povidone-iodide can affect the viability of the thermally injured cells and should also be avoided. Dr. Oracle Cu3 cream® containing copper tripeptide-1, EGF (epidermal growth factor) and bFGF (basic fibroblast growth factor) is applied, [8,9] upon which Vaseline® gauze is placed and dry gauze fixed with adhesive plasters. The dressing is not to be removed for 10 to 13 days. Whenever the adhesive plaster becomes unstable, it is to be replaced and stabilized without detaching the underlying Vaseline gauze. [1]

2. Keeping the cascade on: As is well known, the regenerative cascade recedes as time goes by. The non-ablative laser and fractional laser are good treatment options to choose for the purpose of keeping the regenerative cascade from receding, if treatment sessions are scheduled appropriately.

D) Non-ablative laser: After washing the patient's face, a topical anesthetic cream is applied on the scar, which is then occluded with plastic wrap for at least 30 minutes. Smooth Beam® (1450nm) treatment is performed at 12.5J/cm2 (6mm spot size) and 25msec of cooling spray. The beam overlaps 20-30%. After the first pass of shots, an ice bag is applied to relieve the pain for about 30 seconds, after which the second pass of shots is performed. Lastly, the ice bag is reapplied, intermittently, over a 1 to 2 minute period to relieve pain.

E) Fractional laser: After washing the patient's face, a topical anesthetic cream is applied on the scar, which is then occluded with plastic wrap for at least 30 minutes. Ablative fractional laser (10600nm) with air-cooling is performed at appropriate parameters depending on the state of the scar. The energy needs to be increased up to the level the skin can bear by closely observing the region being treated. In cases of using non-ablative fractional laser (1540nm, Starlux®), air-cooling is not necessary. Three passes of 70mJ/mB with the XD hand piece for each treatment session leaves less down time, less discomfort and less chance of adverse effects than ablative fractional lasers. The outcomes also seem to be better with same number of treatment sessions. (personal experience) [10-12] After each treatment session, Dr. Oracle Cu3 cream® is applied to the treated region and the patient is advised to apply the cream as frequently as possible (at least 3 times a day). Topical treatment will not only facilitate the tissue's recovery [8,9] from fractional thermal damage, but also provide lubrication on the surface to protect from mechanical insults, which can affect the viable tissue around MTZ's (microscopic treatment zone) adversely.

Textural Scars

Textural scars are literally flat or protrude minimally above the level of the surrounding normal skin. [2,4,5]

Sculpting: It may be considered unnecessary to sculpt textural scars which, by definition, are flat and lack acute angled margins or an irregular surface. However, it is better to sculpt first except for a few cases. Sculpting can minimize a mass of scar tissue buried in normal tissue or reduce the mass to a minimal size, which makes the texture of the affected area more congruent to adjacent unaffected skin. If it is clear the amount of scar tissue is not significant, the sculpting procedure can be skipped. [4] However, sculpting and/or subcision are indispensable if the scar is depressed when smiling or frowning.

In the areas other than the face, where pilosebaceous units are fewer in number, sculpting is not recommended with few exceptions.

Keeping the cascade on: Same as atrophic scars. [4]

The fractional laser makes the epithelium replaced anew proportionally. This property is believed to improve the texture of the treated area even without sculpting. [1,4]

Fibroproliferative Scars (FPS)

The ultimate goal for scar treatments is to make the scarred area look just like the unaffected skin around it. To achieve this goal in cases of FPS, there are a few treatment steps that need to be mentioned. First, the protruding mass must be flattened. Thereafter, the texture and color need to be made congruent with the surrounding unaffected skin. In addition to these three steps, recurrence must be prevented. If there are symptoms of pruritus or pain, these need to be controlled simultaneously. (Table 1)

Table 1. Stages of FPS treatments

Stage 1: Prevention of primary occurrence of FPS	
Stage 2: Volume (protrusion) reduction	+ Symptomatic treatments (pruritus or pain)
Stage 3: Texture correction	
Stage 4: Color correction	
Stage 5: prevention of recurrence	

Source: Journal of US-China Medical Science (ISSN 1548-6648), Vol. 8, Issue 6, June 2011, pp.321–334, David Publishing Company, USA. Reprinted with permission.

Above all of these, the prevention of primary occurrence of FPS is most important. In cases that have a predilected location or past history of FPS, preventive measures are in order. Even when there are no indications predicting whether or not the wound would develop into FPS, any preventive measure after injury is uniformly justified, even when the incidence of FPS at a specific area is known to be minimal. According to the author's experience, Improving FPS to a satisfactory level is much more time and labor intensive than NHS.

1. Contour Correction (Volume Reduction)

The first stage of treatment is volume reduction. It is known that cryosurgery[13], intralesional injections of steroids or/and antimitotic drugs [14], sculpting with ablative lasers, and pulsed-dye lasers [15] are effective. Surgical resection [16] and sculpting with ablative lasers are the fastest ways to reduce the volume, but they are accompanied by an extremely high recurrence rate. [17]

Excessive bleeding can blur the operation site when one sculpts FPS with the Er:YAG laser. The CO_2 laser causes less bleeding but usually has a higher chance of post-inflammatory hyperpigmentation (PIH) and deeper residual thermal injury zones. [18,19] However, if several sessions of pulsed dye laser (PDL, 595nm, 5.5J/Cm2, 0.45ms, 10mm spot size, V-Beam®) treatments with two to three week intervals followed within two weeks after surgical revision or sculpting with ablative lasers, the recurrence rate can be held down and the scars can be kept flat. The end point of the PDL lasers is more important than parameters of the PDL. If the scar turns slightly more reddish, it is a sign that the treatment is proceeding in an optimal fashion.

If preceding surgical revision or ablative laser treatment is inappropriate, pulsed dye laser with the same parameters as mentioned above, with or without local injections of steroids or antimitotic agents, need to be repeated every two to four weeks until satisfactory volume reduction is achieved.

2. Texture Correction

This stage of treatment can be handled just like textural scars. However, the operator must be aware of the possibility of the recurrence of protrusion. Once early signs of protrusion are noticed, a pulsed dye laser is recommended as the first choice to reduce volume, vasculature and recurrence.

3. Color Correction

Colors that need to be corrected during or after correction of texture are redness and/or brown (sometimes, dark brown) pigmentation such as PIH. Redness is caused by excessive vasculature in the scar area. As the diameters of the targeted vasculature are small, pulse duration of 0.45msec, which is less than the relaxation time of a 0.1-mm-diameter vessel at a depth of 1.1 to 1.5mm [20], will work to reduce the redness. The author prefers PDL (595nm, spot size of 10mm) at the setting of 3.5-4.5J/Cm2 with 0.45msec, 6.5J/Cm2 with 3msec, or 7J/Cm2 with 6msec. These parameters need to be adjusted appropriately depending on the state of the lesion under the practitioner's responsibilities.

Regarding brown pigmentation, the same parameters of IPL or laser toning (low fluence, large spot size, multiple passed Q-switched 1064nm Nd:YAG laser) as those for melasma, would work. [21,22] Color corrections need to be discussed under a separate chapter to go into greater detail because different types of target chromophores from the correction of the contour must be considered. [1,3]

What should be addressed first, texture or color correction? The author's recommendation is to first deal with texture correction. Texture correction can cause redness or brown pigmentation or make existing dyschromia worse as a side effect, especially in certain ethnic groups. [23] However, if the patient is not as concerned about texture but rather the color, or the color affects aesthesis more, one may skip or postpone the texture correction.

4. Prevention of Recurrence

If there are no signs of protrusion during the treatments for color and texture, the chance of recurrence will not be high. Preventive measures will mainly be topical agents, [24] among which the author prefers silicone ointment or onion extract if there are no signs of protrusion. However, the patient must visit the doctor as soon as possible when finding early signs of protrusion. [17] Either intralesional injections and/or a pulsed dye laser treatment would be a good choice when a patient complains of early signs of protrusion. [20,25-28]

Facial Atrophic Post-Acne Scars (FAPS) [3]

It appears that the same treatment protocol for NHS can be applied to FAPS. However, there are two characteristics that make FAPS a separate entity. These characteristics are the reasons why ablative laser resurfacing is known to be effective for FAPS but is associated with an undesirable side effect profile, a lengthy recovery period and a risk of infection, as well as potential pigmentary alterations. [4,29]

1. FAPS, Densely Congregated Atrophic Scars [3,4]

If FAPS are sculpted down first, the excessive epidermal component can easily be removed, which leaves few pilosebaceous units or long-lived interfollicular epithelial stem cells [8,9] from which regeneration ensues. This also places too great a distance between adjacent unaffected skin and adnexal structures resulting in an increase in the risk of hypopigmentation or further scarring. (Figure 2)

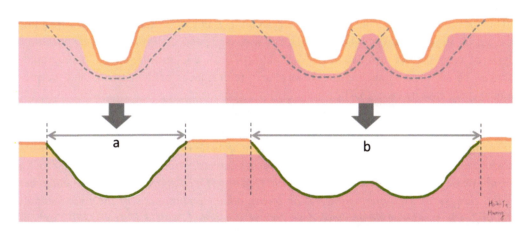

Figure 2. a<b If congregated atrophic scars are sculpted down, the excessive epidermal component can easily be removed and leaves little epidermal tissue from which regeneration ensues or makes too much distance between epidermal tissues thus increasing the risk of hypopigmentation or scarring. Source: Journal of US-China Medical Science (ISSN 1548-6648), Vol. 8, Issue 6, June 2011, pp.321–334, David Publishing Company, USA., and "Combination Treatments of Facial Arophic Post-Acne Scars in Asians: Retrospective Analysis of 248 Pairs of Pre- and Post-Treatment Photographs" awarded with Antoni de Gimbernat International Prize in November 2010. Modified and reprinted with permission.

2. FAPS, Deep and Narrow [3,4]

If this type of scar is sculpted in the first place, an excessive amount of normal tissue must be removed and the depth of sculpting can be excessive, increasing the risk of hypopigmentation or further scarring. (Figure 3) This means the operator cannot sufficiently re-contour the scar to avoid side effects. In other words, the operator has to stop sculpting long before he reaches the desired contour.

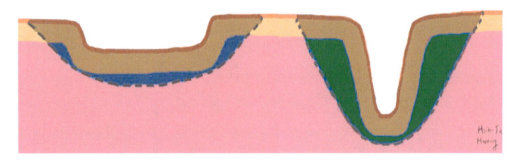

Figure 3. Blue area < green area: the depth and the amount of tissues removed increase as depth to opening diameter ratio increases. Source: Journal of US-China Medical Science (ISSN 1548-6648), Vol. 8, Issue 6, June 2011, pp.321–334, David Publishing Company, USA., and "Combination Treatments of Facial Arophic Post-Acne Scars in Asians: Retrospective Analysis of 248 Pairs of Pre- and Post-Treatment Photographs" awarded with Antoni de Gimbernat International Prize in November 2010. Modified and reprinted with permission.

These two problems can be solved if sculpting is performed after the atrophic scars are made shallower with other treatments; the operator can then re-contour with more confidence and bring about a better outcome by sculpting sufficiently down to the desired contour with less chance of side effects, removing less amount of normal tissue.

This difference was demonstrated statistically in the author's article on FAPS. [3] In this article, an ideal combination treatment protocol was suggested on the basis of the statistical analysis of retrospective evaluation of 248 pairs of pre- and post-treatment photographs, which can be adjusted depending on the diverse circumstances of the patients and the pre-treatment state, case by case. [3,4]

This retrospective study analyzing 248 pairs of pre- and post-treatment photographs [3] of 148 Asian patients (Fitzpatrick's skin type III–IV, 45 males, 103 females, 15.5 to 49.5 years of age (average age: 28.5 years old), more than 6 months' treatments) who were treated by multiple operators demonstrated that the combination of fractional laser (FR), subcision (SB), CROSS (CR), and smooth beam (SM) produced significantly better outcomes than did the use of FR only (p=0.000), or of the other combinations of the four methods (p=0.000). FR produced better outcomes when combined with CR (p=0.000), or SM (p=0.001), or CR+SM (p=0.000), or CR+SB (p=0.000), than when used alone. There were no significant differences between the combinations of FR+CR, FR+CR+SM and FR+CR+SB (p>0.05). However, these three combinations produced significantly better outcomes than did FR+SM (p<0.01). If FR+SB+CR+SM is combined with ablative laser treatment (CS), it improved the outcomes further (p=0.000). This study also demonstrated that the temporal location of the ablative laser sculpting in the treatment protocols affects the outcomes. An independent variable t-test was done to compare the effectiveness of the two groups; in one group ablative laser sculpting was performed prior to other treatments and in the other group laser sculpting was performed after sessions of other treatments (fractional laser, non-ablative laser, CROSS and/or etc.). There were significant differences between these two groups (p<0.05), as the latter group brought about better outcomes than the first group. Inter-operator difference also was statistically analyzed in each of the above-mentioned groups. [3] One of the operators who followed the sculpting procedure as described in the author's previous article [1] on non-hypertrophic scars brought about statistically better outcomes (p<0.05) than the other operators.[3]

The Modified Quantitative Scar Grading System (MQSG) that revealed differences in baselines or pre-treatment status from patient to patient, were reflected in the statistical analysis. [3] The quantitative global scarring grading system [30] proposed by Dr. Goodman and Dr. Baron was incorporated into the MQSG. [3]

Procedures that can prime the regenerative cascade need to be placed first in the treatment protocol. CR and SB ought to be performed on the same day reducing downtime, as an initial treatment to prime the regenerative cascade. If these would be carried out on separate days, the patient would suffer two periods of downtime. It is speculated that the severity of the downtime would not increase synergistically, because CR affects the outer surface of the dermis while SB treats the other aspect of the dermis. If three procedures (CR, SB, and FR) are performed on the same day, three periods of downtime can be condensed into one. However, there is also a risk that the severity of the downtime would be excessively increased because FR, like CR, also affects the outer surface of the dermis.

In cases of FAPS of which the scars are all shallow and acute angle margined atrophic scars, ablative laser sculpting can be considered for the initial treatment. However, as FAPS are mixture of atrophic scars of pleomorphism and cases with shallow and acute angle margined scars only are rarely encountered; sculpting procedures are scheduled later in most cases.

In considering statistical analysis, the following is recommended as an ideal treatment protocol. After a one-day procedure of CR and SB, an alternate treatment of SB and FR every 3 to 4 weeks (OTI[1]; Optimal Temporal Treatment Interval)[3] could be done for several sessions of treatments, depending on the responses to the treatments.

Thereafter, CS should be done when acute angle margined atrophic scars are still noticeable, even though the depth of the atrophic scars have become significantly shallower. This is because these types of scars accumulate make-up and sunscreen lotion and the projection of their margins casts a dark shadow on the bottom. [6] If CS is done afterwards, the area of sculpting can also be reduced because some atrophic scars improve satisfactorily without CS. A few more sessions of SB and FR is recommended after CS, because additional treatments of SB and FR should improve the outcomes. [1]

Patients presenting FAPS as a chief complaint need to be informed that two staged treatments are required because there are two different kinds of chromophores involved. The first stage would be correction of the contour of the scar and the second stage would be correction of dyschromia, which may arise not only from acne but also from laser scar treatments. This matter would best be discussed under a separate heading. [3]

In the first stage of the treatment, even though sun avoidance and sun protection must be advised, PIH may be risked and needs a separate treatment plan in order to achieve satisfactory re-contouring in some Asians, because of the high incidence of PIH in this ethnic group. [23] While reduction of fluence can decrease the incidence and severity of dyschromia, it also decreases the effectiveness of the laser treatments. [3]

An evidence case revealed that variolous (pockmark) scars could be treated successfully with the same treatment protocols as FAPS as variolous scars also are collection of small pleomorphic and atrophic scars. (Figure 4)

---

[1] OTI is defined as the temporal interval between treatment sessions that allows each treatment to cause the most improvement. This value was calculated using quadratic curve equation.

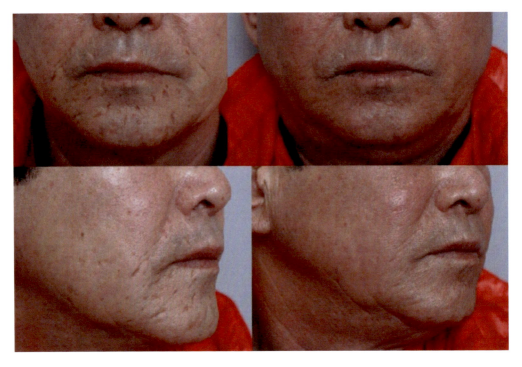

Figure 4. Pre- and Post-Treatment Photographs, 62 year old male, FAPS (pockmarks)

Combination of Lasers and Surgical Scar Revision (CLT + SSR)

Non-Hypertrophic Scars (NHS)

A case that was published in 2009 [1] gives strong evidence that SSR (Surgical Scar Revision) and the CLT (Combination Laser Treatment) are compensatory to each other, in cases where SSR was performed one year prior to CLT. (Figure 5) In addition to this, Nouri et al showed laser treatments of surgical scars starting on the suture removal day are effective. [28]

Table 2.

INDICATIONS ON SSR BEFORE CLT
Absolute indication
Land mark distortion
Relative indications
Functional impairment
Extensive area

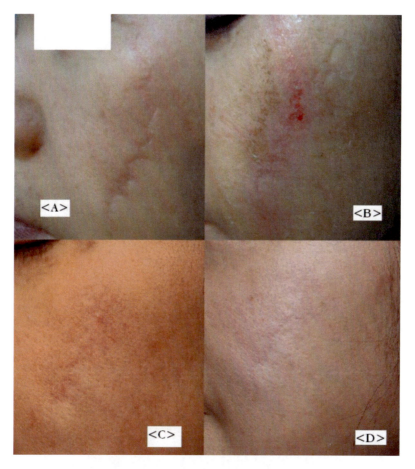

Figure 5. 46 years old, female, NHS (post-surgical), A: Pre-treatment state (3 Feb. 2007), B: Immediate after removal of occlusive dressing (14 Feb. 2007), C: After alternate sessions of non-ablative laser and fractional laser (11 Oct. 2007), D: Long-term follow-up (5 July 2012).

Indications regarding which kind of scars need surgical scar revision prior to CLT and which kind of scars would be better improved with CLT only have yet to be determined. However, a few can be proposed. Landmark distortion can be an absolute indication for SSR first, (Figure 6) while functional impairment and extensive area would be relative indications. SSR is indicated when the scar contractures limit the motion of a joint, [31] however, in certain cases, CLT alone can improve the range of motion of a joint. (Figure 7) For cases of extensive area involvement, skin graft or flap is necessary but when impossible or inappropriate, CLT would be the best remaining option. [4] (Table 2).

Fibroproliferative Scars (FPS)

Despite of the high recurrence rate, FPS can be excised out with following PDL treatment sessions (595nm, 5.5J/Cm2, 0.45ms, 10mm spot size, V-Beam®) within 2 weeks after stitch out by the indications above mentioned. [28] When the volume is reduced to the level with the surrounding unaffected skin and shows no signs of recurring protrusion, textural correction and the subsequent procedures would be commenced as mentioned previously.

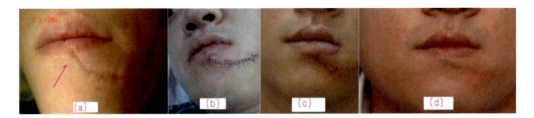

Figure 6. Land mark distortion can be an absolute indication for surgical revision first, while functional impairment and extensive area would be relative indications. Source: Journal of US-China Medical Science (ISSN 1548-6648), Vol. 8, Issue 6, June 2011, pp.321–334, David Publishing Company, USA. Reprinted with permission.

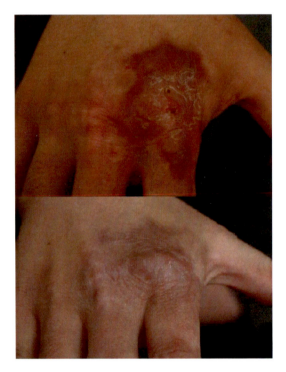

Figure 7. 23 year old male presented keloid with limitation of motion on second MP joint of left hand. Limitation of motion was recovered without SSR. Source: Journal of US-China Medical Science (ISSN 1548-6648), Vol. 8, Issue 6, June 2011, pp.321–334, David Publishing Company, USA. Reprinted with permission.

FAPS

There are reports that surgical revision followed by additional laser skin resurfacing improved FAPS [32]. Therefore, further study on the combinations of surgical revision and the treatment options mentioned above, as well as newly developed devices, need to be carried out for FAPS. [3,32,33]

Burn Scars

Even though the cause of the scar is a burn, it can be included in the classification of NHS or FPS, if the size of the burn scar is smaller than a certain size and the original burn wound is less than a certain depth as described in the "Classification of Scars: Conventional and New" chapter. These scars can be treated following the treatment protocols for each class.

However, for other types of burn scars, research is needed to develop a new subclassification system and combination treatment protocols for each subclassification.

Acknowledgments

Some of the figures, tables and descriptions presented in this chapter were used under the generous permission from David Publishing Company (EL Monte, CA, USA) and Antoni de Gimbernat Foundation (Cambrils, Spain) to which the author ceded the copy right of "Combination Treatments of Facial Atrophic Post-Acne Scars in Asians: Retrospective Analysis of 248 Pairs of Pre- and Post-Treatment Photographs" as awarded with Antoni de Gimbernat International Prize in November, 2010.

Many thanks go to Mr. Hsu-Ju Huang, who made the diagrams of this chapter artistically.

References

[1] Lee Y. Combination treatment of surgical, post-traumatic and post-herpetic scars with ablative lasers followed by fractional laser and non-ablative laser in Asians. *Lasers in surgery and* medicine 2009; 41(2):131-140.

[2] Lee Y. *Combination Laser Treatments and Classification of Scars.* International Scar Meeting in Tokyo 2010. Tokyo, Japan; 2010.

[3] Lee Y. *Combination Treatments of Facial Atrophic Post-Acne Scars in Asians: Retrospective Analysis of 248 pairs of Pre- and Post-Treatment Photographs.* Awarded with Antonie de Gimbernat International Prize. Cambrils, Spain: Antoni de Gimbernat Foundation; 2010.

[4] Lee Y. Combination Treatments and Classification of Scars. *US-China Medical Science* 2011; 8(6):321-334.

[5] Lee Y. Combination Laser Treatments and Classification of Cutaneous Scars. *Journal of Wound Technology* 2012; 15:45-46.

[6] Kadunc BV, Trindade de Almeida AR. Surgical treatment of facial acne scars based on morphologic classification: a Brazilian experience. *Dermatol Surg* 2003; 29(12):1200-1209.

[7] Khatri KA, Ross V, Grevelink JM, Magro CM, Anderson RR. Comparison of Erbium:YAG and Carbon Dioxide Lasers in Resurfacing of Facial Rhytides. *Arch Dermatol* 1999; 135(4):391-397.

[8] Shirakata Y, Kimura R, Nanba D, Iwamoto R, Tokumaru S, Morimoto C, Yokota K, Nakamura M, Sayama K, Mekada E, Higashiyama S, Hashimoto K. Heparin-binding

EGF-like growth factor accelerates keratinocyte migration and skin wound healing. *J Cell Sci* 2005; 118(Pt 11):2363-2370.

[9] Werner S, Smola H, Liao X, Longaker MT, Krieg T, Hofschneider PH, Williams LT. The function of KGF in morphogenesis of epithelium and reepithelialization of wounds. *Science* 1994; 266(5186):819-822.

[10] Lupton JR, Williams CM, Alster TS. Nonablative laser skin resurfacing using a 1540 nm erbium glass laser: a clinical and histologic analysis. *Dermatol Surg* 2002; 28(9):833-835.

[11] Fournier N, Dahan S, Barneon G, Rouvrais C, Diridollou S, Lagarde JM, Mordon S. Nonablative remodeling: a 14-month clinical ultrasound imaging and profilometric evaluation of a 1540 nm Er:Glass laser. *Dermatol Surg* 2002; 28(10):926-931.

[12] Fournier N, Dahan S, Barneon G, Diridollou S, Lagarde JM, Gall Y, Mordon S. Nonablative remodeling: clinical, histologic, ultrasound imaging, and profilometric evaluation of a 1540 nm Er:glass laser. *Dermatol Surg* 2001; 27(9):799-806.

[13] Har-Shai Y, Brown W, Labbe D, Dompmartin A, Goldine I, Gil T, Mettanes I, Pallua N. Intralesional cryosurgery for the treatment of hypertrophic scars and keloids following aesthetic surgery: the results of a prospective observational study. *The international journal of lower extremity wounds* 2008; 7(3):169-175.

[14] Wang XQ, Liu YK, Qing C, Lu SL. A review of the effectiveness of antimitotic drug injections for hypertrophic scars and keloids. *Annals of plastic surgery* 2009; 63(6):688-692.

[15] Alster TS, Williams CM. Treatment of keloid sternotomy scars with 585 nm flashlamp-pumped pulsed-dye laser. *Lancet* 1995; 345(8959):1198-1200.

[16] Ogawa R. Keloids as a serious disease such as malignancy. *Plastic and reconstructive surgery* 2008; 122(3):993-994.

[17] Bouzari N, Davis SC, Nouri K. Laser treatment of keloids and hypertrophic scars. *International journal of dermatology* 2007; 46(1):80-88.

[18] Cho SI, Kim YC. Treatment of atrophic facial scars with combined use of high-energy pulsed CO2 laser and Er:YAG laser: a practical guide of the laser techniques for the Er:YAG laser. *Dermatol Surg* 1999; 25(12):959-964.

[19] Newman JB, Lord JL, Ash K, McDaniel DH. Variable pulse erbium:YAG laser skin resurfacing of perioral rhytides and side-by-side comparison with carbon dioxide laser. *Lasers in surgery and medicine* 2000; 26(2):208-214.

[20] McCraw JB, McCraw JA, McMellin A, Bettencourt N. Prevention of unfavorable scars using early pulse dye laser treatments: a preliminary report. *Annals of plastic surgery* 1999; 42(1):7-14.

[21] Ho SG, Yeung CK, Chan NP, Shek SY, Kono T, Chan HH. A retrospective analysis of the management of acne post-inflammatory hyperpigmentation using topical treatment, laser treatment, or combination topical and laser treatments in oriental patients. *Lasers in surgery and medicine;* 43(1):1-7.

[22] Cho SB, Park SJ, Kim JS, Kim MJ, Bu TS. Treatment of post-inflammatory hyperpigmentation using 1064-nm Q-switched Nd:YAG laser with low fluence: report of three cases. *J Eur Acad Dermatol Venereol* 2009; 23(10):1206-1207.

[23] Chan HH, Manstein D, Yu CS, Shek S, Kono T, Wei WI. The prevalence and risk factors of post-inflammatory hyperpigmentation after fractional resurfacing in Asians. *Lasers Surg Med* 2007; 39(5):381-385.

[24] Zurada JM, Kriegel D, Davis IC. Topical treatments for hypertrophic scars. *Journal of the American Academy of Dermatology* 2006; 55(6):1024-1031.

[25] Gaston P, Humzah MD, Quaba AA. The pulsed tuneable dye laser as an aid in the management of postburn scarring. *Burns* 1996; 22(3):203-205.

[26] Reiken SR, Wolfort SF, Berthiaume F, Compton C, Tompkins RG, Yarmush ML. Control of hypertrophic scar growth using selective photothermolysis. *Lasers in surgery and medicine* 1997; 21(1):7-12.

[27] Liew SH, Murison M, Dickson WA. Prophylactic treatment of deep dermal burn scar to prevent hypertrophic scarring using the pulsed dye laser: a preliminary study. *Annals of plastic surgery* 2002; 49(5):472-475.

[28] Nouri K, Jimenez GP, Harrison-Balestra C, Elgart GW. 585-nm pulsed dye laser in the treatment of surgical scars starting on the suture removal day. *Dermatol Surg* 2003; 29(1):65-73; discussion 73.

[29] Chapas AM, Brightman L, Sukal S, Hale E, Daniel D, Bernstein LJ, Geronemus RG. Successful treatment of acneiform scarring with CO2 ablative fractional resurfacing. *Lasers in surgery and medicine* 2008; 40(6):381-386.

[30] Goodman GJ, Baron JA. Postacne scarring--a quantitative global scarring grading system. *Journal of cosmetic dermatology* 2006; 5(1):48-52.

[31] Ogawa R. The most current algorithms for the treatment and prevention of hypertrophic scars and keloids. *Plastic and reconstructive surgery* 2010; 125(2):557-568.

[32] Jacob CI, Dover JS, Kaminer MS. Acne scarring: a classification system and review of treatment options. *Journal of the American Academy of Dermatology* 2001; 45(1):109-117.

[33] Whang KK, Lee M. The principle of a three-staged operation in the surgery of acne scars. *Journal of the American Academy of Dermatology* 1999; 40(1):95-97.

Chapter 13

Recommended Treatment Protocols

Yongsoo Lee[*]
Oracle Dermatology Clinic, Soe-gu, Daejeon, South Korea

Abstract

In this chapter, the author describes his normal procedures in dealing with patients' complaints regarding scars. He will share treatment protocols and describes his typical treatment timelines and how he uses the Y. Lee scar classification system.

He will also give practical tips such as laser fluences, pulse durations, spot sizes, treatment intervals and the suggested number of passes of laser irradiations that are usually required are concisely delineated.

To set up a successful treatment plan and be able to tell the patient about the prognosis of the scar treatment, the scar must first be classified. As the Y.Lee classification is based upon the morphology, natural behavior and the responses of the scars to the treatment, compare the presented scar to the classification system. In order for this to be accomplished, information on the presented scar needs to be collected during the first examination.

History Taking

1. Date of Injury:
    Many patients do not remember the exact date or sometimes even the year of the injury, especially, when the scar is old. However, it is necessary to determine when the injury occurred. If the scar is not yet mature, corresponding measures including pulsed dye laser treatments need to be implemented. (See chapter 12)
2. Mode of Injury:

---

[*] Email: exusia@naver.com; Fax: +82-42-825-0289; Office: +82-42-488-8975; Mobile: +82-10-8824-0026.

It is very important to check whether or not it is a burn scar. If it is a burn scar, the medical record of the first examination of the burn injury must be reviewed to check the nature of the original injury—its depth and extensiveness. (See chapter 11)

Physical Examination

1. The contour and distribution of the scars need to be checked.
2. Associated symptoms need to be investigated to determine if there is any pain, itching and/or functional impairment.
3. Try to move the scar around parallel to the surface holding both sides with two fingers or make the patient smile or frown to check if the tethering scar tissue anchors the affected area to the underlying structure.
4. The color of the scar must be documented and correction of dyschromia should be included in the treatment plan. *Dyschromia treatment can be postponed until the contour treatment is concluded. However, if the patient desires and the circumstance is relevant, color treatment can be scheduled simultaneously.*
5. It is essential that a pre-treatment photograph be taken. *This photograph is the most important record of all the medical records of the scar treatments. If this photograph is missing, regardless of how many post-treatment photographs may be taken, they would be useless.*

Diagnosis

1. Exclude the possibility that the lesions are attributable to similar-looking diseases. [1]
2. Determine which classification would best describe the scar.

Treatment Plan

1. Set up an appropriate treatment protocol by utilizing Y.Lee classifications.
2. Align the schedule with the patient's calendar if the patient cannot follow an ideal schedule. *Greater compliance of patients can be acquired because some patients are able to accept some downtime if it means a quick response, but others would prefer to avoid recovery time, despite the slow response to treatment. In some cases, prolonged downtime is acceptable during certain time periods, such as vacations. However, many patients often feel that even the slightest trace of treatment must be camouflaged with cosmetics during working hours. Therefore, better compliance to treatment can be achieved by optimizing treatment schedules to meet the circumstances of diverse patients. This would be the way for practitioners to be good guides toward the goal of aesthetic improvement for the patient [2] and one of the best ways to achieve maximum improvements.*

Evaluations

1. Post-treatment photographs need to be taken every six months.
2. Check
   A. the improvements,
   B. if a change of treatment plan is necessary, and
   C. Whether or not further treatments are necessary.
3. As scars rarely heal to the level of unaffected skin, the patient's opinion is important. If he/she is satisfied with the improvement, treatments may be concluded. Or, if not, additional treatment sessions can be contracted.

Data Accumulation and Research

As long-term follow up is necessary to accumulate data for further research, it would be best to take photographs even without treatment schedules every 6 months or so, and patients need to be educated appropriately about managing their scars.[1]

Treatment Protocol for Each Class of Scars

Non-hypertrohic Scars

1. Day #1:
   A. Sculpting with ablative lasers (pulsed CO_2 and Er:YAG)
   B. Occlusive dressing
2. Day #2~#9:
   A. Stabilization of adhesive plasters without detaching the underlying Vaseline gauze. (See chapter 12)
   B. The follow up visit for the plaster stabilization does not have to be every day. Usually five-day intervals between follow up visits are sufficient; however, the patient needs to be advised to schedule a visit whenever the plaster becomes unstable and before it detaches.
3. Day #10~#13:
   A. Attempt to remove the occlusive dressing. If it sticks to the skin, soak it with normal saline for ten to fifteen minutes in order not to cause pinpoint bleeding after its removal.
   B. Postpone the occlusive dressing removal for three additional days if it does not detach, even after normal saline soaking and replace the plasters only.
4. 1 week after dressing removal:
   A. Begin alternate treatment of non-ablative laser and fractional laser every 2 weeks, starting with non-ablative laser.
5. 20 weeks after dressing removal:
   A. Evaluate with a post-treatment photograph
   B. Consult the patient to determine if further treatment is necessary

C. Include subcision for further treatment sessions, if the scar gets more depressed when smiling or frowning.
   D. Make an appointment for long-term follow up if no more contracts are made.
6. Evaluation

   It is best to make appointments for long-term follow up in 6 months or for color treatments (see the color correction section for FPS) as color correction can be made if the outcome is satisfactory.

Textural Scars

1. Day #1:
   A. Sculpting with ablative lasers is usually necessary for textural scars, however, this may be unnecessary in a few cases.
   B. Or, subcision can be necessary if the scar is depressed when smiling, frowning or movement along the surface with two fingers.
2. Day #10~#13: Remove dressing in same manner as non-hypertrophic scars cases.
3. 1 week after dressing removal:
   A. Begin alternate treatments of non-ablative laser and fractional laser every 2 weeks starting with a non-ablative laser.
4. 20 weeks after commencement of alternate treatments of non-ablative lasers and fractional lasers:
   A. Evaluation with post-treatment photographs and pre-treatment photographs
   B. Consult the patient if further treatment would be necessary. Include additional subcision for next treatment sessions, if the scar becomes more depressed when smiling, frowning or movement along the surface with two fingers.
   C. Make an appointment for long-term follow up or for dyschromia treatments.

Fibroproliferative Scars

1. Diagnosis:
   A. Exclude the possibility that the lesion is attributable to similar-looking diseases.
   B. Check if there are symptoms of pruritus and/or pain. If any, appropriate symptomatic treatment need to be combined with the treatments below.
   C. Check if there are functional impairments
   D. Select mode of volume reduction
2. *STEP 1: Volume Reduction*
   A. Options for the Initial Treatments for Volume Reduction
      i. Surgical resection [3,4]
      ii. Sculpting with ablative lasers [5,6]
      iii. Radiation (See chapter 7)
      iv. Pulsed dye laser [7]
      v. Local injections of steroids and/or antimitotics [8]
      vi. Cryosurgery [9]
      vii. Combinations of the above

B. Cases of Volume Reduction by Surgical Resection
   i. 1 week after all the stitches are taken out:
      1. 3 to 5 sessions of pulsed dye laser, every 2 to 3 weeks.
      2. If early signs of protrusion are seen, additional sessions of pulsed dye laser need to be scheduled.
C. Cases of Volume Reduction by Laser Ablation
   i. 1 week after removal of occlusive dressing:
      1. at least 5 sessions of pulsed dye laser, every 2 to 3 weeks
      2. If there are early signs of protrusion, additional sessions of pulsed dye laser need to be scheduled.
D. Cases of Volume Reduction by Cryosurgery
   i. 1 week after spontaneous disappearance of crusts
      1. Schedule at least 5 sessions of pulsed dye laser every 2 to 3 weeks, if additional cryo-treatments are unnecessary.
      2. If early signs of protrusion are evident, additional sessions of pulsed dye laser need to be scheduled.
E. Cases of Volume Reduction by PDL with or without local injections
   i. Pulsed dye laser + local injections
      1. Every 2 weeks until significant volume reduction is achieved.
      2. Every 3 to 4 weeks without local injections until flattened. *If steroidal local injections are administered excessively, depression or atrophy can occur.*
   ii. Pulsed dye laser only
      1. Every 2 weeks until significant volume reduction is achieved.
      2. Every 3 to 4 weeks after significant volume reduction.

3. *STEP 2: Texture Correction*
   A. Alternate treatments of non-ablative laser and fractional laser every 2 weeks or fractional laser only every 3 to 4 weeks are recommended.
   B. Operators must be aware of the possibility of the recurrence of protrusion. Once early signs of protrusion are noticed, go back to the procedures for volume reduction. *Pulsed dye laser is recommended for the first choice to reduce vasculature and early signs of protrusion.*

4. *STEP 3: Color Correction* [10,11]
   A. Two types of color disorder are possible.
      i. Redness
         1. Pulsed dye laser 595nm, one pass, every 3 weeks with one of the following settings:
            A. 4.5J/cm^2, 0.45msec, spot size of 10mm,
            B. 6J/cm^2, 3msec, spot size of 10mm
            C. 7J/cm^2, 6msec, spot size of 10mm
         2. Or, long pulse Nd:YAG, 532nm, 6.5-7.7J/cm2, 20-25msec, two passes, every 3 weeks
      ii. Brown pigmentation [12,13]
         1. Low fluence Q-switched Nd:YAG (Neodymium-Doped Yttrium Aluminum Garnet) laser, 1064nm
            A. Dark brown: 10Hz, 2.1-2.7J/cm2, 8mm spot size, multiple passes,

with PTP mode on, every week.
- B. Light brown: 10Hz, 4.9J/cm2 or 5.1J/cm2, 6mm spot size, multiple passes, with PTP mode on, every week.
- C. When dark brown pigmentation lightens after sessions of treatments, the parameters can set as for light brown pigmentations.
   2. IPL can be a helpful tool for brown discoloration if the operator is comfortable with IPL with the same parameters as melasma.
5. *Prevention of recurrence*
   A. Topical agents [14]: with no signs of protrusion
      i. silicone ointment or
      ii. onion extract
   B. Early signs of protrusion: follow the protocol of volume reduction depending on the size of the protrusion. [15-19]
6. Appointment for a long term follow-up if there is no sign of protrusion for a considerable period of time.

FAPS (Facial Atrophic Post-Acne Scars)

1. Diagnosis: Check the contour of the scars to determine the initial treatment.
   A. If the majority of the scars are narrow and deep in comparison to the opening of the scar, subcision and CROSS are recommended for the initial treatment. [2]
   B. When the majority of the scars are shallow with acute angled margins, sculpting is recommended for the initial treatment.
2. Treatments:
   A. If subcision and CROSS were chosen as initial treatments, fractional laser can be done on the same day to reduce downtime. If these were to be carried out on separate days, the patient would suffer three periods of downtime. [2]
   B. Sculpting techniques can be the same as that of non-hypertrophic scars and the occlusive dressing need to be followed.
   C. 2 weeks after CROSS/subcision or one week after removal of occlusive dressing. An alternate treatment of non-ablative and fractional laser treatments with 2 to 3 week interval can be initiated. Non-ablative laser is recommended first after re-epithelialization is completed but not yet as healthy as the unaffected skin.
   D. Every 2 to 3 months CROSS can be combined with the non-ablative laser or fractional laser to facilitate regeneration at the base of depressed scars.
   E. Evaluation:
      i. After several sessions of alternate treatment of non-ablative laser and fractional laser, photographs need to be taken and compared to pre-treatment photographs.
      ii. If the depth of deep and narrow scars becomes sufficiently shallower, sculpting procedure can be scheduled, which would be followed by alternate treatment sessions of non-ablative laser and fractional laser as previously described. Otherwise, repetition of previous treatments is recommended until they become significantly shallower.

iii. An appointment for long term follow up or for treatments for color correction (see the color correction section for FPS) can be made if the outcome is satisfactory.

Burn Scars

If the burn scar is less than certain size and the original burn wound is less than a certain depth, treatment protocols can follow those of non-hypertrophic scars or fibroproliferative scars. However, for other types of burn scars, there is a need to develop a new subclassification system and combination treatment protocols for each subclassification.

References

[1] Ogawa R. The most current algorithms for the treatment and prevention of hypertrophic scars and keloids. *Plastic and reconstructive surgery* 2010; 125(2):557-568.

[2] Lee Y. *Combination Treatments of Facial Atrophic Post-Acne Scars in Asians: Retrospective Analysis of 248 pairs of Pre- and Post-Treatment Photographs.* Awarded with Antonie de Gimbernat International Prize. Cambrils, Spain: Antoni de Gimbernat Foundation; 2010.

[3] Ogawa R. Keloids as a serious disease such as malignancy. *Plastic and reconstructive surgery* 2008; 122(3):993-994.

[4] Bouzari N, Davis SC, Nouri K. Laser treatment of keloids and hypertrophic scars. *International journal of dermatology* 2007; 46(1):80-88.

[5] Cho SI, Kim YC. Treatment of atrophic facial scars with combined use of high-energy pulsed CO2 laser and Er:YAG laser: a practical guide of the laser techniques for the Er:YAG laser. *Dermatol Surg* 1999; 25(12):959-964.

[6] Newman JB, Lord JL, Ash K, McDaniel DH. Variable pulse erbium:YAG laser skin resurfacing of perioral rhytides and side-by-side comparison with carbon dioxide laser. *Lasers in surgery and medicine* 2000; 26(2):208-214.

[7] Alster TS, Williams CM. Treatment of keloid sternotomy scars with 585 nm flashlamp-pumped pulsed-dye laser. *Lancet* 1995; 345(8959):1198-1200.

[8] Wang XQ, Liu YK, Qing C, Lu SL. A review of the effectiveness of antimitotic drug injections for hypertrophic scars and keloids. *Annals of plastic surgery* 2009; 63(6):688-692.

[9] Har-Shai Y, Brown W, Labbe D, Dompmartin A, Goldine I, Gil T, Mettanes I, Pallua N. Intralesional cryosurgery for the treatment of hypertrophic scars and keloids following aesthetic surgery: the results of a prospective observational study. *The international journal of lower extremity wounds* 2008; 7(3):169-175.

[10] Lee Y. Combination Treatments of Facial Atrophic Post-Acne Scars in Asians: Retrospective Analysis of 248 pairs of Pre- and Post-Treatment Photographs. *Cambrils, Spain: Antoni de Gimbernat Foundation;* 2010.

[11] Lee Y. Combination treatment of surgical, post-traumatic and post-herpetic scars with ablative lasers followed by fractional laser and non-ablative laser in Asians. *Lasers in surgery and medicine 2009*; 41(2):131-140.

[12] Ho SG, Yeung CK, Chan NP, Shek SY, Kono T, Chan HH. A retrospective analysis of the management of acne post-inflammatory hyperpigmentation using topical treatment, laser treatment, or combination topical and laser treatments in oriental patients. *Lasers in surgery and medicine;* 43(1):1-7.

[13] Cho SB, Park SJ, Kim JS, Kim MJ, Bu TS. Treatment of post-inflammatory hyperpigmentation using 1064-nm Q-switched Nd:YAG laser with low fluence: report of three cases. *J Eur Acad Dermatol Venereol* 2009; 23(10):1206-1207.

[14] Zurada JM, Kriegel D, Davis IC. Topical treatments for hypertrophic scars. *Journal of the American Academy of Dermatology* 2006; 55(6):1024-1031.

[15] Gaston P, Humzah MD, Quaba AA. The pulsed tuneable dye laser as an aid in the management of postburn scarring. *Burns* 1996; 22(3):203-205.

[16] Reiken SR, Wolfort SF, Berthiaume F, Compton C, Tompkins RG, Yarmush ML. Control of hypertrophic scar growth using selective photothermolysis. *Lasers in surgery and medicine* 1997; 21(1):7-12.

[17] McCraw JB, McCraw JA, McMellin A, Bettencourt N. Prevention of unfavorable scars using early pulse dye laser treatments: a preliminary report. *Annals of plastic surgery* 1999; 42(1):7-14.

[18] Liew SH, Murison M, Dickson WA. Prophylactic treatment of deep dermal burn scar to prevent hypertrophic scarring using the pulsed dye laser: a preliminary study. *Annals of plastic surgery* 2002; 49(5):472-475.

[19] Nouri K, Jimenez GP, Harrison-Balestra C, Elgart GW. 585-nm pulsed dye laser in the treatment of surgical scars starting on the suture removal day. *Dermatol Surg* 2003; 29(1):65-73; discussion 73.

In: Scars and Scarring
Editor: Yongsoo Lee

ISBN: 978-1-62808-005-6
© 2013 Nova Science Publishers, Inc.

Chapter 14

Striae Distensae

J. A. Savas[1]*, J. Ledon[1], K. Franca[1], A. Chacon[1] and K. Nouri[2]

[1]Mohs and Laser Unit
University of Miami Miller School of Medicine
Department of Dermatology and Cutaneous Surgery
Miami, Florida
[2]Dermatology, Ophthalmology & Otolaryngology
Louis C. Skinner, Jr., M.D. Endowed Chair in Dermatology
Richard Helfman Professor of Dermatologic Surgery
University of Miami Medical Group
Sylvester Comprehensive Cancer Center/University of Miami Hospital and Clinics
Mohs, Dermatologic & Laser Surgery
Surgical Training
Department of Dermatology & Cutaneous Surgery
University of Miami Leonard M. Miller School of Medicine
Sylvester Comprehensive Cancer Center, Mohs/Laser Unit
Miami, FL, USA

Abstract

Striae distensae are linear depressions in the skin that appear perpendicular to areas of increased skin tension. Striae are most commonly the result of changes in skin tension secondary to rapid fluctuations in weight and increases in muscle mass or height. They also appear frequently on the abdomen during pregnancy and in this context are referred to as striae gravidarum. Striae may also be the result of endogenous hypercortisolism like that seen in Cushing's syndrome or disease as well as exogenous hypercortisolism secondary to prolonged administration of systemic or topical corticosteroids.

---

* Email: jsavas@med.miami.edu.

Regardless of the cause, clinically, striae appear initially as raised linear reddish/purple lesions that gradually progress to pale, wrinkled depressions in the skin.

This chapter will address the pathophysiology and risks associated with the development of striae in the context of the above conditions as well as review preventive measures and known treatments. Finally, the chapter will conclude with a discussion on the future directions of the treatment of striae distensae and its subtypes.

Introduction

Striae distensae (SD) or "stretch marks" are a common, well-recognized dermatologic condition affecting patients of all ages, genders, and ethnicities. Clinically, striae appear as multiple, linear, light-colored, atrophic depressions perpendicular to areas of skin that have been exposed to excessive and progressive stretch. Striae most commonly involve the outer aspects of the thighs and the lumbosacral region in boys, and the thighs, upper arms, buttocks, and breasts in girls [1]. They are generally acquired after rapid changes in weight (loss or gain), height (e.g. a growth spurt during puberty), or muscle mass (e.g. weight lifting). Striae also commonly occur during pregnancy, in which case they are referred to as striae gravidarum. Additionally, striae may be the result of endogenous or exogenous hypercortisolism, often complicating Cushing's disease or syndrome as well as systemic and topical steroid administration.

This chapter will address the pathophysiology and risks associated with the development of striae in the context of the above conditions as well as review preventive measures and known treatments. Finally, the chapter will conclude with a discussion on the future directions of the treatment of striae distensae and its subtypes.

Pathogenesis

Striae distensae are characteristic of several clinical conditions, both chronic and acute, with very distinct pathophysiology, making it difficult to determine their true etiology. Initially, most authors were able to agree that mechanical stretch served as the nidus for striae formation however striae were subsequently observed in chronic conditions devoid of stretching forces such as rheumatic fever, typhoid fever, and tuberculosis. This suggested that nutritional deficiency or general debility might be a contributing factor. Moreover, striae were discovered to be a common side effect of steroid excess, further challenging the "skin stretch" hypothesis [2].

While the pathophysiology of striae distensae has still yet to be fully elucidated, several theories have been proposed. It has been suggested that infection or inflammation trigger the release of a so-called "striatoxin" that damages tissue and creates linear atrophic depressions [3]. Mechanical forces from weight gain or growth that generate progressive stretch creating small intradermal tears have been identified as a potential etiology, however there is no consistent causal relationship between growth and the appearance of striae. The absence of striae gravidarum in pregnancy in women with Ehlers-Danlos syndrome and their presence as a general feature of Marfan syndrome suggest that genetic factors play a key role in determining the propensity of an individual to develop striae [4]. Furthermore, gene analyses have revealed a diminished expression of collagen and fibronectin genes in involved tissue, further supporting a role for genetic susceptibility [5].

In the simplest of terms, striae are a form of dermal scarring and their clinical and histologic stages closely parallel those of scar remodeling. For whatever reason, dermal collagen ruptures or separates and the resulting gap is replaced with newly formed collagen that orients itself in the direction of local stress forces [2]. Irrespective of the underlying pathology that may incite a cascade of uncertain events, a final common pathway results in the breakdown and tearing of the dermal matrix, which manifests itself clinically as striae distensae.

Clinical Presentation

Regardless of the context in which they appear, the evolution of striae follow a predictable clinical course. Early, active striae may be pruritic and appear pink to red to violaceous in color. Striae in this stage are referred to as "striae rubra". Over time, they become white or skin-colored depressions with fine wrinkling, closely resembling a scar. Striae in this stage are classified as "striae alba" and are considered permanent. It has been postulated that an early inflammatory response associated with vasodilation that subsides with time, underlies their clinical transformation from a pink raised lesion to their eventual scar-like appearance [6].

The histologic appearance of striae distensae also varies depending on the age of the lesion. A deep and superficial perivascular lymphocytic infiltrate with occasional eosinophils and dilated venules with edema of the upper dermis are characteristic of newly acquired striae. Late-stage striae are significant for scant, elongated collagen bands concentrated within the upper third of the reticular dermis and arranged parallel to the surface of the skin. In the "terminal" stages of striae distensae, there is a thinning of the epidermis due to blunting of the rete ridges and a paucity of collagen and elastic fibers [2,7].

Clinical Conditions Associated with Striae Distensae

Changes in Weight, Height, and Muscle Mass

Striae distensae commonly occur in patients who have recently undergone rapid changes in weight. A common cutaneous manifestation associated with obesity, striae appear perpendicular to areas exposed to sustained and progressive stretching. One study cited the incidence of striae distensae in children with moderate-to-severe obesity as high as 40%. In children with a longer duration of obesity, this percentage was even higher [8]. In a study of 76 obese adults, striae distensae were the most prevalent dermatologic condition, affecting 68.4% of patients. Moreover, the presence of striae was directly correlated with the degree of obesity [9].

When distinguishing striae distensae associated with obesity from those secondary to Cushing's, SD in obese individuals are generally lighter, narrower, and less atrophic [10].

While striae distensae are more commonly found in obese individuals or those who have rapidly gained weight, the presence of SD in patients with anorexia nervosa, while rare, has also been reported [11,12]. Clinically SD in anorexia nervosa are indistinguishable from SD due to other causes. In addition, cases of acquired striae distensae have also been reported in cachectic states such as tuberculosis or typhoid.

Striae distensae also appear during puberty, a time characterized by accelerated growth in height, weight, and muscle mass. The overall incidence of SD during puberty has been reported as approximately 25-35% [13]. Similarly, SD are a common cutaneous finding on the shoulders and in the axilla of body builders, even in the absence of anabolic steroid use.

Pregnancy

Striae gravidarum (SG) are a subtype of striae distensae that appear during pregnancy. The true incidence has yet to be defined; however, studies have reported that anywhere between 50% and 90% of pregnancies are complicated by the appearance of striae gravidarum. The abdomen, breasts, and thighs are most commonly affected and their presence incites considerable anxiety for those affected.

It was initially thought that baseline maternal obesity or the degree of weight gain during pregnancy was associated with an increased risk for the development of striae gravidarum, but current evidence remains conflicted on the issue. Many have abandoned the idea that mechanical stretch is responsible for striae because studies have failed to find a relationship between growth in abdominal girth in pregnant women and the formation of SD [14]. A survey-based study found that a personal history of breast or thigh striae, family history of striae, and race (non-white) are statistically significant predictors of the development of striae during pregnancy [1].

An association between serum relaxin levels and the incidence of SG has also been investigated. Serum relaxin levels that are lower than normal may potentially contribute to SG formation due to decreased elasticity of connective tissue. Studies conducted have revealed that women who acquire stretch marks after 36 weeks gestation have lower serum relaxin levels than pregnant women who do not develop striae. However, there was no correlation found between severity of SG and levels of serum relaxin suggesting that the relationship between the two requires further consideration [15].

Prevention of Striae Gravidarum

Various topical preparations, over the counter and otherwise, have been advertised as effective for the prevention of SG but unfortunately, the efficacy of these solutions does not play out in the evidence-based literature. Anecdotal evidence advocates the use of cocoa butter lotion or olive and other assorted oils applied topically for the prevention of striae gravidarum; however, several controlled studies have not been able to corroborate the efficacy of these topical massage therapies and they are currently not recommended as a preventive measure. [16-18] Several studies, including double-blinded, randomized, placebo-controlled trials, have investigated the efficacy of cocoa butter lotion for the prevention of striae gravidarum, however it appears that topical application of cocoa butter does not reduce the likelihood of developing striae gravidarum [19]. A recent Cochrane level review supported these findings, concluding that no high-quality evidence exists to support the use of any topical preparations for the prevention of striae gravidarum [20].

On the other hand, hydrant creams such as trofolastin with the active ingredient *Centella asiatica* extract, verum (menthol) cream, and alphastria cream, composed of hyaluranoic acid, have all demonstrated some efficacy in decreasing the incidence of the development of striae gravidarum and may be beneficial [21].

Hypercortisolism

Cutaneous side effects of excess cortisol are well-documented in the literature, and include steroid-induced acne, hirsutism, atrophy, acanthosis nigricans, ecchymoses, pigmentary changes, and arguably the most striking: abdominal violaceous striae. Endogenous disease that causes derangements in the hypothalamic-pituitary-adrenal (HPA) axis as well as the administration of systemic or topical glucocorticosteroids results in excess circulating cortisol. High steroid hormone levels have been shown to have a catabolic effect on the activity of fibroblasts as well as decrease the deposition of collagen in the dermal matrix leading to structural instability of connective tissue [22]. Striae distensae that are the result of elevated cortisol levels are generally violaceous in color, larger and more diffuse with a propensity for the abdomen and flexural and intertriginous areas. Unlike the other corticosteroid-induced cutaneous effects, striae distensae are not completely reversible upon discontinuation of corticosteroid therapy or treatment of the underlying disease [23].

Treatment

While striae may become less conspicuous over time, they rarely resolve without intervention. Even with intervention, improvement rather than complete resolution is a more realistic goal and this should be stressed to patients prior to the initiation of treatment. As is true for most conditions, treatment of striae in the early, active phase seems to result in the greatest improvement. Once striae reach a mature, static phase, they are significantly more resistant to treatment and most interventions result in disappointing outcomes.

To date there remains no treatment that consistently offers improvement in the appearance of striae distensae. The first treatment modality to provide reliable results was tretinoin cream, but other topical agents, laser and light therapies, radiofrequency devices and others have also been employed, albeit with variable outcomes.

Topical Agents

Early intervention of striae rubra with topical tretinoin cream has been shown to provide favorable results, however in the more well established striae alba, outcomes have been less successful. In a double-blind, randomized, vehicle controlled trial, Kang and colleagues [24] found that treating early, clinically active striae with 0.1% topical tretinoin cream resulted in marked improvement in clinical appearance after only 2 months in patients affected by striae of varying etiologies.

Glycolic acid (GA), a topical alpha hydroxyl acid commonly used in rejuvenation, peeling, and photoaging, has also been applied to the treatment of striae distensae. In vivo and in vitro studies have demonstrated that GA may have a stimulatory effect on collagen production by fibroblasts, a mechanism that would be beneficial in the treatment of striae distensae, however, there is a lack of controlled trials able to demonstrate the clinical efficacy of GA for this indication. Further studies are needed to elucidate the role of topical GA in the prevention or treatment of striae distensae [21].

Trichloracetic acid (TCA), similar to GA has been used safely at low concentrations for superficial peels; however, at higher concentrations, the incidence of scarring increases, thus limiting its use. A handful of studies have reported improvement in the texture and color of stretch marks using concentrations between 15% and 20% for repeated chemexfoliation to the level of the papillary dermis at one-month intervals [21].

Lasers and Light Therapies

Topical agents provide inconsistent results in striae rubra and have proven to have little to no value for the treatment of striae alba. Inspired by the success of lasers for the treatment of scars and rhytides, these devices have been applied to the treatment of striae distensae in the hopes of achieving similar efficacy. The usefulness of these laser and light sources may lie in their ability to produce energy that selectively targets oxyhemoglobin, in the case of striae rubra, or possibly through the effects of laser-induced changes in collagen and elastin formation.

308nm Excimer Laser

The 308nm xenon-chloride excimer laser emits light energy close to that of narrow-band ultraviolet-B (UVB) light and is used primarily for the treatment of psoriasis and hypopigmentary disorders such as vitiligo. The excimer laser offers increased efficacy over traditional phototherapy through its ability to deliver higher fluences with greater precision in less time [21]. The 308nm excimer laser has been used successfully in a handful of studies for temporary re-pigmentation of late-stage hypopigmented striae alba. Histologically, the treated striae demonstrated increased melanin content and hypertrophy of melanocytes after treatment with the excimer laser. Unfortunately no improvement in skin atrophy was documented [25,26].

Pulsed Dye Laser (585nm)

Early in their clinical course, striae rubra are characterized by dilated vessels, which can serve as a selective target for the pulsed dye laser (PDL). The pulsed dye laser has been shown to significantly improve the appearance of striae rubra when used at low fluences. While PDL may effectively reduce the erythema of early, active striae, striae alba demonstrate almost no clinically apparent change after treatment with PDL [27,28]. McDaniel and colleagues proposed that the 585nm PDL may increase fibroblast activity resulting in an increased production of collagen and elastin, thus promoting favorable scar remodeling [27].

Pulsed dye lasers have also been used in conjunction with radiofrequency (RF) devices due to a reported synergistic effect on neocollagenesis [29]. Preliminary studies have shown significant improvement in the overall appearance of SD in the majority of patients who underwent RF ablation with subsequent PDL therapy. Furthermore, all 37 subjects treated using this modality had darker skin phototypes and only one case was complicated by transient hyperpigmentation [30]. While further studies are needed, RF may be a useful adjunct to laser treatment of SD.

1,064nm Neodyium: Yittrium-Aluminum-Garnet Laser (Nd:YAG)

The 1,064nm Nd: YAG laser is well-established for the treatment of vascular lesions and has also demonstrated the ability to induce dermal collagen formation when used to treat facial rhytides [31]. The combination of vascular selectivity and collagen induction have proven beneficial in the treatment of immature striae rubra in patients with skin phototypes II-IV [32]. The longer wavelength effectively lowers the laser's selectivity for melanin, resulting in less epidermal damage when compared to other devices. This translates into an overall more favorable side effect profile and importantly, allows this laser to be safely and effectively used in darkly complexioned patients.

Fractional Photothermolysis

Fractional photothermolysis (FP) is a fairly new concept in laser therapy that was developed to overcome the adverse effects associated with ablative laser resurfacing and the diminished efficacy of non-ablative lasers [33]. Fractional laser resurfacing can be delivered in either an ablative or non-ablative mode. These laser devices produce focused laser energy that is delivered in a microarray pattern, producing small columns of tissue destruction in the epidermis and dermis called microscopic treatment zones (MTZs), with intervening islands of healthy tissue. Within these cones of destruction, the induction of tissue remodeling and synthesis of new collagen and elastic fibers occurs. The surrounding unaffected, healthy tissue serves as a structural scaffolding as well as provides nutritional support for the treated zones offering the advantage of significantly reduced healing times [34].

The difference between ablative and non-ablative FP lies in the balance between the complete vaporization of columns of tissue (ablative) versus thermal injury with residual epidermal necrotic debris (non-ablative). The non-ablative technique achieves only minimal efficacy and requires multiple treatment sessions over an extended period of time while the fractional ablative technique boasts superior efficacy, albeit with more procedure-related discomfort, post-operative erythema, and recovery time [35].

Recently, fractional photothermolysis has shown promising efficacy in the treatment of atrophic acne scars. Given the clinical and histologic similarity of striae to atrophic scars, comparable outcomes could theoretically be achieved in SD.

Fractional Ablative Devices vs. Non-ablative Devices

The three ablative wavelengths used for fractional ablative laser resurfacing are the 10,600nm CO_2 laser, the 2,940nm erbium:yttirum-aluminum-garnet (Er:YAG) laser, and the 2,790nm yttrium: sapphire; garnet (YSSG) laser. The difference between theses three devices is the ratio of thermal injury to ablation achieved [35]. The device primarily used for fractional non-ablative laser resurfacing is the 1,550m erbium: glass (Er:Glass) laser [35].

Studies show that both ablative and non-ablative fractional laser resurfacing are both safe and effective for the treatment of striae rubra and striae alba, with some studies suggesting greater efficacy in striae alba. However, to date, neither modality has been distinguished as superior to the other [36].

Adverse effects associated with FP, ablative or non-ablative, are generally mild and most commonly include transient erythema and edema as well as post-inflammatory hyperpigmentation. Dyschromia is more frequently a complication of the ablative technique, particularly the CO_2 fractional ablative laser, and should therefore be avoided in patients with Fitzpatrick skin types IV through VI [36].

Intense Pulsed Light (IPL):

Intense pulsed light (IPL) is a form of noncoherent, polychromatic light energy delivered in wavelengths between 400nm and 1200nm. The broad spectrum available with IPL makes it an ideal device for the treatment of various dermatologic conditions such as telangiectasia, vascular malformations, lentigines, acne, poikiloderma of Civatte, as well as photoaging, and the removal of unwanted hair.

Previous studies have demonstrated that IPL induces neo-collagen formation and potentially improves epidermal atrophy and dermal elastosis, a feature that has recently been exploited for the treatment of SD. [37] Investigation of this modality demonstrated that five IPL treatments at two week intervals could result in both clinical and microscopic improvement of abdominal striae alba. While IPL offers the advantage of little to no downtime after treatment, post-inflammatory hyperpigmentation complicated up to 40% of cases and therefore larger studies are needed to corroborate the safety in striae distensae [37].

Special Considerations in Darkly Complexioned Patients:

Unfortunately, the use of lasers for scars in patients with skin phototypes IV –VI may result in an unacceptable potential for persistent erythema, scarring, and hyperpigmentation and should therefore be avoided or used with great caution [38]. Jimenez and colleagues suggested that the use of PDL to treat striae rubra should be limited to patients with Fitzpatrick skin phototypes II to IV [28]. Another study comparing the 585nm pulsed dye laser and the short-pulsed CO_2 laser reported an unacceptable potential for persistent erythema, scarring and hyperpigmentation and recommended that both lasers should be used with extreme caution or avoided altogether in patients with phototypes IV to VI [38]. Furthermore, treatment of striae with the 1,450nm diode laser should be avoided in similarly complexioned individuals [39].

Other Modalities Used in the Treatment of Striae Distensae

Microdermabrasion

Resurfacing with aluminum oxide has become a popular treatment for acne scars, dyspigmentation, and fine wrinkles. It appears that microdermabrasion exerts a molecular effect on epidermal signal transduction pathways, ultimately resulting in dermal remodeling [40]. One promising Egyptian study enrolled 20 patients with SD and treated half the body with five sessions of microdermabrasion at one-week intervals, while striae on the other half of the body served as a control. The majority of patients showed overall good to excellent improvement in treated striae, with striae rubra showing a greater response than striae alba. Furthermore, biopsy and special assay evaluation showed an upregulation of type I procollagen mRNA [41].

Future Directions

Microneedling

A small pilot study performed in Korea evaluated the efficacy and safety of a disk microneedle system for the treatment of SD. A total of 16 patients (skin phototypes III and IV) with both striae rubra and alba were enrolled and received three treatments at four-week intervals. All 16 patients reported at least minimal to moderate improvement and side effects were limited to mild pain, erythema, and pinpoint bleeding. Histologic evaluation revealed increased dermal collagen and a normalization of the pattern of dermal elastic fibers [42]. Future studies comparing microneedling to currently accepted treatments are needed to substantiate the utility of this therapeutic option.

Combined Platelet-Rich Plasma and Intradermal Radiofrequency

Intradermal radiofrequency devices have recently been developed that are capable of delivering high fluences directly to the dermis. These devices were initially developed as a way to enhance filler delivery by passing the filler material through a needle electrode. A small cohort of Asian patients with late-stage striae distensae (duration between 5 and 22 years) were treated with this same device, however in place of filler material, autologous platelet-rich plasma was injected into the dermis.

Platelet-rich plasma has a well-documented favorable effect on wound healing through platelet-mediated secretion of growth factors and other metabolites that positively influence wound regeneration and repair [43]. After three sessions of intradermal RF combined with autologous platelet-rich plasma, all patients showed a satisfactory clinical response with 42% experiencing excellent or marked improvement. The procedure was well tolerated and transient bruising was the only significant adverse effect reported [44].

References

[1] Chang AL, Agredano YZ, Kimball AB. Risk factors associated with striae gravidarum. *Journal of the American Academy of Dermatology* 2004;51:881-5.

[2] Arem AJ, Kischer CW. Analysis of striae. *Plastic and reconstructive surgery* 1980;65:22-9.

[3] F K. Seitrag zur atiologie und pathogenese der stria cutis distensae. *Archives of Dermatology and Syphilology* 1925;149:667.

[4] Burrows NP LC. Disorders of connective tissue. In: Burns T BS, Cox N, Griffith C, ed. Text Book of Dermatology: *Blackwell Science*; 2004:46-7.

[5] Lee KS, Rho YJ, Jang SI, Suh MH, Song JY. Decreased expression of collagen and fibronectin genes in striae distensae tissue. *Clinical and experimental dermatology* 1994;19:285-8.

[6] Watson RE, Parry EJ, Humphries JD, et al. Fibrillin microfibrils are reduced in skin exhibiting striae distensae. *The British journal of dermatology* 1998;138:931-7.

[7] Ackerman AB CN, Sanchez J, Guo Y, et al. An algorithmic method based on pattern analysis. In: Histologic diagnosis of inflammatory skin diseases. 2nd ed. Baltimore: Williams and Wilkins; 1997:734-6.

[8] Hsu HS, Chen W, Chen SC, Ko FD. Colored striae in obese children and adolescents. Zhonghua Minguo xiao er ke yi xue hui za zhi [Journal] *Zhonghua Minguo xiao er ke yi xue hui* 1996;37:349-52.

[9] Boza JC, Trindade EN, Peruzzo J, Sachett L, Rech L, Cestari TF. Skin manifestations of obesity: a comparative study. *Journal of the European Academy of Dermatology and Venereology : JEADV* 2012;26:1220-3.

[10] Angeli A, Boccuzzi G, Frajria R, Bisbocci D. [Adrenal gland function test in the differential diagnosis of sthenic obesity with pink striae]. *Folia endocrinologica* 1970;23:566-78.

[11] Strumia R. Skin signs in anorexia nervosa. Dermato-endocrinology 2009;1:268-70.

[12] Tyler I, Wiseman MC, Crawford RI, Birmingham CL. Cutaneous manifestations of eating disorders. *Journal of cutaneous medicine and surgery* 2002;6:345-53.

[13] Ammar NM, Rao B, Schwartz RA, Janniger CK. Adolescent striae. *Cutis; cutaneous medicine for the practitioner* 2000;65:69-70.

[14] Osman H, Rubeiz N, Tamim H, Nassar AH. Risk factors for the development of striae gravidarum. *American journal of obstetrics and gynecology* 2007;196:62 e1-5.

[15] Lurie S, Matas Z, Fux A, Golan A, Sadan O. Association of serum relaxin with striae gravidarum in pregnant women. *Archives of gynecology and obstetrics* 2011;283:219-22.

[16] Mallol J, Belda MA, Costa D, Noval A, Sola M. Prophylaxis of Striae gravidarum with a topical formulation. A double blind trial. *International journal of cosmetic science* 1991;13:51-7.

[17] Wierrani F, Kozak W, Schramm W, Grunberger W. [Attempt of preventive treatment of striae gravidarum using preventive massage ointment administration]. *Wiener klinische Wochenschrift* 1992;104:42-4.

[18] de Buman M, Walther M, de Weck R. [Effectiveness of Alphastria cream in the prevention of pregnancy stretch marks (striae distensae). Results of a double-blind study]. *Gynakologische Rundschau* 1987;27:79-84.

[19] Osman H, Usta IM, Rubeiz N, Abu-Rustum R, Charara I, Nassar AH. Cocoa butter lotion for prevention of striae gravidarum: a double-blind, randomised and placebo-controlled trial. *BJOG : an international journal of obstetrics and gynaecology* 2008;115:1138-42.

[20] Brennan M, Young G, Devane D. Topical preparations for preventing stretch marks in pregnancy. *Cochrane Database Syst Rev* 2012;11:CD000066.

[21] Elsaie ML, Baumann LS, Elsaaiee LT. Striae distensae (stretch marks) and different modalities of therapy: an update. *Dermatologic surgery : official publication for American Society for Dermatologic Surgery* [et al] 2009;35:563-73.

[22] Uitto J, Teir H, Mustakallio KK. Corticosteroid-induced inhibition of the biosynthesis of human skin collagen. *Biochemical pharmacology* 1972;21:2161-7.

[23] Buchman AL. Side effects of corticosteroid therapy. *Journal of clinical gastroenterology* 2001;33:289-94.

[24] Kang S, Kim KJ, Griffiths CE, et al. Topical tretinoin (retinoic acid) improves early stretch marks. *Archives of dermatology* 1996;132:519-26.

[25] Goldberg DJ, Sarradet D, Hussain M. 308-nm Excimer laser treatment of mature hypopigmented striae. *Dermatologic surgery : official publication for American Society for Dermatologic Surgery* [et al] 2003;29:596-8; discussion 8-9.

[26] Goldberg DJ, Marmur ES, Schmults C, Hussain M, Phelps R. Histologic and ultrastructural analysis of ultraviolet B laser and light source treatment of leukoderma in striae distensae. *Dermatologic surgery : official publication for American Society for Dermatologic Surgery* [et al] 2005;31:385-7.

[27] McDaniel DH. Laser therapy of stretch marks. *Dermatologic clinics* 2002;20:67-76, viii.

[28] Jimenez GP, Flores F, Berman B, Gunja-Smith Z. Treatment of striae rubra and striae alba with the 585-nm pulsed-dye laser. *Dermatologic surgery : official publication for American Society for Dermatologic Surgery* [et al] 2003;29:362-5.

[29] Zelickson BD, Kist D, Bernstein E, et al. Histological and ultrastructural evaluation of the effects of a radiofrequency-based nonablative dermal remodeling device: a pilot study. *Archives of dermatology* 2004;140:204-9.

[30] Suh DH, Chang KY, Son HC, Ryu JH, Lee SJ, Song KY. Radiofrequency and 585-nm pulsed dye laser treatment of striae distensae: a report of 37 Asian patients. *Dermatologic surgery : official publication for American Society for Dermatologic Surgery* [et al] 2007;33:29-34.

[31] Goldberg DJ, Samady JA. Intense pulsed light and Nd:YAG laser non-ablative treatment of facial rhytids. *Lasers in surgery and medicine* 2001;28:141-4.

[32] Goldman A, Rossato F, Prati C. Stretch marks: treatment using the 1,064-nm Nd:YAG laser. *Dermatologic surgery : official publication for American Society for Dermatologic Surgery* [et al] 2008;34:686-91; discussion 91-2.

[33] Geronemus RG. Fractional photothermolysis: current and future applications. *Lasers in surgery and medicine* 2006;38:169-76.

[34] Fisher GH, Geronemus RG. Short-term side effects of fractional photothermolysis. *Dermatologic surgery : official publication for American Society for Dermatologic Surgery* [et al] 2005;31:1245-9; discussion 9.

[35] Alexiades-Armenaka M, Sarnoff D, Gotkin R, Sadick N. Multi-center clinical study and review of fractional ablative CO2 laser resurfacing for the treatment of rhytides, photoaging, scars and striae. *Journal of drugs in dermatology* : JDD 2011;10:352-62.

[36] Yang YJ, Lee GY. Treatment of Striae Distensae with Nonablative Fractional Laser versus Ablative CO(2) Fractional Laser: A Randomized Controlled Trial. *Annals of dermatology* 2011;23:481-9.

[37] Hernandez-Perez E, Colombo-Charrier E, Valencia-Ibiett E. Intense pulsed light in the treatment of striae distensae. *Dermatologic surgery : official publication for American Society for Dermatologic Surgery* [et al] 2002;28:1124-30.

[38] Nouri K, Romagosa R, Chartier T, Bowes L, Spencer JM. Comparison of the 585 nm pulse dye laser and the short pulsed CO2 laser in the treatment of striae distensae in skin types IV and VI. *Dermatologic surgery : official publication for American Society for Dermatologic Surgery* [et al] 1999;25:368-70.

[39] Tay YK, Kwok C, Tan E. Non-ablative 1,450-nm diode laser treatment of striae distensae. *Lasers in surgery and medicine* 2006;38:196-9.

[40] Karimipour DJ, Kang S, Johnson TM, et al. Microdermabrasion: a molecular analysis following a single treatment. *Journal of the American Academy of Dermatology* 2005;52:215-23.

[41] Abdel-Latif AM EA. Treatment of striae distensae with microdermabrasion: a clinical and molecular study. *JEWDS* 2008:24-30.

[42] Park KY, Kim HK, Kim SE, Kim BJ, Kim MN. Treatment of striae distensae using needling therapy: a pilot study. *Dermatologic surgery : official publication for American Society for Dermatologic Surgery* [et al] 2012;38:1823-8.

[43] Anitua E, Andia I, Ardanza B, Nurden P, Nurden AT. Autologous platelets as a source of proteins for healing and tissue regeneration. *Thrombosis and haemostasis* 2004;91:4-15.

[44] Kim IS, Park KY, Kim BJ, Kim MN, Kim CW, Kim SE. Efficacy of intradermal radiofrequency combined with autologous platelet-rich plasma in striae distensae: a pilot study. *International journal of dermatology* 2012;51:1253-8.

Chapter 15

Research on Scar Treatments

Yongsoo Lee[*]
Oracle Dermatology Clinic, Soe-gu, Daejeon, South Korea

Abstract

In this chapter, it is the author's intention to postulate future scar treatment possibilities by demonstrating present practices which are of dubious nature in scar treatment research, along with solutions to overcome these significant issues.

In scar treatment research, the prospective randomized, controlled, double blind study design is virtually impossible. Why such study designs are thought to be impossible and how this seeming impossibility can possibly be overcome will be offered in this chapter. In addition, the author will seek to demonstrate other difficulties encountered during data collection, data management and the statistical analysis, giving alternate means of successfully managing data and its analysis.

The difficulties considered as a dubious practice in scar treatment research need to be identified and solutions must be provided in order for modern scar treatment to make significant and needed progress in the future.

In the field of laser scar treatments, many new devices have saturated the market in recent years along with a number of articles demonstrating their effectiveness in the form of statistical analysis.

This type of evaluations is vital and essential to measure the capabilities of a new device and as the first step of introducing novel devices into medical practice. However, in such circumstances, it is necessary to remind one of the fundamental questions to clinicians of any medical field, 'Is this statistical validity also significant clinically?' [1]

---

[*] Email: exusia@naver.com. Fax: +82-42-825-0289; Office: +82-42-488-8975; Mobile:+82-10-8824-0026.

Study Design

There are two types of articles on laser scar treatments. Some of them attempt to show a certain device is effective in treating scars or skin rejuvenation by statistical analysis (DE type article); on the other hand, others attempt to demonstrate how much the scarred area of the skin is improved aesthetically (AI type article) by a device or certain treatments. The difference between these two types of articles comes from the study design. DE type articles frequently employ measuring devices to measure the height and redness of scars and, sometimes, histologic measurements. [2,3] AI type articles try to measure aesthetic improvement by evaluators' opinions as scores of improvement; frequently, the objects of measurements are pre- and post-treatment photographs. The evaluators are medical doctors, nurses or sometimes the patients themselves who received the treatments. There are articles double purposed to measure the effectiveness of a device and, at the same time, aesthetic improvement of the patients by employing multiple means of assessments. [4] Besides the measuring methods, the differences are also found in the way variables are statistically analyzed.

Ideal Study Design

The soundest type of study design is the **prospective randomized controlled double blinded study**, in which patients are randomly assigned to a study category (such as clinical treatment or control), and are then followed forward in time (making it a prospective study) and the outcome is assessed. [1]

1. Randomized & controlled: Sample members need to be allocated to treatment groups by chance alone to avoid selection bias. [1] The probability of influence by unanticipated biases diminishes as the sample size grows larger. [1]
2. Double blinded or double masked: Humans involved in the study do not know the allocation of the sample members, so that they cannot influence measurements. The investigator cannot judge, even subconsciously, a greater improvement in a patient receiving the treatment the investigator prefers. Often, both the investigator and the patient are able to influence measurements, in which case both might be masked; such a study is termed double-masked or double-blinded study. [1]
3. Prospective: The study group and control group are followed forward in time and the outcome is assessed. [1]

Dificulties in Scar Treatment Study

Difficulties in Establishing Sound Study Designs in Scar Treatment Research

1. Randomly allocate patients to control group or study group

A) Control group need to have all the characteristics of the experimental group except the treatment under study. [1] The difficulties in scar treatment study design are as follows.
   i. No identical scars exist.
   ii. Even split face [5] are not identical enough to the other half [6] (Figure 1)

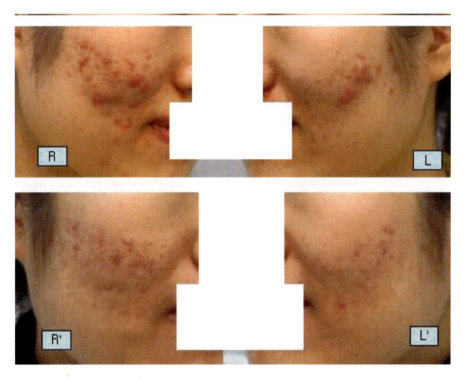

Figure 1. Pre- (Oct. 2006) and post- treatment (Dec. 2006) photographs of acne on face. As acne itself is not identically on each side of the face, FAPS are never be identical on both sides of the face. As R and L (acne) are not identical, R' and L' (FAPS) are not identical on both sides of the face. Source: "Combination Treatments of Facial Arophic Post-Acne Scars in Asians: Retrospective Analysis of 248 Pairs of Pre- and Post-Treatment Photographs" awarded with Antoni de Gimbernat International Prize in November 2010. Courtesy of Antoni de Gimbernat Foundation.

   iii. Split scar study design do not provide a sound enough control group as symmetrical and large enough scars, half part of which can serve as a control are rarely encountered. [7,8]

   It is an excellent and much more reliable study design to place considerable space between the control side and the treatment side in split scar study design. There is no data regarding how far they need to be separated in order not to influence the control side. [7,8]
B) Without an adequate control group (i.e., a group of scars that has all the characteristics of the treated scars except the treatment under study) random allocation is obviously impossible and meaningless even if it were possible.
2. In a double-blinded study, both the investigator and the patients who receive the treatments do not know the allocation of the sample members. [1]

A) As placebo laser treatment is impossible, everyone who participated in the study is not blinded.
   B) However, the evaluators can be blinded easily if individuals who are not involved in the research are asked to evaluate the outcomes, even though those who provide the treatment cannot be blinded.
   C) Patients' evaluations of outcomes
      i. If patients' evaluations were employed to a scar treatment study, the evaluators of the study are not blinded either.
      ii. A patient's evaluation and a doctor's evaluation can be significantly different [9,10], because patients can have different levels of expectation and there may be different standards from patient to patient, which tend to be subjective. This subjectivity also comes from being not blinded.
3. Prospective Study

   It is ideal to follow the study group and control group forward in time and the outcome is assessed. [1] However, this type of study design can require a prohibitively long time to gain a study result in scar treatment research. Frequently, it requires many months or sometimes years, to acquire sufficient data for a strong conclusion. Considering typical four- week treatment intervals of laser scar treatments, it is premature to make conclusions with a few months of observations, especially, in fibroproliferative scars (keloids and hypertrophic scars) cases, as they are notorious for their recurring tendencies.

Difficulties in Data Management

1. Sampling

   It is not easy to collect a large number of scar samples for a scar treatment research project. Small sample sizes in the scar treatment study are caused mainly by the reality that it is hard to find same type of scars in similar state (heterogeneous pre-treatment states) [6] and scar treatments take many months, or sometimes, years to collect sound data for strong conclusions. If it were possible, it would have taken years to collect large size of sample cases.
2. Collecting Raw Data
   A) There is no better way to evaluate the aesthetic improvement of a patient than by comparing pre- and post-treatment photographs. It would be ideal to compare the pre- and post-treatment state of a patient but it is impossible because no one can precisely remember their pre-treatment state six months prior or longer, exactly as it was.
   B) In addition to this, a photograph can be affected by many factors and provide biases during those time periods. It is impossible to take photographs under exactly the same conditions after many months or years later, even if a room without a window is dedicated for the photo and the same lighting system were used, because even the light bulbs can get old and may radiate a different quality and strength of light than many months before.

3. Measurements

As both effectiveness of a device and aesthetical improvement of a patient are continuous variables, accuracy can be affected greatly by precision of instruments or methods for measuring data. [1]

    i. Scales for measurement:
        1. The absence of standardized valid measures of scarring and treatment outcome is a major barrier to drawing strong conclusions in scar treatment researches. [11]
            A) To measure the effectiveness of a device:

When the purpose of a study is to measure the effectiveness or the characteristics of a device, it is good to use instruments to measure the depth, height and redness of scars. Even in such cases, the evaluators need to be individuals who are not involved in the research project.

            B) To measure the improvement of the aesthesis:

However, the improvement measured by such a device is not always directly related to the patient's aesthetic improvement. [6,10] Even when the height or redness of a scar is decreased to a significant degree, the scar may still be noticeable and annoy the patient. [12] Thus, It is necessary to employ an evaluation system that reflects the improvement of the aesthetic state of a scar when the purpose of the study is to determine how much the treatments or devices affected the aesthesis of patients. [10]

    ii. Confounding factor:
        1. Dyschromia of the scar can be a challenging factor when evaluating the improvement of the scar contour, and the contour of the scar can be a confounding factor when evaluating improvement in dyschromia, even if evaluators were asked not to consider changes in the conditions other than that of concern so that the scores would represent the improvement of the contour or dyschromia only. [6]
        2. Grading pre-treatment state
            A) Patients' grading of pre-treatment status also is not recommended as determination of disease load in terms of patient's perception of severity is intrinsically imperfect, due to varying subjectivity among individuals. [13] This subjectivity also comes from their not being blinded evaluators.
            B) Differences between the perspectives of evaluators [10]
        3. The different conditions of photographs at the time of pre-treatment photography and post-treatment photography.

Difficulties in Statistical Analysis

1. Variables:

A dubious, yet common practice, is treating continuous variables as categorical variables to assess the aesthetic improvement of scar treatments

[9,11,14], where the intervals of the classes or cutoff points between the classes were determined by custom, arbitrary and varied from study to study. [6,10,11] For example, if the class intervals were defined as excellent (over 80% improvement), fair (over 70% improvement), and good (over 60%) and so on, there is no rationale to define class intervals in this way because some can consider 90% improvement excellent while some consider 80% excellent. [10] Consequently, the true relationship between variables are meant to be obscured. [11]

2. Purpose of Statistical Analysis

Many times, the purpose of the statistical analysis is not clear. There can be two kinds of purposes in the statistical analysis of scar treatment studies. One is to demonstrate how much improvement has been made from the base line (i.e., pre-treatment state), and the other is to clarify how closely the treatment improved the scars to the unaffected state. [6,10]

Solutions to the Difficulties

Study Design

Two major obstacles to establishing the ideal study design in scar treatments research are lack of control groups and placebo treatments. These two factors make it impossible to allocate patients randomly to a control group or a study group and, consequently, to make it double blinded study. If these two factors could be compensated for, the study design would be closer to an ideal one.

1. Control group [6]
   A. unaffected skin around the scar as control: 'How closely improved is it to the normal skin?'

      If unaffected skin around the scar is employed as control to which the pre- and post-treatment states are compared, the measurements would represent how closely the scar improved to the normal skin after treatments.

      If the evaluators are asked to rate 0% when there was no difference between the pre-treatment photograph and the post-treatment photograph and to rate 100% when there is no difference between the treated region and the adjacent unaffected skin, [10] the scores assessed by the evaluators represent how much the scarred skin appearance approached that of normal skin. [6]

   B. Pre-treatment state as control: 'How much improvement has there been from the baseline?'
      1. If the pre-treatment state is employed as control, the measurements would represent how much improved from the baseline (pre-treatment state) after treatments. [6]
      2. Overcoming the heterogeneity of pre-treatment state:

If pre-treatment states are scored depending on the severity of each scar and the evaluation scores comparing pre- and post-treatment states are weighted by pre-treatment severity scores, the pre-treatment state of scars can serve as a control group despite their heterogeneity. [6]
2. Double blinded study

Because placebo treatments are virtually impossible in laser scar treatments, operator and the patients cannot be blinded. However, evaluators can be easily blinded if those who evaluate the treatment outcomes did not participate in the study. Patients' evaluations need to be avoided because they intrinsically have biases as previously mentioned, in addition to their not being blinded to treatments. Also, avoid operators' evaluations because they are not blinded to the treatments, either. [1] For the scientific research to be valid, at least one side ought to be blinded.

3. Prospective study

As retrospective study design is useful in situations in which the outcomes being studied either have a very small incidence, which would require a vast sample, or are very long developing, which would require a prohibitively long time to gain a study result, [1] retrospective study design is frequently used for scar treatments research. [11]
   A. However, retrospective studies typically have poorer data quality than prospective ones [11] due to the following reasons:
      i. The diagnosis of scarring is based on clinical assessments recorded in chart reviews. This method of assessment suffers in that the reporting practices of individual clinicians vary considerably. [11]
      ii. Interrater reliability of diagnosing scarring is not available. [11]
      iii. Both the validity and reliability of the measurement of the scarring are not demonstrated [11].
   B. Sound retrospective study design requires meticulous medical records. In order to make the medical record meticulous and useful in retrospective studies standardized valid measures of scarring and the treatment outcomes are imperative. [11]
   C. As retrospective studies typically have poorer data quality than prospective ones, [11] it is recommended that a prospective study be designed whenever possible, despite the aforementioned difficulties.

Data Management

1. Sampling
   A. Small sample size: 'The Bigger the Sample, the Stronger the Statistical Conclusions' [1]
      i. In scar treatment studies, it is not easy to collect significant number of sample cases due to the reasons previously mentioned. When it is impossible to have large enough sample size, Wilcoxon signed rank test, Wilcoxon rank sum test, Kruskal Wallis test, Friedman Test or Spearman's rank correlation

can be taken into consideration. However, as these non-parametric tests do not sufficiently reflect information contained in the data; this is especially true when interval scales are reduced to ordinal scales. Parametric tests are recommended whenever applicable. [15]

 ii. It is virtually impossible to collect homogenous groups of sample cases because the pre-treatment state of scars are never identical. [6] This reality makes it more difficult to have large samples. However, this difficulty can be overcome to a certain degree by having the evaluators' scores weighted with the severity of pre-treatment state. [6]

2. Collecting Raw Data

 In order to take photographs under the most similar conditions of many months or years before, the settings of the camera must not be changed once they are set. These must include shutter speed, aperture opening, lighting system and especially, the white balance also must be maintained as they are for many years.

3. Measurements

 A. Scales for measurement: As there are neither standardized valid measures nor any measuring device [11] for aesthetic improvement, scales for evaluation of aesthetic improvement after treatments need to be set by the study designers. The most information containing variable type is ratio scales which generally behave like continuous data and may not be separated out. [1]

  If we ask evaluators to score 0 to 10 points, the scores are likely to be like *.0 or *.5 points. However if we ask the evaluators to give scores 0 through 100, this would provide more freedom to give, for example, something like 53% or 97% improvement rather 5.5 or 9.5 points. This would make the evaluation scores behave more like continuous variables. The narrower the evaluation range becomes, the variable behaves more like discrete variables, which contain less information. In this context, we need to employ a broad and convenient scoring range. A percentile scale (0 to 100%) evaluation scale is recommended as a 0 to 10 points scale system may limit the evaluators' freedom to provide more elaborate information about the relationship between independent variables and dependent variables. A percentile system, therefore, would represent improvement more elaborately so that more information could be provided in the raw scores given by the evaluators.

 B. Confounding factor:

  1. The confounding factors previously mentioned can be overcome to a certain degree by taking multiple evaluators or measurements and comparing these measurements statistically. Evaluations with no statistical differences will be included in the next step of statistical analysis and the others should be considered outliers and disregarded. [6,10]

  2. A patient's evaluation and a doctor's evaluation can be significantly different, [6,10] because patients can have different levels of expectation and there may be different standards from patient to patient, which tend to be subjective. [9,10] Patients not being blinded to the treatments also is one of the causes of their subjectivity. Therefore, patients' evaluations are not

recommended to be used as measurements.
- C. Grading pre-treatment state
    1. Patients' grading of pre-treatment state is not recommended as determination of disease load in terms of their perception of severity is intrinsically imperfect, due to varying subjectivity among individuals. [13] This subjectivity also comes from the patients not being blinded.
    2. In order to reflect the severity of the pre-treatment state to the statistical analysis,
        - A. scar grading systems are necessary such as the Modified Quantitative Scar Grading System (MQSG) [6] or the Quantitative Global Scarring Grading system. [16]
        - B. Or a group of blinded professional evaluators need to give scores of ratio scales on the pre-treatment states and these evaluations of the pre-treatment states need to be statistically compared. [6,10] As there can be differences between perspectives of professionals, use the evaluation scores of evaluators that show no significant statistical differences to each other.
4. Statistical Analysis
    - A. Variables
        - i. It is recommended to use a ratio scale, just as the evaluators scored and not to reduce the variables from ratio scale to ordinal scale because we can lose information. [1,6,10,11]
        - ii. However, there is a rationale to reduce, for example, age (ratio scale) to age group (ordinal scale), because there are obvious physiologic differences between age groups, such as the pre-pubertal age group (<15 years of age) has obvious differences to the post-pubertal age group (≥15 years of age) due to hormonal activity. In addition, ordinal variables of age groups are usually used as independent variables, but not dependent variables, as improvement percentages in some of scar treatment studies. [6,10]
    - B. Purpose of statistical analysis
        The purpose of statistical analysis must be clarified before designing a study as described in the control group section.

Acknowledgments

Some of the figures, tables and descriptions presented in this chapter were used under the generous permission from Antoni de Gimbernat Foundation (Cambrils, Spain) to which the author ceded the copy right of "Combination Treatments of Facial Atrophic Post-Acne Scars in Asians: Retrospective Analysis of 248 Pairs of Pre- and Post-Treatment Photographs" as awarded with Antoni de Gimbernat International Prize in November, 2010.

References

[1] Riffenburgh RH. *Statistics in Medicine* New York, NY, USA: Elsevier Academic Press. 2006.

[2] Chan HH, Wong DS, Ho WS, Lam LK, Wei W. The use of pulsed dye laser for the prevention and treatment of hypertrophic scars in chinese persons. *Dermatol Surg* 2004; 30(7):987-994; discussion 994.

[3] Hambleton J, Shakespeare PG, Pratt BJ. The progress of hypertrophic scars monitored by ultrasound measurements of thickness. *Burns* 1992; 18(4):301-307.

[4] Seo KY, Yoon MS, Kim DH, Lee HJ. Skin rejuvenation by microneedle fractional radiofrequency treatment in Asian skin; Clinical and histological analysis. *Lasers in surgery and medicine*; 44(8):631-636.

[5] Alster TS, McMeekin TO. Improvement of facial acne scars by the 585 nm flashlamp-pumped pulsed dye laser. *J Am Acad Dermatol* 1996; 35(1):79-81.

[6] Lee Y. *Combination Treatments of Facial Atrophic Post-Acne Scars in Asians: Retrospective Analysis of 248 pairs of Pre- and Post-Treatment Photographs.* Awarded with Antonie de Gimbernat International Prize. Cambrils, Spain: Antoni de Gimbernat Foundation; 2010.

[7] Nouri K, Jimenez GP, Harrison-Balestra C, Elgart GW. 585-nm pulsed dye laser in the treatment of surgical scars starting on the suture removal day. *Dermatol Surg* 2003; 29(1):65-73; discussion 73.

[8] Alster TS, Williams CM. Treatment of keloid sternotomy scars with 585 nm flashlamp-pumped pulsed-dye laser. *Lancet* 1995; 345(8959):1198-1200.

[9] Chua SH, AngP, Khoo LS, Goh CL. Nonablative 1450-nm diode laser in the treatment of facial atrophic acne scars in type IV to V Asian skin: a prospective clinical study. *Dermatol Surg* 2004; 30(10):1287-1291.

[10] Lee Y. Combination treatment of surgical, post-traumatic and post-herpetic scars with ablative lasers followed by fractional laser and non-ablative laser in Asians. *Lasers Surg Med* 2009; 41(2):131-140.

[11] Lawrence JW, Mason ST, Schomer K, Klein MB. Epidemiology and impact of scarring after burn injury: a systematic review of the literature. *J Burn Care Res;* 33(1):136-146.

[12] Kadunc BV, Trindade de Almeida AR. Surgical treatment of facial acne scars based on morphologic classification: a Brazilian experience. *Dermatol Surg* 2003; 29(12):1200-1209.

[13] Goodman GJ, Baron JA. Postacne scarring: a qualitative global scarring grading system. *Dermatol Surg* 2006; 32(12):1458-1466.

[14] Cho SI, Kim YC. Treatment of atrophic facial scars with combined use of high-energy pulsed CO2 laser and Er:YAG laser: a practical guide of the laser techniques for the Er:YAG laser. *Dermatol Surg* 1999; 25(12):959-964.

[15] Jong-Gu Park S-JJ, Tae-Yong Lee, *Woong-Soep Park.* SPSSWIN을 이용한 보건통계학 (Biomedical Statistics by SPSSWIN): Gye-Chuk Publishers. 2003.

[16] Goodman GJ, Baron JA. Postacne scarring--a quantitative global scarring grading system. *J Cosmet Dermatol* 2006; 5(1):48-52.

[17] Lee Y. *Combination Laser Treatments and Classification of Scars.* International Scar Meeting in Tokyo 2010. Tokyo, Japan; 2010.
[18] Lee Y. *Combination Treatments and Classification of Scars.* US-China Medical Science 2011; 8(6):321-334.
[19] Lee Y. Combination Laser Treatments and Classification of Cutaneous Scars. *Journal of Wound Technology* 2012; 15:45-46.

Index

#

1,064nm Neodyium Yittrium-Aluminum-Garnet Laser (NdYAG), 17, 18, 23, 24, 166, 177, 192, 200, 207, 210, 217, 221
1,550m erbium glass (Er Glass) laser, 217
10,600-nm CO_2 fractional laser, 18
1064-nm Q-switched neodymium yttrium-aluminum-garnet (NdYAG) laser, 17
1450-nm diode laser, 18, 19, 24, 177, 232
1450-nm diode lasers, 19
1550-nm Er-doped fractional photothermolysis, 18
2,790nm yttrium sapphire, 217
2,940nm erbium yttirum-aluminum-garnet (ErYAG) laser, 9, 15, 16, 17, 174, 178, 188, 189, 192, 200, 205, 209, 217, 232
308nm Excimer Laser, 216
308nm xenon-chloride excimer laser, 216
5 isoforms of the GPx selenoprotein, 71
585-nm PDL, 16, 17, 19
5-Fluorouracil (5-FU), 12, 22, 151, 152
810-nm diode laser, 18

β

β-rays, 123, 124

γ

γ-rays, 123, 124

A

ablation, 10, 15, 54, 144, 175, 176, 217
ablative, 4, 14, 17, 18, 19, 23, 24, 145, 155, 171, 174, 175, 176, 177, 178, 185, 188, 189, 190, 191, 192, 193, 194, 195, 197, 199, 201, 205, 206, 207, 208, 210, 217, 218, 221, 222, 232
ablative fractional CO_2 laser, 14
ablative fractional photothermolysis (AFP), 175
ablative laser sculpting, 194, 195
ablative lasers, 4, 17, 174, 175, 176, 185, 191, 192, 199, 205, 206, 210, 217, 232
acanthosis nigricans, 215
acatalamic mice, 70
accordion effect, 134
acetylsalicylic acid (ASA), 143
acne, 4, 5, 6, 7, 9, 10, 11, 16, 17, 18, 19, 20, 21, 23, 24, 25, 29, 32, 33, 35, 36, 37, 47, 124, 146, 147, 148, 149, 154, 155, 156, 157, 159, 162, 163, 166, 167, 168, 178, 182, 183, 195, 199, 200, 201, 210, 215, 217, 218, 225, 232
acne scars, 5, 7, 16, 17, 18, 19, 20, 21, 23, 24, 25, 29, 35, 147, 149, 155, 157, 159, 162, 163, 166, 167, 168, 178, 199, 201, 217, 218, 232
actin filaments, 111
actinic keratoses, 10, 21
actin-rich fibroblasts (myofibroblasts), 5, 45, 46, 59, 60, 67, 78, 81, 84, 85, 105, 111
activator protein-1 (AP-1), 58, 61, 83, 164
adhesion kinase, 50, 55, 78, 100, 104
adipocytes, 69, 86
adnexal structures, 193
adventitial fibroblasts, 66
adverse effects, 14, 141, 142, 143, 147, 152, 153, 187, 188, 190, 217
aesthesis, x, 192, 227
aging, ix, 69, 75, 76, 77, 95, 98
alginates, 111
allantoin, 142
allergic contact dermatitis, 14
Allium cepa, 142, 160
alpha hydroxyl acid, 216
alpha-smooth muscle actin, 54, 101
alphastria cream, 215

anabolic steroid, 214
anger, 28, 29, 31, 49
angioedma, 154
angiofibromas, 10
angiogenesis, 44, 59, 62, 70, 77, 92, 98, 111
angiotensin II (AngII), 58, 62, 67, 70, 76, 80, 83, 88
anorexia nervosa, 214, 220
anti-fibrotic therapies, 60
anti-inflammatory, 12, 74, 96, 142, 143, 158, 160
antimitotic drugs, 191
antioxidant enzyme, 63, 68, 69, 70, 71, 75, 77, 81, 89
antioxidant responsive element (ARE), 58, 75, 83
antioxidant vitamins, 76
anxiety, 25, 26, 27, 28, 29, 30, 32, 33, 214
apoptosis, 5, 46, 50, 55, 59, 60, 63, 65, 67, 71, 72, 74, 76, 79, 82, 85, 88, 90, 91, 92, 94, 95, 96, 100, 143, 151, 152, 164
apurinic/apyrimidinic endonuclease/redox effector factor-1 (APE/Ref-1), 58, 61, 79
arbutin, 16
ascorbate, 71, 89
ascorbic, 16, 89
assessment, 8, 9, 20, 21, 22, 35, 105, 123, 128, 163, 186, 229
atherosclerosis, 74, 75, 85
ATP generation, 65
ATP-synthase, 65
atrophic, 4, 5, 6, 7, 9, 10, 15, 16, 17, 18, 19, 21, 23, 24, 41, 110, 111, 131, 132, 148, 153, 154, 155, 156, 157, 162, 163, 166, 167, 177, 178, 180, 181, 182, 188, 191, 193, 194, 195, 200, 209, 212, 213, 217, 232
atrophic scars, 10, 15, 16, 17, 18, 19, 23, 24, 110, 131, 132, 153, 154, 155, 156, 167, 178, 180, 181, 182, 191, 193, 194, 195, 217
atrophy, 4, 5, 7, 15, 126, 144, 150, 152, 166, 207, 215, 216, 218
autoimmune diseases, 74
autologous fat, 156
avoidant/numbing symptoms, 27
azelaic, 16, 188

B

BCG vaccination, 48
benzoic acid, 148
bFGF (basic fibroblast growth factor), 190
bilirubin, 64, 68, 72, 73, 74, 76, 85, 91, 92, 95, 96
biliverdin, 58, 64, 72, 73, 74, 92, 94, 95, 96
biliverdin reductase, 58, 72, 94, 95
bioinformatics, 99, 102
biologically effective doses (BEDs), 125
bleomycin, 12, 63, 70, 81, 105, 151, 153, 164, 166

bleomycin-induced lung fibrosis, 70
bleomycin-induced pulmonary fibrosis, 63, 81
blush, 158
body dysmorphic disorder, 32
Borges' relaxed skin tension line (RSTL), 132, 133
Botulinum toxin A, 159
bovine collagen, 154, 156, 166
boxcar, 7, 16, 29, 153, 154
brachytherapies, 123, 124
breast cancer, 127
broad-band contractures, 131, 132
broken line effect, 134
bronzer, 158
bupivacaine, 151
burn scars, 25, 34, 80, 160, 184, 185, 199, 209
burn severity, 27
burns, 4, 5, 11, 27, 33, 34, 35, 72, 78, 80, 103, 158, 161, 167, 184, 186

C

cachectic, 214
calcipotriol, 143, 160
calcium channel blockers, 150
calcium hydroxyapatite, 153, 155
calcium hydroxylapatite, 155, 167
camouflage, 140, 157
cancer, 34, 49, 53, 54, 65, 70, 74, 75, 79, 104, 127, 128, 129, 154, 164, 166
carbon dioxide (CO2) laser, 9, 14, 15, 16, 17, 18, 20, 22, 23, 167, 172, 174, 178, 189, 192, 200, 201, 205, 209, 217, 218, 221, 222, 232
carbon monoxide (CO), 22, 58, 72, 73, 74, 85, 91, 92, 93, 94, 221
carboxyhemoglobin, 58, 74
carcinogenesis, 124, 127, 128
cardiac fibroblasts, 67, 70, 80, 84, 87, 88
cardiomyocytes, 69, 70, 87
catalase, 58, 64, 68, 70, 72, 76, 77, 87, 88
categorical variables, 227
CD3+ T cells, 143
cefaclor, 146
celecoxib, 143, 161
cell adhesion molecules, 111
cell proliferation, 42, 44, 45, 67, 70, 83, 84, 99, 111
cell-matrix communication, 100
cellular redox balance, 58, 63, 69, 73
Centella asiatica, 215
chemexfoliation, 216
chemical exfoliation,, 10
chemical peels, 4, 10, 11, 19, 21, 139, 140, 150, 162
chemical reconstruction of skin scars (CROSS), 21, 148, 162, 187, 194, 208

chemoattractant protein-1, 50, 100
chemokine, 77, 100
chemotaxis, 43, 51
chemotherapeutic agents, 150
chemotherapy agent, 12
chest wall keloid, 128
chikenpox, 47
chondroitin sulfate, 6
chromophores, 172, 173, 174, 176, 180, 192, 195
chronic granulomatous disease, 58, 66, 82
c-Jun N-terminal kinases (JNK), 48, 58, 61
classification of scars, 8
clotting factors, 43, 44
CO_2 laser, 14, 15, 16, 17, 18, 20, 22, 23, 174, 178, 189, 192, 200, 209, 217, 218, 221, 222, 232
coagulation, 11, 18, 43, 44, 66, 72, 110, 148, 175
cocoa butter lotion, 214
cognitive behavioral therapy, 31, 32
cognitive-behavioral methods, 32, 37
coherence, 171, 172
Coherent UltraPulse, 15
collagen, 4, 5, 7, 10, 11, 15, 16, 17, 18, 20, 22, 44, 45, 46, 47, 48, 50, 52, 53, 54, 59, 60, 62, 67, 70, 73, 77, 80, 84, 87, 100, 101, 102, 105, 111, 141, 142, 143, 145, 147, 149, 150, 151, 152, 153, 154, 155, 156, 158, 159, 163, 164, 165, 166, 167, 168, 172, 174, 175, 213, 215, 216, 217, 218, 219, 220, 221
collagen biosynthesis, 101
collagen fibers, 5, 18, 45, 47, 175
collagen induction therapy, 11
collagenase, 6, 9, 22, 45, 111, 152, 165
collagen-glycosaminoglycan copolymers, 159
collagen-producing fibroblasts, 101
collimation, 171
combination laser treatment, 185, 196, 199, 233
combination therapy, 152
Combined Platelet-Rich Plasma and Intradermal Radiofrequency, 219
complement system, 57
complications, 10, 13, 16, 17, 66, 74, 75, 76, 77, 96, 97, 112, 126, 167
computer pattern generator (CPG) scanning device, 15
concealer, 158
confounding factor, 77, 227, 230
connective tissue growth factor (CTGF), 100, 176, 178
contact dermatitis, 14, 116, 119, 142
continuous data, 230
continuous variables, 227, 230
Continuous-Wave (CW), 160, 164, 167, 172, 178, 219, 222

contour, 132, 174, 175, 188, 189, 192, 193, 194, 195, 204, 208, 227
Contractubex®, 142
contractures, 4, 5, 8, 34, 47, 52, 131, 133, 135, 136, 160, 197
control group, 224, 225, 226, 228, 229, 231
copper tripeptide-1, 190
CO-releasing molecules (CO-RMs), 73
Corticoid injections (triamcinolone acetonide 10 mg / 40 mg), 11
corticosteroid ointment, 119
corticosteroid(s), 100, 110, 119, 131, 132, 142, 143, 150, 160, 215, 221
cortisol, 30, 215
cosmetics, 204
Cre/loxP recombinase, 101
cross-linking of collagen, 60
cryogen cooling spray, 17
cryosurgery, 12, 139, 140, 144, 145, 161, 191, 200, 209
Cryosurgery (or cryotherapy, cryoablation), 4, 8, 16, 19, 144, 145, 150, 151, 152, 153, 161, 166, 206, 207
cryosurgery needles, 145
cryotherapy, 4, 8, 16, 19, 144, 145, 150, 151, 152, 153, 161, 166
cyclooxygenase-2 (COX-2), 143
cytochrome c oxidase, 74, 82, 94
cytochrome P450, 64
cytochromes, 72
cytokine IL-6, 77
cytokines, 5, 43, 45, 48, 59, 60, 67, 76, 78, 100, 110, 141, 143, 147
cytoskeleton, 54, 111
cytosolic Cu/Zn-dependent SOD1, 69
cytosolic enzyme, 71

D

data management, 223
data quality, 229
decorin, 152
de-epithelialization, 15
defocused, 173
dependent variables, 230, 231
depigmentation, 118, 126, 136
depression, 25, 26, 27, 28, 29, 30, 31, 32, 35, 36, 37, 38, 188, 207
dermabrasion, 4, 10, 15, 19, 21, 23, 31, 145, 156
dermal deformity, 188
dermaroller, 149, 162
desmosomes, 148
despair, 31

detachment, 28, 145
diabetes, 47, 65, 69, 74, 75, 76, 77, 80, 86, 95, 96, 97, 98
diabetes mellitus, 74, 75, 76, 80, 86, 95, 97
diamond fraise, 10, 145
discomfort, 6, 17, 25, 29, 33, 141, 187, 188, 190, 217
discrete variables, 230
disfigurement, 26, 30, 32, 33, 34, 36, 37, 188
dissociative flashback, 28
doctor-patient relationship, 26
donor site morbidity, 136
dopamine, 33
dot peeling, 18, 23
double-blinded study, 142, 224, 225
downtime, 18, 174, 175, 187, 188, 195, 204, 208, 218
Duox1-2, 66
dyschromia, 180, 192, 195, 204, 206, 227
dyskeratosis, 151
dyspigmentation, 150, 151, 155, 159, 218

E

E3 ubiquitin ligase, 49
earlobe keloid, 128, 165
ecchymoses, 215
Ectropion, 16
effectiveness, 18, 19, 22, 36, 123, 124, 141, 146, 153, 159, 165, 178, 186, 187, 188, 194, 195, 200, 209, 223, 224, 227
efficacy, 9, 18, 22, 99, 105, 125, 140, 141, 142, 143, 144, 145, 146, 152, 154, 156, 158, 160, 165, 166, 175, 187, 188, 214, 215, 216, 217, 218, 219
EGF (epidermal growth factor), 43, 84, 190, 200
Ehlers-Danlos syndrome, 212
elastic fiber, 6, 213, 217, 219
elastic garments, 141
elastin, 100, 103, 216
Electrical Stimulation, 159
electron-beams, 123, 124
endogenous antioxidant systems, 62
endogenous antioxidants, 74
endothelial, 43, 44, 45, 51, 59, 64, 66, 69, 72, 83, 86, 87, 88, 90, 91, 92, 94, 95, 96, 97, 101, 104, 109, 111, 116, 151, 165
endothelial cells, 45, 59, 66, 69, 72, 83, 86, 91, 96, 101, 109, 111, 116
endothelial nitric oxide synthase, 64, 87
energy density, 13, 14
epidermal nevi, 10
epidermis, 9, 10, 15, 17, 18, 42, 47, 72, 90, 113, 132, 145, 147, 174, 175, 213, 217
epidermolysis, 145

epithelial cells, 62, 67, 70, 85, 88, 90, 111
epithelization, 43, 72, 77, 111
equibiaxial strain, 50
Erbium yttrium-aluminum-garnet (ErYAG) laser, 15, 16, 17, 174, 178, 188, 189, 192, 200, 209, 232
ERK, 48, 50, 58, 84
erythrocytes, 69, 74, 86
estrogen, 7
ethnic groups, 172, 192
excess relative risk (ERR), 127
excision, 16, 22, 125, 126, 143, 144, 152, 155, 156
extracellular matrix (ECM), 41, 42, 44, 45, 46, 48, 49, 52, 54, 58, 59, 60, 62, 63, 67, 70, 99, 100, 103, 111, 141, 151, 164
extracellular matrix metalloproteinase inducer, 58, 70
extracellular matrix remodeling, 141
extracellular peroxidases, 67
extracellular SOD3, 69
exudate, 111
eyelid grafts, 135

F

facial rejuvenation, 11, 176
fascia, 47, 113, 114, 133, 159
Fenton chemistry, 65, 73
ferritin, 64, 68, 73, 75, 96
ferrous iron, 75
Fetal wound healing, 62
Fibrillar collagen, 102, 105
fibrin, 59
fibroblast growth factor, 43, 44, 190
fibroblast precursors, 101
fibroblast-matrix interactions, 100
fibroblasts, 5, 43, 44, 45, 46, 48, 49, 50, 52, 53, 54, 55, 59, 60, 66, 67, 70, 71, 73, 78, 80, 84, 85, 87, 88, 93, 100, 101, 104, 105, 109, 111, 116, 145, 151, 152, 164, 165, 215, 216
fibroblast-specific hypoxia-inducible factor-1 alpha, 101
fibroblast-specific protein-1, 101
fibrogenesis, 60, 67, 72, 73, 78, 84, 101, 102, 103
fibrogenic factors, 60
fibronectin, 44, 51, 70, 81, 100, 111, 165, 213, 220
fibroplasia, 48
fibroproliferation, 100, 101, 102
Fibroproliferative Scars (FPS), 166, 181, 182, 185, 191, 192, 197, 199, 206, 209
fibrosis, 12, 14, 17, 26, 49, 50, 53, 54, 55, 60, 62, 63, 65, 67, 68, 70, 71, 73, 75, 78, 80, 81, 84, 85, 87, 88, 91, 99, 100, 101, 102, 103, 104, 105, 106, 127, 158

fillers, 16, 31, 140, 150, 153, 154, 155, 156, 157, 166, 167
flap, 92, 120, 133, 134, 136, 137, 178, 197
flow dopplers, 8
fluence, 172
foam compression, 117
foam(s), 91, 111, 117, 119
focal adhesion kinase (FAK), 50, 78, 100
focal length, 173
follicles, 174
folliculitis, 47
foreign body granuloma, 154, 156
foundation, 157, 158
fractional laser(s), 18, 23, 24, 171, 175, 176, 178, 185, 189, 190, 191, 194, 197, 199, 205, 206, 207, 208, 210, 217, 218, 232
Fractional Photothermolysis, 178, 217
free fatty acids, 76
free radical nitric oxide, 64
free radical-induced peroxidation, 74
Friedman Test or Spearman's rank correlation, 229
full thickness skin graft, 134, 135
functional impairments, 206

G

galvanic skin responses (GSR), 30
garments, 117, 119, 141
Gaussian cross-sectional power density pattern, 173
Gel sheet, 119
gelatin, 45
gelatinases, 45
general debility, 212
genetic factors, 29, 110, 212
Gilberts, 74
glucation end-products (AGE), 58, 76
glucocorticosteroids, 215
glucose 6-phosphate dehydrogenase (G6PD), 58, 68, 85, 86, 87
glutathione (GSH), 58, 64, 68, 71, 77, 85, 86, 88, 89, 90, 95
glutathione disulfide, 58, 64, 68
glutathione peroxidase (GPx), 58, 64, 68, 70, 71, 72, 77, 86, 88, 89, 90
glutathione reductase, 58, 64, 68
glycolic, 10, 11, 16, 21, 147, 148, 149, 162, 163
glycolic acid, 10, 11, 21, 147, 148, 162, 163, 216
glycoproteins, 100
glycosaminoglycan, 5, 22, 142, 159, 165, 168
glycosaminoglycan synthesis, 142
glycosaminoglycans, 100
GPx enzymes, 70, 71
granulation, 4, 5, 45, 72, 78

granulation tissue, 5, 45, 72, 78
granulomas, 156
growth factor(s), 41, 42, 43, 44, 45, 48, 49, 51, 53, 54, 57, 59, 60, 62, 68, 71, 78, 83, 84, 85, 88, 90, 92, 100, 103, 110, 111, 151, 164, 165, 176, 178, 190, 200, 219
GSH-dependent enzyme, 71
guanylyl cyclase, 58, 73
guilt, 31

H

H_2O_2, 58, 60, 64, 66, 67, 68, 69, 70, 71, 73, 74, 190
hallucinations, 28
heart failure, 69, 84
heat shock protein-47, 101
helper T cells, 101
hematocytes, 42
heme, 57, 58, 64, 65, 68, 70, 72, 73, 74, 75, 90, 91, 92, 93, 94, 95, 96
heme oxygenase (HO), 58, 64, 90, 91, 92, 93, 95, 96
heme proteins, 57, 90
hemoglobin, 9, 58, 72, 74, 172, 176
hemolytic anemia, 69
hemoproteins, 57, 72, 74
hemostasis, 43, 44, 66
heparin, 142
heparinoid, 109, 117, 119
herpes simplex virus, 146, 154, 166
hirsutism, 215
histopathology, 181
homeostasis, 48, 59, 64, 65, 68, 75, 76, 80, 82, 97
hormones, 68, 85, 110, 111
Hospital Depression and Anxiety Scale, 30
human collagen, 153
hyaluronic acid, 5, 153, 154, 157, 166, 167
hyaluronic acid derivatives, 153
hyaluronidase, 6, 154, 157
hydration, 11, 141
hydrocolloids, 111
hydrogels, 104, 111
hydrogen peroxide, 58, 60, 64, 79, 82, 89, 93
hydroquinone, 14, 16
hydroxyl radical, 58, 60
hydroxyproline, 73
hyper-arousal symptoms, 27
hyperbilirubinemia, 74
hyperglycemia, 63, 65, 76, 86
hyperinflammation, 66
hyperpigmentation, 9, 14, 16, 21, 148, 151, 152, 162, 172, 175, 178, 188, 192, 200, 210, 217, 218
hypertension, 62, 69, 80, 81, 84, 86, 88, 110

hypertrophic, 4, 5, 6, 7, 8, 9, 11, 12, 13, 14, 16, 17, 19, 20, 22, 30, 32, 33, 34, 36, 41, 46, 47, 48, 50, 52, 54, 55, 60, 62, 69, 86, 102, 103, 104, 105, 109, 110, 111, 112, 113, 117, 118, 120, 123, 124, 128, 129, 131, 132, 133, 137, 140, 141, 143, 144, 145, 148, 149, 150, 151, 152, 153, 155, 158, 159, 160, 161, 164, 165, 167, 180, 181, 185, 186, 194, 200, 201, 206, 208, 209, 210, 226, 232
hypertrophic scars, 4, 5, 6, 11, 12, 13, 14, 16, 19, 20, 22, 30, 32, 36, 41, 46, 47, 50, 52, 54, 62, 69, 86, 103, 104, 109, 110, 112, 113, 117, 118, 120, 123, 124, 128, 129, 131, 132, 133, 140, 141, 143, 144, 145, 148, 149, 150, 151, 152, 153, 155, 158, 159, 160, 161, 164, 165, 167, 180, 181, 185, 186, 194, 200, 201, 206, 208, 209, 210, 226, 232
hypnosis, 32, 37
hypopigmentary, 216
hypopigmentation, 9, 11, 16, 17, 144, 145, 149, 152, 193
hypothalamic-pituitary-adrenal (HPA) axis, 215
hypoxia, 58, 61, 62, 76, 94, 101, 111
hypoxia inducible factor-1 (HIF-1), 58, 61, 73, 104

I

iatrogenic Cushing's syndrome, 151
ice pick, 7, 16, 17, 153, 159
idiopathic pulmonary fibrosis, 60, 67, 78, 84, 158
illusions, 28
imiquimod, 140, 143, 160
immune cells, 111
immunogenicity, 154, 155, 156
immunomodulator, 143
immunomodulatory, 74
immunosuppressive agents, 110
incidence, 6, 9, 16, 128, 129, 145, 153, 191, 195, 213, 214, 215, 216, 229
incision lines, 132
indication, 142, 149, 197, 198, 216
infection, 7, 9, 10, 16, 77, 111, 112, 153, 154, 156, 193, 212
inflammation, vii, 4, 7, 9, 11, 20, 42, 43, 44, 45, 47, 48, 51, 53, 54, 59, 60, 62, 66, 67, 73, 74, 76, 77, 80, 81, 83, 90, 91, 92, 96, 98, 99, 100, 104, 109, 110, 111, 112, 116, 117, 148, 154, 212
inflammatory cascade, 100
inflammatory cell(s), 4, 44, 45, 57, 59, 60, 62, 66, 77, 99, 101, 110
inflammatory mediators, 5, 62, 66, 67, 72, 73, 147
inflammatory signaling, 50, 55, 104
injections, 11, 12, 19, 31, 54, 69, 112, 163, 164, 167, 191, 192, 193, 200, 206, 207, 209
insulin-like growth factor (IGF), 49

integrin, 43, 50, 54, 78, 83
integrins, 51, 101, 111
intense pulsed light (IPL), 18, 218
interferon, 22, 54, 58, 67, 89, 143, 152, 165
interferon (INF)γ, 58, 67
interferon-alpha 2b, 152
interferon-α, 143
interleukin, 58, 67, 98, 102, 151, 165
interleukin (IL)-1, 67
interleukin-6, 98, 151, 165
interpersonal therapy, 32
interrater reliability, 20
interstitial fibrosis, 63, 70
intracellular mechanosensor, 101
intracellular water, 174
intracheal zymosan, 66
intradermal or subdermal fillers, 153
intralesional agents, 139, 140, 150, 159
Intralesional Cryotherapy, 145
intralesional propranolol, 159
intra-lesional therapy, 4
intrusive recollections, 27
ion channels, 111
IPL (intense pulsed light), 18, 172, 192, 208, 218
iron, 58, 64, 65, 68, 72, 75, 82, 85, 91, 96
iron regulatory protein (IRP), 58, 75
irradiance, 173
ischemic necrosis, 156
isotretinoin, 9, 10, 21

J

JNK and p38 pathways, 48

K

keloids, 4, 5, 6, 9, 12, 13, 14, 19, 20, 22, 23, 30, 32, 36, 41, 46, 47, 48, 49, 52, 54, 86, 100, 103, 109, 110, 112, 113, 118, 120, 123, 124, 125, 126, 127, 128, 129, 131, 132, 133, 136, 140, 141, 143, 144, 145, 146, 149, 150, 152, 153, 159, 160, 161, 164, 165, 168, 176, 178, 180, 181, 185, 186, 200, 201, 209, 226
keratinocyte, 51, 67, 71, 73, 90, 92, 104, 200
Keratinocyte growth factor (KGF), 43, 44, 200
keratinocyte(s), 5, 42, 44, 45, 51, 59, 67, 70, 71, 72, 73, 78, 83, 87, 89, 90, 92, 93, 101, 104, 143, 174, 200
kidney mesangial cells, 67
Kirschner wire, 135
knockout (KO) of Nox2, 67
kojic, 16

Kruskal Wallis test, 229
Kupffer cells, 62

L

lactic acid, 10, 147, 148, 149, 153, 154, 155, 166
Landmark distortion, 197
Langer line, 132
Langerhans cells, 143
LASER, 171
laser vaporization, 15, 22
Laser-Assisted Skin Healing (LASH) technique, 19
laser-tissue interaction, 171, 172, 174
lentigines, 218
leptin, 76
lidocaine, 12, 13, 147, 151, 156, 163
limited photothermal effect, 15
linear contractures, 131, 132
lipid peroxidases, 64
lipid peroxidation, 70, 71, 74, 77, 81, 90, 95, 142
lipopolysaccharide (LPS), 59, 66, 67, 83, 84
liposomal lidocaine, 13
liposuction, 156
local flaps, 136
local necrosis, 154
long pulse, 207
low density lipoprotein (LDL), 59, 74, 85, 90, 95
Luxar NovaPulse, 15

M

macrolide, 152
macrophages, 5, 43, 44, 48, 51, 59, 62, 66, 71, 72, 77, 89, 91, 101, 104
make-up, 157, 158, 188, 195
malignancy, 111, 200, 209
malignant changes, 127
Marfan syndrome, 212
mast cell, 7, 145
matrix metalloproteinase (MMP), 45, 46, 48, 53, 58, 59, 70, 88, 102, 105
maturation phase, 45
measurements, 8, 17, 159, 224, 228, 230, 231, 232
mechanical forces, 52, 54, 99, 100, 109, 111, 112, 113, 116, 119, 120, 132
mechanobiology, 42, 50
mechanoreceptors, 111
mechanosensors, 111
mechanotransduction pathway, 50
medium, 111, 147, 172
melanin, 8, 9, 14, 109, 117, 118, 172, 216, 217
melanin indices, 8

melanosomes, 145
melasma, 18, 192, 208
membrane type-MMPs, 45
mesangial cells, 60, 67, 84
metal binding proteins, 68
metalloproteinases, 45, 46, 51, 53
methylxanthine, 159
microarray pattern, 217
microdermabrasion, 11, 21, 139, 140, 145, 146, 150, 162, 218, 222
microneedling, 4, 11, 19, 21, 31, 139, 140, 149, 150, 162, 163, 219
microscopic thermal treatment zones, 18
microscopic treatment zones (MTZs), 175, 217
migration of keratinocytes, 5, 44
minocycline, 159, 167
mitochondrial electron transport chain, 65
mitochondrial Mn-dependent SOD2, 69
mitochondrial or nuclear DNA, 65
mitochondrial respiration, 63, 74
mitochondrial respiratory chain, 64, 82
mitogen, 44, 53, 59, 61, 84, 85
mitogen-activated protein kinase (MAPK), 53, 59, 61, 84, 85
mitomycin C, 152, 165
Modified Quantitative Scar Grading System (MQSG), 195, 231
Mohs defects, 10
moisturizer, 119, 157
monoamine oxidase, 33
Monoamine Oxidase Inhibitors, 33
monochromaticity, 171
monocyte chemoattractant protein-1 (MCP-1), 50, 100
monocytes, 43, 44, 59, 66, 104
morphology, x, 100, 179, 180, 181, 183, 184, 203
MTZ's (microscopic treatment zone), 175, 190, 217
multiple z-plasties, 133, 134
multi-protein complexes, 65
myofibroblasts, 5, 45, 46, 59, 60, 67, 78, 81, 84, 85, 105, 111

N

NADPH oxidase (Nox), 59, 62, 64, 66, 68, 69, 80, 81, 82, 83, 84, 86, 87, 96, 97
narrow-band ultraviolet-B (UVB), 216
necrosis, 11, 15, 44, 59, 67, 83, 127, 133, 144, 148, 151, 152, 154, 156, 157
NEDD4, 49
negative pressure, 159, 168
neocollagenesis, 149, 174, 217
neovascularization, 44, 73, 92

neurodegeneration, 65, 74, 89
neutrophils, 5, 43, 44, 59, 62, 66
NF-E2-related factor 2 (Nrf2), 59, 61, 75, 83, 92, 94, 96
NF-κB, 59, 61, 62, 66, 68, 76
nitric oxide (NO), 59, 64, 71, 81, 83, 84, 87, 89, 96, 97
non- or minimally invasive treatment, 139, 140, 157
non-ablative FP (NAFP), 175
non-ablative lasers, 4, 17, 174, 175, 206, 217
non-comedogenic, 157
non-hypertrophic scars, 194, 206, 208, 209
non-occlusive bandage, 13
non-parametric tests, 230
Non-Steroidal Anti-Inflammatory Drugs (NSAIDs), 143
Noradrenegic and Specific Serotonergic Antidepressants, 33
norepinephrine, 33, 38
Norepinephrine Reuptake Inhibitors, 33
Norepinephrine-Dopamine Reuptake Inhibitors, 33
normotrophic, 4, 5, 41
Nox1-5, 66
Nox-generated ROS, 65, 67
Nrf2-Keap1 complex, 61
nuclear factor κB (NF-κB), 59, 61, 62, 66, 68, 76
nutritional deficiency, 212
nylon, 113

O

obesity, 213, 214, 220
occlusion, 141, 143, 154
occlusive dressing, 16, 190, 197, 205, 207, 208
olive, 214
onion extract, 11, 22, 142, 192, 208
onion-extract gels, 140
operating distance, 173
ordinal scale(s), 230, 231
organic peroxides, 71
osteopontin, 48, 53
osteoporosis, 77
ovary cells, 69
overcorrection, 154, 155, 156
oxidative phosphorylation system, 65
oxyhemoglobin, 172, 216

P

p47phox, 66, 67, 83
p53, 61
palisading granulomas, 154

panatrophy, 4, 5
paraffin, 153
parameters, xi, 12, 30, 143, 171, 172, 173, 176, 190, 192, 208
parametric tests, 230
Parkinson, 65
pathological scars, 46, 110, 111, 113, 131, 132, 133
pathological wound healing, 64, 75
PDL, 12, 13, 14, 16, 17, 19, 175, 192, 197, 207, 216, 217, 218
peak power, 172
peels, 4, 10, 11, 16, 19, 21, 139, 140, 147, 148, 149, 150, 162, 163, 216
penetration, 16, 22, 145, 147, 163, 173
pentose phosphate pathway, 64, 68
Pentoxifylline, 159
Perceived Stress Scale, 30
perforator flaps, 136
perforator pedicled propeller flap, 136, 137
Pericytes, 101
periodontal diseases, 77
perioperative scar management, 110
peri-orbital rhytides, 18
peritoneal fibrosis, 70, 88
peroxidases, 64, 67, 72, 88, 89
peroxidation, 68, 70, 71, 74, 77, 81, 89, 90, 95, 142
Peroxiredoxins (Prdx), 59, 64, 71, 72
peroxynitrite, 64, 71
petechiae, 17
petroleum jelly, 13
phagocytic cells, 62, 155
phagocytosis, 43
Pharmacological Therapy, 31
photoaging, 216, 218, 221
photocoagulate, 16
photography, 9, 227
photon(s), 105, 123, 124, 171
phototherapy, 216
pigmentary alterations, 13, 193
pigmentary changes, 146, 156, 215
pigmentation, 8, 47, 109, 112, 117, 118, 126, 142, 147, 161, 192, 207, 208, 216
pilosebaceous units, 184, 191, 193
pinpoint bleeding, 143, 205, 219
Pirfenidone, 158
placebo, 37, 142, 143, 160, 214, 220, 226, 228, 229
planimetric z-plasty, 133
Plasmodium falciparum malaria, 69
platelet-derived growth factor (PDGF), 43, 44, 48, 51, 53, 84, 100
platelet-rich plasma, 219
platelets, 43, 44, 66, 94, 222
pliability, 8, 159

pockmarks, 183, 196
poikiloderma of Civatte, 218
polydioxanone sutures, 113
polyethylene gel sheet, 117, 119
polyethylene gel sheets, 119
polylactic acid, 154, 167
poly-l-lactic acid, 153, 154, 155
polymethylmethacrylate, 153, 156
polyol pathway, 76
polypropylene, 113
polyurethane films, 119
population inversion, 171
post-inflammatory hyperpigmentation (PIH), 172, 175, 178, 192, 195, 200, 210, 218
post-operative bruising, 14
post-traumatic stress disorder, 25, 26, 27, 31, 32, 34
power density, 173
pox scars, 146
precursor, 6
prefocused, 173
pregnancy, 6, 110, 119, 211, 212, 214, 220
preoperative assessment, 110
preserved particulate fasica lata, 159
pressure dressings, 11, 141
pressure therapy, 8, 140, 158, 160
presynaptic alpha-2 adrenergic receptors, 33
prilocaine, 13
primary radiation therapy, 124
procollagen, 101, 219
procollagenase, 151, 164
pro-fibrotic factor, 60
prognosis, 30, 180, 185, 203
proliferation, 6, 12, 41, 42, 43, 44, 45, 49, 59, 60, 62, 63, 67, 70, 73, 81, 83, 84, 99, 100, 104, 110, 111, 116, 142, 150, 151
pro-oxidant enzymes, 58
Propionibacterium acnes, 29
prospective study, 28, 224, 226, 229
protein kinase C (PKC), 59, 61
pseudofrosting, 148
psoriasis, 9, 216
psoriatic skin, 72
psychodynamic psychotherapy, 32
psychodynamic therapy, 32
psychological preatment, 26, 31
psychopathological responses, 27
psychopharmacological agents, 32
psychopharmacological treatment(s), 26, 31
psychosocial rehabilitation, 26
psychotherapeutic, 32, 37
puberty, 6, 212, 214
pulse duration, 17, 174, 176, 189, 192, 203
pulse width, 172, 174

Pulsed-dye laser(s) (PDL), 12, 13, 14, 16, 17, 19, 175, 192, 197, 207, 216, 217, 218
Punch excisions, 16
punch grafts, 16
Purpura, 13
purpuric, 14

Q

Q-switched, 17, 23, 166, 172, 177, 192, 200, 207, 210
QualiFibro questionnaire, 30
QualiFibro/Cirurgia Plástica-UNIFESP, 30
quality of life, 4, 25, 26, 30, 32, 33, 34, 36
Quantitative Global Scarring Grading system, 231
quercetin, 142

R

radiation, vii, 8, 27, 47, 70, 72, 87, 89, 98, 100, 111, 123, 124, 125, 126, 127, 128, 129, 131, 132, 136, 171, 172, 176, 185, 206
radiofrequency (RF) devices, 215, 217, 219
randomized controlled double blinded study, 224
ratio scales, 230, 231
raw data, 226, 230
reactive nitrogen species, 59, 64
reactive oxygen species (ROS), 57, 59, 60, 61, 62, 63, 64, 65, 66, 67, 68, 69, 70, 71, 72, 73, 74, 75, 76, 77, 80, 81, 82, 83, 84, 85, 88, 94, 96
reclusion, 25
recontouring, 15
redox balance, 58, 63, 68, 69, 73, 77
redox-sensitive cysteine residues, 61
redox-sensitive histone deacetylases (HDACs), 61
reenactment, 28
re-epithelialization, 5, 10, 16, 18, 44, 45, 174, 175, 189, 208
re-epithelialization (epidermal regeneration), 44
relaxation techniques, 32
relaxin, 214, 220
remodeling, 4, 5, 16, 17, 18, 42, 43, 45, 46, 47, 48, 59, 62, 66, 67, 79, 81, 84, 99, 100, 101, 102, 110, 117, 141, 142, 174, 176, 177, 200, 213, 216, 217, 218, 221
remodeling phase, 5, 45, 46, 59, 117
renal cortical cells, 69
renal fibrosis, 60, 70, 88
renin-angiotensin system, 76
residual thermal damage, 15, 174, 176, 189
residual thermal injury, 174, 192
retinoic, 16, 142, 221

retinoic acid, 142, 221
retrograde response, 65, 74, 82
retrospective study design, 229
rheumatic fever, 212
rhinophyma, 10
rhytides, 18, 23, 177, 200, 209, 216, 217, 221
risk of scarring, 4, 29
roentgen, 123, 124
rolling, 7, 16, 29, 153, 155
ROS detoxification, 57, 72, 77
rosacea-like eruptions, 156

S

salicylic acid, 10, 21, 147, 148, 157, 162
sample size, 224, 226, 229
sampling, 226, 229
sandpaper, 145
scanning device, 15
scar classification, x, 47, 179, 180, 203
scar contractures, 34, 131, 133, 134, 136, 197
Scar Grading System, 195, 231
scar maturation, 109, 117, 118, 141
scar prophylaxis, 141
scar revision, 20, 22, 112, 118, 131, 132, 178, 187, 197
scarring grading system, 195, 201, 232
scattering, 154, 173
sculpting, 166, 174, 175, 188, 189, 190, 191, 192, 193, 194, 195, 205, 206, 208
seborrheic keratoses, 10
secondary radiation carcinogenesis, 124
selection bias, 224
Selective Photothermolysis, 173
Selective Serotonin Reuptake Enhancers, 33
Selective Serotonin Reuptake Inhibitors, 32
self-consciousness, 26, 34
self-esteem, 25, 26, 29, 30, 33, 34
self-hypnosis, 32
semi-occlusive silicone-based ointments, 11
serotonin, 33, 37, 38
Serotonin -Norepinephrine Reuptake Inhibitors, 33
serotonin receptors, 33
Sharplan FeatherTouch, 15
shear force, 111
silicone, 11, 12, 16, 22, 36, 117, 119, 140, 141, 143, 153, 155, 157, 159, 160, 167, 186, 192, 208
silicone gel sheet, 12, 117
silicone sheeting compression, 16
silicone sheeting,, 140
single nucleotide polymorphisms (SNPs), 49, 110
skin closure tape, 117
skin flaps, 131, 132, 136

skin graft(s), 131, 132, 134, 135, 136, 137, 146, 197
skin grafting, 134
skin resurfacing, 18, 23, 146, 177, 198, 200, 209
skin tension, 41, 49, 120, 132, 137, 211
skin test, 154
sleep disturbance, 30
Smooth Beam®, 190
social interaction, 25, 26, 29, 33
social phobia, 26, 32
socioeconomic group, 26
soft silicone tape, 117
soft tissue augmentation, 10, 153, 155, 166, 167
soft-tissue coagulation, 18
solar elastosis, 10, 177
solar protection, 14
spontaneous emission of radiation, 171
stellate cells, 58, 60, 62, 67, 80, 81, 84
stem cells, 101, 102, 104, 105, 193
sterile abscesses, 154
stigmatization, 26, 30
stimulated emission, 171
stretch marks, 6, 22, 212, 214, 216, 220, 221
stretch tension, 125
striae alba, 7, 14, 213, 215, 216, 218, 219, 221
striae distensae, 4, 5, 6, 7, 14, 20, 211, 212, 213, 214, 215, 216, 218, 219, 220, 221, 222
striae gravidarum, 211, 212, 214, 215, 219, 220
striae rubra, 7, 213, 215, 216, 217, 218, 219, 221
striatoxin, 212
stromal cells, 42
stromelysins, 45
study design, 223, 224, 225, 226, 228, 229, 230
study group, 224, 226, 228
subcision, 11, 16, 18, 23, 146, 150, 155, 159, 163, 191, 194, 206, 208
subcision (subcutaneous incisionless surgery), 18
subcutaneous fibrosis, 127
subcutaneous/fascial tension reduction sutures, 113
subscision, 155, 187
substance abuse, 26
sun avoidance, 195
sun protection, 188, 195
superoxide, 59, 60, 64, 65, 67, 82, 84, 87, 88
superoxide anion, 59, 60
superoxide dismutase(s) (SODs), 67, 69, 70, 71
surgical adhesive, 118
surgical resection, 191, 206
surgical scar revisions, viii, 187, 196
surgical site infections (SSIs), 112, 113
surgical tapes, 109, 117
suture marks, 113, 133
suture techniques, 112, 113, 133

sutures, 113, 115, 116, 117, 118, 119, 120, 132, 133, 135, 137
suturing technique, 109, 112, 113
syringomas, 10

T

tacrolimus, 152, 165
target chromophores, 174, 176, 180, 192
tarsorrhaphy, 135
tattoo removal, 10
telangiectasia, 127, 218
telangiectasis, 127
tenascin, 100
tensile strength, 4, 5, 46, 143
tension, 4, 6, 41, 49, 52, 54, 100, 104, 111, 112, 113, 114, 116, 119, 120, 125, 131, 132, 133, 136, 137, 159, 211
tension line, 49, 132
teratogenicity, 142
tethering scar tissue, 188, 204
tetrameric heme protein, 70
textural scars, 181, 190, 192, 206
texture, 4, 8, 11, 15, 17, 47, 188, 191, 192, 207, 216
the 1064 nm NdYAG laser, 154
the non-ablative 1540-nm Erglass fractional laser, 18
Thermal Relaxation Time (TRT), 173, 174
thickness skin grafts, 134, 135
thioredoxin, 71
three-layered sutures, 113, 133
thyroid cancer, 127
tie-over fixation, 135
timidity, 25
tissue formation, 5, 42, 44, 47, 73, 77, 144
tissue remodeling, 18, 42, 47, 66, 217
topical agents, 19, 109, 117, 140, 144, 192, 215
topical anesthetic cream, 147, 188, 190
topical anesthetic cream (EMLA), 147, 188, 190
topical antibiotics, 14
topical corticosteroids, 140, 142, 211
topical steroid creams, 14
topical therapies, 22, 139, 140, 144, 160
topical treatments, 11
topical vitamin preparations, 140
Tram-tracking, 150
tranexamic acid, 109, 117, 118
transforming growth factor-beta 1 (TGF-b1), 60, 151
transforming growth factors (TGF)-β, 100
transgenic knockout mice, 101
transverse electric modes (TEMs), 173
tretinoin, 215, 221
tretinoin cream, 215
Triamcinolone, 150
trichloracetic acid, 216
trichloroacetic acid, 10, 18, 23, 147, 148, 162
Tricyclic Antidepressants, 33
trofolastin, 215
tuberculosis, 212, 214
tubulointerstitial fibrosis, 70
tumor necrosis factor-alpha (TNFα), 67
Tyndall effect, 154, 166
type I collagen, 17, 45, 164
type III collagen, 46
type-1 hemochromatosis, 65
typhoid, 212, 214
typhoid fever, 212
typical locations for hypertrophic scars, 6
tyrosines, 61

U

ubiquinone, 65
ulceration, 37, 127, 141, 150, 152
urea ointments, 109, 117, 119
UV light, 73

V

vaporization, 15, 22, 174, 217
variables, 9, 13, 80, 224, 227, 228, 230, 231
varicella infection, 153
variolous (pockmark) scars, 195
variolous scars, 195
vascular endothelial growth factor, 43, 51, 83, 151, 165
Vascular Endothelial Growth Factor (VEGF), 5, 43, 44, 51, 66, 70, 83, 93, 151, 165
vascular malformations, 218
vascular smooth muscle cells, 66, 67
vascularity, 4, 14, 101, 176, 180
vasculature, 157, 192, 207
Vaseline, 109, 117, 119, 190, 205
vasoconstriction, 57, 72, 93
V-Beam®, 192, 197
Verapamil, 151, 152, 165
verum (menthol) cream, 215
vimentin, 23, 101
vinculin, 50
visual numeric scales, 30
vitamin A, 142
vitamin C, 68, 85, 89
vitamin E, 142
vitamin E, 142
vitamin toxicity, 142
vitamins B2, B6 and C, 109, 117

vitiligo, 216

W

wavelength, 172, 174, 175, 217
Wilcoxon rank sum test, 229
Wilcoxon signed rank test, 229
wire brushes, 10, 145
Wnt pathway, 49
wound contraction, 44, 51
wound dehiscence, 127
wound dressings, 111, 112, 119
wound fibrosis, 101, 102
wound healing, 4, 5, 6, 8, 9, 11, 16, 17, 18, 19, 21, 41, 42, 43, 44, 45, 47, 48, 50, 51, 52, 53, 57, 59, 60, 62, 63, 64, 65, 66, 67, 68, 69, 70, 71, 72, 73, 75, 76, 77, 78, 80, 83, 86, 87, 90, 91, 92, 93, 96, 98, 99, 100, 101, 103, 105, 110, 111, 112, 116, 117, 119, 141, 146, 164, 176, 186, 200, 219
wound repair mechanism, 174
w-plasties, 131, 132
wrinkle line, 132

X

xanthine oxidoreductase, 64
X-rays, 123, 124

Z

z-plasties, 131, 132, 133, 134